Office Management
of Obesity

Office Management
of Obesity

George A. Bray, MD
Boyd Professor, Pennington Biomedical Research Center
Louisiana State University
Baton Rouge, Louisiana

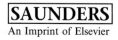
An Imprint of Elsevier

SAUNDERS
An Imprint of Elsevier

The Curtis Center
Independence Square West
Philadelphia, PA 19106

OFFICE MANAGEMENT OF OBESITY   ISBN 0-7216-0647-4

Notice

Medicine is an ever-changing field. Standard safety precautions must be followed, but as new research and clinical experience broaden our knowledge, changes in treatment and drug therapy may become necessary or appropriate. Readers are advised to check the most current product information provided by the manufacturer of each drug to be administered to verify the recommended dose, the method and duration of administration, and contraindications. It is the responsibility of the treating physician, relying on experience and knowledge of the patient, to determine dosages and the best treatment for each individual patient. Neither the Publisher nor the author assume any liability for any injury and/or damage to persons or property arising from this publication.

The Publisher

Library of Congress Cataloging-in-Publication Data
Office management of obesity/[edited by] George A. Bray.
    p.   ;   cm.
Consist mostly of articles originally published in Primary care: clinics in office practice.
    Includes bibliographical references.
    ISBN 0-7216-0647-4
    1. Obesity. 2. Primary care (Medicine) 3. Health. I. Bray, George A. II. Primary care.
    [DNLM: 1. Obesity–therapy–Collected Works. 2. Primary Health Care–Collected Works. WD 210 O32 2004]
    RC628.O34 2004
616.3'98–dc22   2003059127

Acquisitions Editor: Rebecca A. Schmidt

Publishing Services Manager: Frank Polizzano

Printed in the United States of America

Last digit is the print number: 9 8 7 6 5 4 3 2 1

Contributors

Jeanine Albu, MD
Obesity Research Center, Columbia University, New York, New York
The Management of the Obese Diabetic Patient

Charles J. Billington, MD
Metabolic/Endocrine Section, Minneapolis VA Medical Center,
Minneapolis, Minnesota
Etiology of Obesity

George L. Blackburn, MD, PhD
Beth Israel Deaconess Medical Center, Boston, Massachusetts
*Surgical Approaches to the Treatment of Obesity: A Practical
Guide for the Covering Physician*

George A. Bray, MD
Pennington Biomedical Research Center, Baton Rouge, Louisiana
Risks of Obesity

Maria L. Collazo-Clavell, MD
Division of Endocrinology, Metabolism and Nutrition, Mayo Clinic,
Rochester, Minnesota
Metabolic Syndrome

Dympna Gallagher, EdD
Department of Medicine and Institute of Human Nutrition, Columbia
University; and Obesity Research Center, St. Luke's-Roosevelt Hospital,
New York, New York
Evaluation of Body Composition: Practical Guidelines

Amy A. Gorin, PhD
Weight Control and Diabetes Research Center, The Miriam Hospital/ Brown Medical School, Providence, Rhode Island
Behavioral Techniques for Treating the Obese Patient

Frank Greenway, MD
Pennington Biomedical Research Center, Baton Rouge, Louisiana
Clinical Evaluation of the Obese Patient

Sandra Hassink, MD, FAAP
Assistant Professor of Pediatrics, Thomas Jefferson University, Philadelphia, Pennsylvania
Problems in Childhood Obesity

David Heber, MD, PhD
University of California Los Angeles Center for Human Nutrition, Los Angeles, California
Herbal Preparations for Obesity: Are They Useful?

Priscilla Hollander, MD, PhD
Baylor University Medical Hospital, Dallas, Texas
Orlistat in the Treatment of Obesity

John M. Jakicic, PhD
Physical Activity & Weight Management Research Center, University of Pittsburgh, Pittsburgh, Pennsylvania
Exercise Strategies for the Obese Patient

Michael D. Jensen, MD
Endocrine Research Unit, Mayo Clinic, Rochester, Minnesota
Metabolic Syndrome

Alexandra Kazaks
Department of Nutrition, University of California, Davis, California
Obesity: Food Intake

Catherine M. Kotz, PhD
Minnesota Obesity Center, Minneapolis VA Medical Center and University of Minnesota, Minneapolis, Minnesota
Etiology of Obesity

Robert F. Kushner, MD

Professor of Medicine, The Feinburg School of Medicine of Northwestern University; and Medical Director, Wellness Institute, Northwestern Hospital, Chicago, Illinois
The Office Approach to the Obese Patient

Allen S. Levine, PhD

Director, Minnesota Obesity Center, Minneapolis VA Medical Center, Minneapolis, Minnesota
Etiology of Obesity

Jennifer C. Lovejoy, PhD

Women's Nutrition Research Program, Pennington Biomedical Research Center, Baton Rouge, Louisiana
The Menopause and Obesity

Janey S.A. Pratt, MD, FACS

Harvard-wide Bariatric Surgery Study Group (HBSSG), Boston, Massachusetts
Surgical Approaches to the Treatment of Obesity: A Practical Guide for the Covering Physician

Nazia Raja-Khan, MD

Obesity Research Center, Columbia University, New York, New York
The Management of the Obese Diabetic Patient

Donna H. Ryan, MD

Pennington Biomedical Research Center, Baton Rouge, Louisiana
Use of Sibutramine to Treat Obesity

Mi-Yeon Song, PhD

Department of Rehabilitation Medicine, Kyung Hee University College of Oriental Medicine, Seoul, Korea; and Obesity Research Center, St. Luke's-Roosevelt Hospital, New York, New York
Evaluation of Body Composition: Practical Guidelines

Judith S. Stern, ScD, RD

Professor of Nutrition and Internal Medicine, Department of Nutrition, University of California, Davis, California
Obesity: Food Intake

Rena R. Wing, PhD

Department of Psychiatry and Human Behavior, The Miriam Hospital/
Brown Medical School, Providence, Rhode Island
Behavioral Techniques for Treating the Obese Patient

Holly Wyatt, MD

Division of Endocrinology, Metabolism, and Diabetes, University
of Colorado Health Sciences Center; and Program Director, CORE,
Denver, Colorado
The Prevalence of Obesity

Preface

This book, *Office Management of Obesity*, originally was published as an issue of the *Primary Care Clinics in Office Practice* devoted to obesity. The original 14 articles from this issue have been expanded to 17 chapters for this book. The additional chapters deal with the control of food intake, metabolic syndrome, and the surgical treatment of obesity.

A book on obesity is timely. In late 2002, the National Center for Health Statistics published data showing that 30.5% of adult Americans are obese and that 64.5% are overweight or obese. These figures have more than doubled in the past two decades to produce what is widely called an epidemic. The World Health Organization recognized this when it entitled its working paper on obesity "Preventing and Managing the Global Epidemic." Obesity is a global problem with a higher prevalence in African-Americans, Hispanic-Americans, and women.

For this book, I have taken the opportunity to showcase the many women who are contributing their research to this problem. They include both senior leaders in the field and members of the next generation of leaders. I often hear that women are not given appropriate opportunities to participate in preparing chapters for such important books; thus I have carefully chosen a group of highly skilled women to write most of the chapters in this book. Where I have included men, it was because a woman was not available or because the man had a very unusual point of view.

Preparation of this book has been a team effort. The authors are to be thanked for the work they did on the original manuscript and subsequent revisions. My tireless administrative assistant, Heather Miller, has used her great knowledge of the English language to make the editorial work go smoothly, and Rebecca Schmidt has served as the editor at Elsevier. As a team, we are proud to present this book for your consideration of obesity, a global epidemic.

CONTENTS

1

Evaluation of Body Composition: Practical Guidelines

Dympna Gallagher

Mi-Yeon Song

The choice of body composition measurements greatly depends on the question being asked. Body composition measurement methods vary in complexity and precision, and range from simple field based methods (anthropometry, bioimpedance analysis) to more technically challenging, laboratory based methods (dual energy x-ray absorptiometry, hydrostatic weighing, air plethysmography, whole-body counting for ^{40}K, deuterium, and bromide dilutions, and magnetic resonance imaging). This chapter focuses on practical guidelines for the evaluation of body composition where access to specialized equipment is unavailable, with special consideration to age, sex, and race related issues.

Skeletal muscle mass

Skeletal muscle mass (SM) represents approximately 40% of body weight in young adults [1]. With increasing age, SM mass decreases to approximately 30% of young values at elderly ages [2]. SM mass represents approximately 60% of the body's cell mass. Two components are usually considered as representative of whole body metabolically active tissue, body cell mass and fat free mass (FFM). FFM is body weight minus fat mass. SM is one of the more difficult components to quantify. Common measurement methods include anthropometry, dual energy X-ray absorptiometry (DXA) derived appendicular skeletal muscle (ASM), and magnetic resonance imaging.

Fat mass or percentage fat

Assuming that the body consists of two compartments, fat and FFM (body weight equals fat plus FFM), the reference percent fat for adults is age-, race-, and sex-dependent. Table 1 shows the percentage of fat values for women and men in three race groups, and stratified by age [3].

Choice of body composition methods

Body mass index

The National Institutes of Health and the World Health Organization recently adopted similar body weight (adjusted for height) guidelines for overweight and obesity [4–6]. The body mass index (BMI = weight in kg/height in m^2) continues to be the most commonly used index of weight status. Normal weight is a BMI between 18.5 kg/m^2 and 25.9 kg/m^2, overweight is a BMI between 25.0 kg/m^2 and 29.9 kg/m^2, and obese is a BMI greater than 30.0 kg/m^2 [6] (see Table 1). Although BMI is not a measure of

Table 1

Predicted percentage body fat by sex and ethnicity based on four-compartment estimates of percentage body fat

Age and BMI	Women			Men		
	African American	Asian	Caucasian	African American	Asian	Caucasian
20 to 39 years						
BMI < 18.5	20	25	21	8	13	8
BMI ≥ 25	32	35	33	20	23	21
BMI ≥ 30	38	40	39	26	28	26
40 to 59 years						
BMI < 18.5	21	25	23	9	13	11
BMI ≥ 25	34	36	35	22	24	23
BMI ≥ 30	39	41	41	27	29	29
60 to 79 years						
BMI < 18.5	23	26	25	11	14	13
BMI ≥ 25	35	36	38	23	24	25
BMI ≥ 30	41	41	43	29	29	31

From Gallagher D, Heymsfield SB, Heo M, et al. Healthy percentage body fat ranges: an approach for developing guidelines based on body mass index. Am J Clin Nutr 2000;72(3):699. Reproduced with permission by the *American Journal of Clinical Nutrition*. © Am J Clin Nutr. American Society for Clinical Nutrition.

Table 2
Classification of overweight and obesity by BMI

	Obesity class	BMI kg/m^2
Underweight		<18.5
Normal		18.5–24.9
Overweight		25.0–29.9
Obesity	I	30.0–34.9
	II	35.0–39.9
Extreme obesity	III	≥40

From Expert panel on the identification, evaluation, and treatment of overweight in adults. Clinical guidelines on the identification, evaluation, and treatment of overweight and obesity in adults; executive summary. Am J Clin Nutr 1998;68:901. Reproduced with permission by the *American Journal of Clinical Nutrition.* © Am J Clin Nutr. American Society for Clinical Nutrition.

body composition, it is commonly considered an index of fatness because of the high correlation between BMI and percentage of body fat in children [7] and adults [8]. The prediction of percentage of body fat in African American (AA), Asian, and Caucasian adults was found to vary by age (higher in older persons), sex (higher in males), and race (higher in As compared with AA and C) [3] as shown in Table 2. The following equation is proposed to estimate percent body fat:

$$\text{Percent Body Fat} = 76.0 - 1097.8 \times (1/\text{BMI}) - 20.6 \times \text{SEX} + 0.053$$
$$\times \text{Age} + 95.0 \times \text{Asian} \times (1/\text{BMI}) - 0.044$$
$$\times \text{Asian} \times \text{Age} + 154 \times \text{SEX} \times (1/\text{BMI}) + 0.034$$
$$\times \text{SEX} \times \text{Age},$$

where multiple R = correlation coefficient, 0.90; SEE = standard error of the estimate, 4.31%; sex = 0 for female and 1 for male; race = codes for race, 1 for Asian, 2 for other races.

No differences in the prediction of percentage of fat from BMI were observed between Hispanic American (HA), European American (EA), and African American men. In women, differences in the percentage of body fat predicted by BMI were observed between HA and EA ($P<0.002$) and AA and HA ($P = 0.020$), but not between AA and EA ($P = 0.490$). At BMIs less than 30 kg/m^2, HA tended to have more body fat than EA and AA, and at BMIs greater than 35 kg/m^2, EA tended to have more body fat than the other groups [9]. Equations for prediction of percent body fat are shown in Table 3.

Anthropometry

For routine clinical use, anthropometric measurements have been preferred because of the ease of measurement and low cost. Waist circumference and the waist-hip ratio measurements are commonly-used surrogates of fat distribution, especially in epidemiology studies. Waist circumference is highly correlated with visceral fat [10,11] and was recently included as

Table 3
Formulas for prediction of percent body fat

	Women	Men
Hispanic	73.175–915.644 (1/BMI)	69.622–1210.938 (1/BMI)
Caucasian	79.145–1105.59 (1/BMI)	64.813–1084.43 (1/BMI)
African American	76.955–1072.573 (1/BMI)	65.832–1146.108 (1/BMI)

Adapted from Fernandez JM, Heo S, Heymsfield RN. Is the prediction of body fat from BMI in Hispanics different from African Americans and European Americans? Am J Clin Nutr 2003;77:71–5. Reproduced with permission by the *American Journal of Clinical Nutrition.* © Am J Clin Nutr. American Society for Clinical Nutrition.

a clinical risk factor in the definition of the metabolic syndrome [12]. Specifically, waist circumferences greater than 102 cm (40 in) in men and 88 cm (35 in) in women are suggestive of elevated risk.

Prediction of percentage fat

Skinfold thicknesses, which estimate the thickness of the subcutaneous fat layer, are highly correlated with percentage of body fat. Because the subcutaneous fat layer varies in thickness throughout the body, a combination of site measures is recommended that reflect upper and lower body distribution. Predictive percent body fat equations that are based on skinfold measures are age-and sex-specific in adults and children. Examples of predictive equations were published by Jackson and Pollock [13], Jackson et al [14] and Durnin and Womersley [15] in adults, and Boileau et al [16] and Bray et al [17] in children. Bray et al [17] reported that the equations by Siri [18] and Lohman et al [19] provided the best estimate of body fat in African Americans and Caucasians (10–12 years); the measurement precision was greater in fatter children compared with leaner children.

Prediction of skeletal muscle mass

Arm, thigh, and calf muscle areas can be estimated based on skinfold thickness and limb circumference measures [20]. In one study, a skinfold-circumference model had higher accuracy than a body weight and height model in predicting total body SM in healthy adult populations [20]. The following two equations are proposed to estimate skeletal muscle. These models were developed and cross-validated in nonobese adults (BMI less than 30 kg/m^2).

Model 1

$$\text{Skeletal muscle mass} = \text{Height} \times [0.00744 \times \text{CAG}^2 + 0.00088 \times \text{CTG}^2 + 0.00441 \times \text{CCG}^2] + 2.4 \times \text{sex} - 0.048 \times \text{age} + \text{race} + 7.8$$

R^2 = the variance explained by the model (ie, 91% or $R^2 = 0.91$); $P<0.0001$; SEE is 2.2 kg; sex is 0 for female and 1 for male; race is -2.0 for Asian, 1.1

for African American, 0 for Caucasian and Hispanic; height is in meters; CAG is skinfold-corrected upper arm girth; CTG is skinfold corrected thigh girth; CCG is skinfold corrected calf girth. All girths are measured in centimeters.

Model 2

$$\text{Skeletal muscle mass} = 0.244 \times \text{BW} + 7.80 \times \text{Height}$$
$$+ 6.6 \times \text{sex} - 0.098 \times \text{age} + \text{race} - 3.3$$

$R^2 = 0.86$, $P < 0.0001$, and SEE is 2.8 kg; sex is 0 for female and 1 for male, race is -1.2 for Asian, 1.4 for African American, and 0 for Caucasian and Hispanic; BW is body weight in kilograms, and height is in meters.

Bioimpedance analysis

Bioimpedance analysis (BIA) is a simple, low-expense, noninvasive body composition measurement method. BIA is based on the electrical conductive properties of the human body [21]. Measures of bioelectrical conductivity are proportional to total body water and the body's components with high-water concentrations, such as fat free and skeletal muscle mass. BIA assumes that the body consists of two compartments, fat and FFM. BIA is best known as a technique for the measurement of percentage of body fat. Compared with multicompartment body composition models, a two-compartment model approach (eg, BIA and anthropometry) produces greater errors when estimating percentage of body fat in children [22] and adults [23]. Table 4 shows selected single frequency BIA equations for predicting FFM in different age groups. We selected equations that were developed in populations diverse in age, sex, and race/ethnicity. No single equation has been validated in all groups.

There is a strong correlation between BIA resistance and skeletal muscle measurements in the arms [24,25] and legs [25,26]. Janssen et al [27] reported that MRI-measured SM mass is strongly correlated with the BIA resistance index (Ht^2/R). The following SM prediction equation was developed from a multiethnic group (Caucasian, Hispanic, and African American) of females (n = 158) and males (n = 230):

$$\text{SM mass (kg)} = [(Ht^2/R \times 0.401) + (\text{sex} \times 3.825)$$
$$+ (\text{age} \times -0.071)] + 5.102$$

Ht^2 = height squared; unit of measurement = cm^2; R is BIA resistance in ohms; sex is 0 for female and 1 for male. $R^2 = 0.86$; SEE = 2.7 kg (9%).

Dual energy x-ray absorptiometry

Dual energy x-ray absortiometry (DXA) provides an important means of quantifying total body and regional fat mass, skeletal muscle mass, and bone

Table 4
Selected single-frequency BIA equations for predicting fat-free mass

Study	Reference method	n	Age (years)	Race/country	Equation	R^2	SEE
Children							
Deurenberg et al [81]	D_b	166	7 to 15	Unknown/Netherlands	$0.406(S^2/R) + 0.36(W^a)$ $+ 5.58(S) + 0.56(Sex^b) - 6.48$	0.97	1.68
Schaefer et al [82]	D_b	59 Men 53 Women	3.9 to 19.3	Unknown/Germany	$0.65(S^2/R) + 0.68(Age) + 0.15$	0.975	1.98
Houtkooper et al [83]	3C	53 Men 41 Women	10 to 14	Caucasian/United States	$0.83(S^2/R) + 4.43$	0.88	2.60
Adults							
Baumgartner et al [84]	4C	35 Men 63 Women	65 to 94	Caucasian/United States	$0.28(S^2/R) + 0.27(W^a) + 4.5(S)$ $+ 0.31\ (Thigh\ C^c) - 1.732$	0.91	2.47
Deurenberg et al [81]	D_b	661	16 to 83	Unknown/Netherlands	$0.34(S^2/R) - 0.127(Age) + 0.273(W^a)$ $+ 4.56(Sex^b) + 15.34(S) - 12.44$	0.93	2.63
Segal et al [85]	D_b	1069 Men	17 to 59	Unknown/United States	$0.0013(S^2/R) - 0.044(R) + 0.305(W^a)$ $- 0.168(Age) + 22.668$	0.89	3.61
Segal et al [86]	D_b	498 Women	17 to 62	Unknown/United States	$0.0011(S^2) - 0.021(R) + 0.232(W)$ $- 0.068(Age) + 14.595$	0.89	2.43

Abbreviations: 3C, three-compartment model; 4C, four-compartment model; D_b, body density; R, resistance; S, stature; Thigh C, thigh circumference; W, body weight.

Adapted from Baumgartner RN. Electrical impedance and total body electrical conductivity. In: Roche AF, Heymsfield SB, Lohman TG, editors. Human body composition. Champaign (IL): Human Kinetics; 1996. p. 92; with permission.

[a]Unit of measurement for weight is kilogram.
[b]Use code 0 for female, code 1 for male.
[c]Unit of measurement for thigh circumference is centimeter.

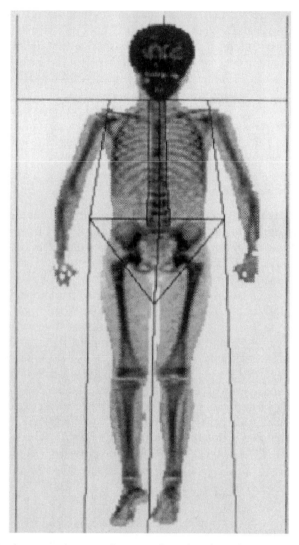

Fig. 1. DXA planogram demonstrating cut-points that determine arm and leg regions. Appendicular skeletal muscle is the sum of lean soft tissue from both arms and legs. (*From* Song MY, Kim J, Horlick M, et al. Prepubertal Asians have less limb skeletal muscle. J Appl Physiol 2002;92(6):2286; with permission.)

mineral mass and density. Using specific anatomic landmarks, the trunk, legs, and arms are identified (Fig. 1). The fat-free soft tissue (ie, nonfat, nonbone mineral mass) of the extremities is largely (approximately 76%) skeletal muscle [28] and is considered ASM mass [29]. DXA- and MRI-measured lower limb SM mass were shown to be highly correlated (r = 0.94, $P < 0.001$) in adults [30] and high correlations were found between DXA-measured ASM and MRI-derived total body skeletal muscle mass in adults (r = 0.98) [31].

Baumgartner et al [32] developed an anthropometric equation for predicting ASM mass in elderly Hispanic and non-Hispanic Caucasian men and women. Sarcopenia was defined as ASM (kg) divided by height^2 (m^2) that is less than two standard deviations below the mean of the young reference group. In the elderly men, the mean ASM/height^2 was approximately 87% of the young group. The corresponding value in women was approximately 80%. Table 5 shows the estimated prevalences of sarcopenia in the same survey sample for each ethnic group, by age and sex [32]. Obese and sarcopenic persons are reported as having worse outcomes than those who are nonobese and sarcopenic [33].

Magnetic resonance imaging

Recent advances in our laboratory strongly support the use of MRI as a reference method for evaluating and monitoring changes over time in whole-body and regional body composition. Because of the expense that is associated with this technique, it does not present as a practical measurement method for use in clinical screening. It should be acknowledged that in vivo measurement in humans of SM mass, total adipose tissue (TAT) mass and its distribution, and masses of several organs is possible. SM and TAT, including total subcutaneous adipose tissue (SAT), visceral adipose tissue (VAT), and intermuscular adipose tissue (IMAT) can be measured using whole-body, multislice MRI. Subjects are placed on the 1.5 T scanner (General Electric, 6X Horizon, Milwaukee, WI) platform with their arms extended above their heads. The protocol involves the acquisition of approximately 40 axial images, 10 mm thickness, at 40 mm intervals across the whole body [34,35]. Image analysis software (Tomovision, Montreal, Canada) is used to analyze images on a PC workstation (Gateway, Madison, WI). MRI-volume estimates are converted to mass using the assumed density of 1.04 kg/L for SM and 0.92 kg/L for adipose tissue [1,34].

Table 5
Prevalance (%) of sarcopenia[a] in the New Mexico Elder Health Survey, by age, sex, and ethnicity, 1993–1995

Age group (years)	Men		Women	
	Hispanic (n = 221)	Non-Hispanic caucasians (n = 205)	Hispanics (n = 209)	Non-Hispanic caucasians (n = 173)
<70	16.9	13.5	24.1	23.1
70 to 74	18.3	19.8	35.1	33.3
75 to 80	36.4	26.7	35.3	35.9
>80	57.5	52.6	60.0	43.2

[a] Appendicular skeletal muscle mass/height^2 (kg/m^2) less than two standard deviations below the mean value for the young adults from the Rosetta Study.
Data from Baumgartner RN, Koehler KM, Gallagher D, et al. Epidemiology of sarcopenia among the elderly in New Mexico. Am J Epidemiol 1998;147(8):760.

The technical error for repeated measurements of the same scan by the same observer of MRI-derived SM, SAT, VAT, and IMAT volumes in our laboratory are 1.9%, 0.96%, 1.97% and 0.65%, respectively.

Visceral adipose tissue

Excess abdominal or visceral adipose tissue (VAT) is recognized as an important risk factor in the development of coronary heart disease [36,37] and noninsulin dependent diabetes mellitus [38,39]. The most accurate measurement of VAT requires imaging techniques (MRI and CT), that are impractical in a clinical setting. Fig. 2 shows cross-sectional images at the L4–L5 level that were acquired in two Caucasian men. Waist circumferences were 85.0 cm and 85.5 cm with corresponding total VAT of 1.5 kg and 3.1 kg, respectively. Despite similar waist circumferences, total VAT was two times higher in one male, which highlights the limitation of using waist circumference as a measure of VAT, given that abdominal SAT is included in the measure.

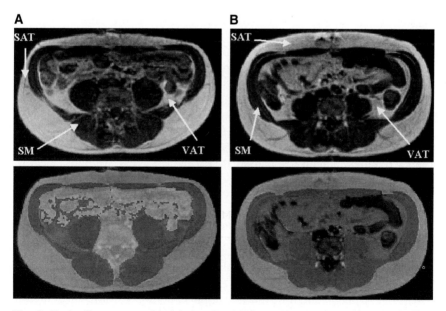

Fig. 2. Single slice, cross-sectional image (by MRI) at the L4–L5 level acquired in two Caucasian men. Total VAT mass was calculated as the sum of approximately 7 slices (10 mm-thick slice and 40 mm between slices) within the visceral cavity. Waist circumference was measured at the midpoint between the lowermost rib (anterior view, approximately 10th rib) and the iliac crest (waist circumference was not measured at a level meant to correspond to the MRI slice taken at L4–L5). (A) Waist circumference = 85.0 cm; VAT = 1.5 kg; age 40 years. (*B*) Waist circumference = 85.5 cm; VAT = 3.1 kg; age 29 years.

Skinfold thicknesses have been used as a continuous variable that grades adiposity or adipose tissue distribution within a study population [40]. Waist circumference and the waist-hip ratio (WHR) are commonly used to predict visceral fat accumulation in epidemiological studies [11,38]. Several investigators argued that simple waist circumference is a better index of variation in VAT than WHR [10,41].

Abdominal fat that is estimated by DXA [42–46] does not differentiate between the intra-abdominal and subcutaneous abdominal depots. DXA has some advantages over CT and MRI as a means of estimating fat distribution, including relative ease of access to systems, simplicity of measurements, relatively low cost, and lower radiation exposure, compared with CT. Regions of interest (ROI) have been identified using DXA. The DXA trunk ROI (CV, coefficient of variation = 0.728%) [47] includes chest, abdomen, and pelvis. Park et al [47] reported that the highest correlation with total VAT by MRI was for single slice VAT area at the level of L4–L5 (r = 0.87).

Intermuscular adipose tissue

A less well-understood adipose tissue depot is that which is located between muscle bundles and is visible by MRI and CT. Recent reports suggested that adipose tissue that is located below the muscle fascia is significantly negatively correlated with insulin sensitivity [48], whereas SAT that is located above the muscle fascia is not correlated with insulin sensitivity. Ryan and Nicklas [49] reported greater midthigh intermuscular adipose tissue (IMAT), lower glucose use, and less insulin sensitivity in African American women, compared with Caucasian women with similar body fatness and maximum oxygen consumption levels. In the elderly, greater IMAT (as suggested by lower skeletal muscle attenuation by CT) is associated with lower specific force production [50]. The most accurate measurement of IMAT requires imaging techniques (MRI and CT) that are impractical in a clinical setting. Currently, there is no surrogate measure of IMAT.

Sex and race difference in body composition in children

Greater limb lean tissue mass was reported in African American children compared with Caucasian children throughout Tanner stages 1 to 5 [51]. Ellis [52] and Ellis et al [53] reported race differences in FFM between 5- to 7-year-old African American and Caucasian children. Sex differences in lean body mass [52–54] were reported from birth throughout childhood; girls have smaller amounts than boys. A recent report from a longitudinal analysis of children followed from Tanner 1 through 5 found that Tanner 1 girls had smaller limb lean mass than boys [55]. Total body bone mineral content (TBBMC) was reported to be lower in Tanner 1 African American, Asian, and Caucasians girls compared with boys [56].

He et al [57] investigated race and sex differences in regional and total body fat mass in prepubertal children (182 boys and 176 girls) using anthropometry and DXA. Subjects were Asian (n = 143), African American (n = 95), and Caucasian (n = 120), ages 5 to 12 years, and were determined to be prepubertal by Tanner staging [58].There were sex differences in body fat distribution in prepubertal children, but the specific characteristics were different for Asians compared with African Americans and Caucasians. Also, there were differences in body fat distribution in Asian children compared with African Americans and Caucasians that varied by sex. This comparison of prepubertal, African American, Asian, and Caucasian children suggested phenotypic differences in fat distribution. Because an android fat pattern corresponds with greater visceral fat accumulation, a question is raised about the associated health risk.

An association between android fat and cardiovascular risk factors, such as blood pressure, was reported in an African American and Caucasian pediatric population [59]. He and colleagues [60] recently investigated these same relationships in a large, cross-sectional pediatric sample (n = 920, ages 5–18 years), according to race, sex, and puberty. Significant positive relationships between systolic and diastolic BP and trunk fat (adjusted for total fat) were seen in boys at all pubertal stages in all three races by DXA and skinfold measurements. In girls, trunk fat was not a significant predictor of BP.

Song et al [61] assessed skeletal muscle mass using DXA in prepubertal children (170 girls, 166 boys). After adjusting for age, height, and body weight: (1) Asian girls and boys had lower amounts of ASM than African Americans ($P < 0.001$); (2) Asian girls had lower amounts of ASM than Caucasian girls ($P = 0.004$); and (3) there was a trend toward less ASM in Asian boys ($P < 0.001$). These findings demonstrated that skeletal muscle mass as a fraction of body weight is lower in Asian children compared with African American and Caucasian children.

Race differences in TBBMC that are adjusted for total body bone area, age, height, and weight were reported in prepubertal African American, Asian, and Caucasian girls and boys. African American children had higher TBBMC than Asian and Caucasian children [56], whereas no differences were found between Asian and Caucasian children.

Sex and race difference in body composition in adults

Using a cross-sectional design, Gallagher et al [62] investigated the influence of age and race on arm skeletal muscle (ArSM), leg skeletal muscle (LSM), and combined ArSM and LSM, which is called total appendicular skeletal muscle. This study was performed on 156 African American and 135 Caucasian women and men ranging in age from 20 to 94 years. Subjects were healthy, ambulatory, and had a BMI that was less than 36 kg/m^2. African American men and women had significantly greater ASM than Caucasian men and women ($P < 0.001$) even after adjusting for body weight, height, age, and skeletal lengths. Results were similar for ArSM and LSM. The results of this study suggested that there is a sex difference in the rate of muscle loss with age. African Americans had greater muscle mass than Caucasians; however, the amount of change with age did not differ significantly between ethnic groups. Ortiz et al [63] matched African American and Caucasian women by body weight, height, and age. ASM was quantified using DXA. They found a significantly ($P < 0.01$) greater ASM in African American women (18.0 ± 3.0 kg versus 15.7 ± 2.2 kg). Body weight, total body fat, and FFM were similar between the two ethnic groups. The implication is that African American women have a relatively smaller visceral organ and nonmuscle tissue compartment than their Caucasian counterparts.

It is well-established that African American men [64], women [65], and children [66] have less VAT relative to TAT than Caucasians. Park et al [67] measured VAT, using whole body MRI, in women (18 Asian American, 36 European American) and men (19 Asian American, 34 European American) with BMI less than 30.0 kg/m^2. Compared with European American women, Asian American women had higher VAT ($P < 0.05$) after adjusting for age and total body fat. No differences were found among the men.

Efforts are ongoing to better understand variations in IMAT as a function of age, race, and level of fatness. We recently investigated whole body IMAT measured by MRI in 185 women (African American, n = 78, BMI 30.0 ± 5.5 kg/m^2; 45.7 ± 16.9 years; Caucasian, n = 107, BMI 24.8 ± 5.2 kg/m^2, 44.0 ± 16.4 years) and 61 men (African American, n = 40, BMI 25.5 ± 3.2 kg/m^2; 46.2 ± 19.1 years; Caucasian, n = 21, BMI 23.3 ± 2.4 kg/m^2, 44.4 ± 20.1 years). After adjusting for TAT, SM, and age, African American men and women had more IMAT and less VAT than Caucasians. When the women were grouped by menopausal status (premenopausal and postmenopausal), IMAT was greater in premenopausal ($P = 0.05$) and marginally greater in postmenopausal ($P = 0.09$) African American women [68]. An additional analysis was conducted on 128 premenopausal women (African American, n = 53, BMI 28.5 ± 5.6 kg/m^2, 36.0 ± 8.1 years; Caucasian, n = 75; BMI 24.3 ± 5.2 kg/m^2, 35.4 ± 8.9 years), none of whom were taking birth control medication. In the total sample, weight ($P = 0.001$), race ($P = 0.09$), and weight ∗ race interaction (interaction between TAT and weight) ($P = 0.02$) explained 66.5% of the variance in IMAT. African Americans had a significantly greater increment in IMAT per kilogram of body weight compared with Caucasians, although at low body weight, IMAT was similar in Caucasians. Findings were similar for TAT. TAT ($P = 0.001$), race ($P = 0.045$), and TAT ∗ race interaction (interaction between TAT and weight) ($P = 0.0007$) explained 72.7% of the variance in IMAT in the total sample. African Americans had a significantly greater increment in IMAT per kilogram of TAT (30 g IMAT/kg TAT in Caucasian versus 49 g IMAT/kg TAT in African American) [69]. Collectively, these studies demonstrate sex and race differences in body composition in children and adults.

Measuring changes in body composition

During the adult life span, body weight generally increases slowly and progressively until about the seventh decade, and thereafter, declines into old age [2,70]. Increased incidences of physical disabilities and comorbidities are likely linked to aging-associated body composition changes. Characterization of the aging processes identified losses in muscle mass, force, and strength, which collectively are defined as "sarcopenia." Little is known about the overall rate at which sarcopenia develops in otherwise healthy elderly subjects, if the rate of progression differs between women and men, and the underlying mechanisms that are responsible for age-related sarcopenia.

We recently completed a longitudinal study where we tested the hypothesis that an accelerated rate of SM loss occurs in the presence of weight stability over a 2-year period. Subjects were 26 healthy, independently-living, ambulatory, elderly, African American women with a mean age at baseline of 75.5 ± 5.1 years. Body composition was measured using repeated multislice MRI and DXA. Despite no significant changes in body weight ($P = 0.62$) or FFM ($P = 0.6$), SM mass ($P = 0.02$) and bone mineral content ($P = 0.03$) decreased and IMAT ($P < 0.001$) and VAT increased ($P = 0.01$) after adjusting for their baseline values. No changes were found in physical performance (200 m walk, 2 min walk), function (chair rise), activity (physical activity scale for the elderly), grip strength, or standing balance. These data demonstrated a disproportionate loss of SM over a 2-year period in healthy, elderly women [71,72].

Summary

The measurement of body composition in the truest sense allows for the estimation of body tissues, organs, and their distributions in living persons without inflicting harm. It is important to recognize that there is no single measurement method that is error-free. Furthermore, bias can be introduced if a measurement method makes assumptions related to body composition proportions and characteristics that are inaccurate across different populations. Some methodologic concerns include hydration of fat-free body mass changes with age and differences across ethnic groups [73]; the density of fat-free body mass changes with age and differences between men and women [74,75]; total body potassium decreases with age [73] and fatness [76] and differences between African Americans and Caucasians [77]; the mass of skeletal muscle differences across race group [63]; and VAT differences across sex [78] and race [67,79,80] groups, independent of total adiposity. These between-group differences influence the absolute accuracy of methods for estimating fatness or FFM that involve the two-compartment model approach. The clinical significance of the body compartment to be measured should be determined before a measurement method is selected, because the more advanced techniques are less accessible and more costly.

References

[1] Snyder WS, Cook MJ, Nasset ES, et al. Report of the Task Group on Reference Men International Commission on Radiological Protection. Oxford: Pergamon; 1975. No. 23.

[2] Forbes GB. Body composition in infancy, childhood, and adolescence. In: Human body composition. NewYork: Springer-Verlag; 1987. p. 125–55.

[3] Gallagher D, Heymsfield SB, Heo M, et al. Healthy percentage body fat ranges: an approach for developing guidelines based on body mass index. Am J Clin Nutr 2000; 72(3):694–701.

[4] World Health Organization. Obesity: preventing and managing the global epidemic. Report of a WHO consultation on obesity. Geneva (Switzerland): WHO; 1998.

[5] U.S. Department of Health and Human Services. Clinical guidelines on the identification, evaluation, and treatment of overweight and obesity in adults: the evidence report. Washington, DC: US DHHS; 1998. Publication #98–4083.

[6] Expert panel on the identification, evaluation, and treatment of overweight in adults. Clinical guidelines on the identification, evaluation, and treatment of overweight and obesity in adults; executive summary. Am J Clin Nutr 1998;68:899–917.

[7] Mei Z, Grummer-Strawn LM, Pietrobelli A, et al. Validity of body mass index compared with other body-composition screening indexes for the assessment of body fatness in children and adolescents. Am J Clin Nutr 2002;75(6):978–85.

[8] Gallagher D, Visser M, Sepulveda D, et al. How useful is body mass index for comparison of body fatness across age, sex, and ethnic groups? Am J Epidemiol 1996;143(3):228–39.

[9] Fernandez JM, Heo S, Heymsfield RN, et al. Is percent body fat differentially related to BMI in Hispanic-, African-, and European-Americans? Am J Clin Nutr 2003;77: 71–5.

[10] Pouliot MC, Despres JP, Lemieux S, et al. Waist circumference and abdominal sagittal diameter: best simple anthropometric indexes of abdominal visceral adipose tissue accumulation and related cardiovascular risk in men and women. Am J Cardiol 1994; 73(7):460–8.

[11] Janssen I, Heymsfield SB, Allison DB, et al. Body mass index and waist circumference independently contribute to the prediction of nonabdominal, abdominal subcutaneous, and visceral fat. Am J Clin Nutr 2002;75(4):683–8.

[12] Expert Panel on Detection, Evaluation, and Treatment of High Blood Cholesterol in Adults. Executive summary of the third report of The National Cholesterol Education Program (NCEP) Expert Panel on Detection, Evaluation, And Treatment of High Blood Cholesterol In Adults (Adult Treatment Panel III). JAMA 2001;285(19):2486–97.

[13] Jackson AS, Pollock ML. Generalized equations for predicting body density of men. Br J Nutr 1978;40(3):497–504.

[14] Jackson AS, Pollock ML, Ward A. Generalized equations for predicting body density of women. Med Sci Sports Exerc 1980;12(3):175–81.

[15] Durnin JV, Womersley J. Body fat assessed from total body density and its estimation from skinfold thickness: measurements on 481 men and women aged from 16 to 72 years. Br J Nutr 1974l;32(1):77–97.

[16] Boileau RA, Wilmore JH, Lohman TG, et al. Estimation of body density from skinfold thicknesses, body circumferences and skeletal widths in boys aged 8 to 11 years: comparison of two samples. Hum Biol 1981;53(4):575–92.

[17] Bray GA, DeLany JP, Harsha DW, et al. Evaluation of body fat in fatter and leaner 10-y-old African American and white children: the Baton Rouge Children's Study. Am J Clin Nutr 2001;73(4):687–702.

[18] Siri WE. Body composition from fluid spaces and density: analysis of methods. 1961. Nutrition 1993;9(5):480–91.

[19] Lohman TG, Slaughter MH, Boileau RA, et al. Bone mineral measurements and their relation to body density in children, youth and adults. Hum Biol 1984;56(4):667–79.

[20] Lee RC, Wang Z, Heo M, et al. Total-body skeletal muscle mass: development and cross-validation of anthropometric prediction models. Am J Clin Nutr 2000;72(3): 796–803.

[21] Baumgartner RN. Electrical impedance and total body electrical conductivity. In: Roche AF, Heymsfield SB, Lohman TG, editors. Human body composition. Champaign (IL): Human Kinetics; 1996. p. 79–109.

[22] Bray GA, DeLany JP, Volaufova J, et al. Prediction of body fat in 12-y-old African American and white children: evaluation of methods. Am J Clin Nutr 2002;76(5):980–90.

[23] Houtkooper LB, Lohman TG, Going SB, et al. Why bioelectrical impedance analysis should be used for estimating adiposity. Am J Clin Nutr 1996;64:436S–48S.

[24] Brown BH, Karatzas T, Nakielny R, et al. Determination of upper arm muscle and fat areas using electrical impedance measurements. Clin Phys Physiol Meas 1988;9(1): 47–55.

[25] Pietrobelli A, Formica C, Wang Z, et al. Dual-energy x-ray absorptiometry body composition model: review of physical concepts. Am J Physiol Endocrinol Metab 1996;271: E941–51.

[26] Nunez C, Gallagher D, Grammes J, et al. Bioimpedance analysis: potential for measuring lower limb skeletal muscle mass. J Parenter Enteral Nutr 1999;23(2):96–103.

[27] Janssen I, Heymsfield SB, Baumgartner RN, et al. Estimation of skeletal muscle mass by bioelectrical impedance analysis. J Appl Physiol 2000;89(2):465–71.

[28] Heymsfield SB, Wang ZM, Baumgartner RN, et al. Human body composition: advances in models and methods. Annu Rev Nutr 1997;17:527–58.

[29] Heymsfield SB, Smith R, Aulet M, et al. Appendicular skeletal muscle mass: measurement by dual-photon absorptiometry. Am J Clin Nutr 1990;52:214–8.

[30] Shih R, Wang Z, Heo M, et al. Lower limb skeletal muscle mass: development of dual-energy x-ray absorptiometry prediction model. J Appl Physiol 2000;89(4):1380–6.

[31] Kim J, Wang Z, Heymsfield SB, et al. Total-body muscle mass: estimation by new dual-energy x-ray absorptimetry method. Am J Clin Nutr 2002;76(2):378–83.

[32] Baumgartner RN, Koehler KM, Gallagher D, et al. Epidemiology of sarcopenia among the elderly in New Mexico. Am J Epidemiol 1998;147(8):755–63.

[33] Morley JE, Baumgartner RN, Roubenoff R, et al. Sarcopenia. J Lab Clin Med 2001; 137(4):231–43.

[34] Janssen I, Ross R. Effects of sex on the change in visceral, subcutaneous adipose tissue and skeletal muscle in response to weight loss. Int J Obes Relat Metab Disord 1999; 23(10):1035–46.

[35] Gallagher D, Kovera AJ, Clay-Williams G, et al. Weight loss in post-menopausal women: no evidence of adverse alterations in body composition. Am J Physiol Endo Metab 2000;279:124–31.

[36] Lapidus L, Bengtsson C, Larsson B, et al. Distribution of adipose tissue and risk of cardiovascular disease and death: a 12 year follow up of participants in the population study of women in Guthenburg, Sweden. BMJ 1984;289:1257–61.

[37] Han TS, van Leer EM, Seidell JC, et al. Waist circumference as a screening tool for cardiovascular risk factors: evaluation of receiver operating characteristics (ROC). Obes Res 1996;6:533–47.

[38] Ohlson LO, Larsson B, Svardsudd K, et al. The influence of body fat distribution on the incidence of diabetes mellitus 13.5 years of follow-up of the participants in the study of men born in 1913. Diabetes 1985;34:1055–8.

[39] Seidell JC, Han TS, Feskens EJ, et al. Narrow hips and broad waist circumferences independently contribute to increased risk of non-insulin-dependent diabetes mellitus. J Intern Med 1997;242:401–6.

[40] Heymsfield SB, Allison DB, Wang Z, et al. Evaluation of total and regional body composition. In: Bray GA, Bouchard C, James WPT, editors. Handbook of obesity. New York: Marcel Dekker Inc; 1998. p. 41–78.

[41] Kekes-Szabo T, Hunter GR, Nyikos I, et al. Anthropometric equations for estimating abdominal adipose tissue distribution in women. Int J Obes Relat Metab Disord 1996; 20(8):753–8.

[42] Schlemmer A, Hassager C, Haarbo J, et al. Direct measurement of abdominal fat by dual photon absorptiometry. Int J Obes 1990;14:603–11.

[43] Svendsen OL, Hassager C, Bergmann I, et al. Measurement of abdominal and intra-abdominal fat in postmenopausal women by dual x-ray absorptiometry and anthrometry: comparison with computerized tomography. Int J Obes 1993;17:45–51.

[44] Taaffe DR, Lewis B, Marcus R. Regional fat distribution by dual-energy x-ray absorptiometry: comparison with anthropometry and application in a clinical trial of growth hormone and exercise. Clinical Science Am J Clin Nutr 1994;87:581–6.

[45] Jensen MD, Kanaley JA, Reed JE, et al. Measurement of abdominal and visceral fat with computed tomography and dual-energy x-ray absorptiometry. Am J Clin Nutr 1995;61(2):274–8.

[46] Treuth MS, Hunter GR, Kekes-Szabo T. Estimating intraabdominal adipose tissue in women by dual-energy X-ray absorptiometry. Am J Clin Nutr 1995;62:527–32.

[47] Park YW, Heymsfield SB, Gallagher D. Are dual-energy x-ray absorptiometry regional estimates associated with visceral adipose tissue mass? Int J Obes Relat Metab Disord 2002;26(7):978–83.

[48] Kelley DE, Goodpaster BH, Storlien L. Muscle triglyceride and insulin resistance. Annu Rev Nutr 2002;22:325–46.

[49] Ryan AS, Nicklas BJ. Age-related changes in fat deposition in mid-thigh muscle in women: relationships with metabolic cardiovascular disease risk factors. Int J Obes Relat Metab Dis ord 1999;23(2):126–32.

[50] Goodpaster BH, Carlson CL, Visser M, et al. Attenuation of skeletal muscle and strength in the elderly: the Health ABC Study. J Appl Physiol 2001;90(6):2157–65.

[51] Sun M, Gower BA, Bartolucci AA, et al. A longitudinal study of resting energy expenditure relative to body composition during puberty in African American and white children. Am J Clin Nutr 2001;73:308–15.

[52] Ellis KJ. Body composition of a young, multiethnic, male population. Am J Clin Nutr 1997;66:1323–31.

[53] Ellis KJ, Abrams SA, Wong WW. Body composition reference data for a young multi-ethnic female population. Appl Radiat Isot 1998;49:587–8.

[54] Butte NF, Hopkinson JM, Wong WW, et al. Body composition during the first 2 years of life: an updated reference. Pediatr Res 2000;47:578–85.

[55] Taylor RW, Gold E, Manning P, et al. Gender differences in body fat content are present well before puberty. Int J Obes Relat Metab Disord 1997;21:1082–4.

[56] Horlick M, Thornton J, Wang J, et al. Bone mineral in prepubertal children: gender and ethnicity. J Bone Miner Res 2000;15:1393–7.

[57] He Q, Horlick M, Thornton J, et al. Sex and race differences in fat distribution among Asian, African-American, and Caucasian prepubertal children. J Clin Endocrinol Metab 2002;87(5):2164–70.

[58] Tanner JM. Growth and adolescence. 2nd edition. Oxford (UK): Blackwell; 1962.

[59] Daniels SR, Morrison JA, Sprecher DL, et al. Association of body fat distribution and cardiovascular risk factors in children and adolescents. Circulation 1999;99(4):541–5.

[60] He Q, Horlick M, Fedun B, et al. Trunk fat and blood pressure in children through puberty. Circulation 2002;105(9):1093–8.

[61] Song MY, Kim J, Horlick M, et al. Prepubertal Asians have less limb skeletal muscle. J Appl Physiol 2002;92(6):2285–91.

[62] Gallagher D, Visser M, De Meersman RE, et al. Appendicular skeletal muscle mass: effects of age, gender, and ethnicity. J Appl Physiol 1997;83(1):229–39.

[63] Ortiz O, Russell M, Daley TL, et al. Differences in skeletal muscle and bone mineral mass between black and white females and their relevance to estimates of body composition. Am J Clin Nutr 1992;55(1):8–13.

[64] Hill JO, Sidney S, Lewis CE, et al. Racial differences in amounts of visceral adipose tissue in young adults: the CARDIA (Coronary Artery Risk Development in Young Adults) study. Am J Clin Nutr 1999;69(3):381–7.

[65] Conway JM, Yanovski SZ, Avila NA, et al. Visceral adipose tissue differences in black and white women. Am J Clin Nutr 1995;61(4):765–71.

[66] Goran MI, Nagy TR, Treuth MS, et al. Visceral fat in white and African American prepubertal children. Am J Clin Nutr 1997;65(6):1703–8.

[67] Park YW, Allison DB, Heymsfield SB, et al. Larger amounts of visceral adipose tissue in Asian Americans. Obes Res 2001;9(7):381–7.

[68] Gallagher D, Kuznia P, Heshka S, et al. Greater infiltration of adipose tissue in muscle of African-Americans compared to Caucasians. FASEB J 2003;14:4.

[69] Harris T, Kuznia P, Heshka S, et al. Variations in muscle adipose tissue infiltration by weight/adipose tissue in premenopausal women. FASEB J 2003;14:4.

[70] Baumgartner RN, Stauber PM, McHugh D, et al. Cross-sectional age differences in body composition in persons 60+ years of age. J Gerontol A Biol Sci Med Sci 1995;50(6): M307–16.

[71] Song MY, Ruts E, Janumala F, et al. Skeletal muscle mass loss in healthy elderly African-American females. FASEB J 2002;16(5):A1024.

[72] Janumala F, Ruts E, Kim J, et al. Skeletal muscle fatty infiltration increases over two years in healthy elderly African-American females. FASEB J 2002;16(4):A230.

[73] Mazariegos M, Wang ZM, Gallagher D, et al. Differences between young and old females in the five levels of body composition and their relevance to the two-compartment chemical model. J Gerontol1994;16(5):M201–8.

[74] Lohman TG. Advances in body composition assessment. Champaign (IL): Human Kinetics Publishers; 1992.

[75] Heymsfield SB, Wang Z, Baumgartner RN, et al. Body composition and aging: a study by in vivo neutron activation analysis. J Nutr 1993;123(2 Suppl):432–7.

[76] Pierson RN Jr, Lin DH, Phillips RA. Total-body potassium in health: effects of age, sex, height, and fat. Am J Physiol 1974;226(1):206–12.

[77] Cohn SH, Abesamis C, Zanzi I, et al. Body elemental composition: comparison between black and white adults. Am J Physiol 1977;232(4):E419–22.

[78] Despres JP, Couillard C, Gagnon J, et al. Race, visceral adipose tissue, plasma lipids, and lipoprotein lipase activity in men and women: the Health, Risk Factors, Exercise Training, and Genetics (HERITAGE) family study. Arterioscler Thromb Vasc Biol 2000;20(8): 1932–8.

[79] Yanovski JA, Yanovski SZ, Filmer KM, et al. Differences in body composition of black and white girls. Am J Clin Nutr 1996;64(6):833–9.

[80] Perry AC, Applegate EB, Jackson ML, et al. Racial differences in visceral adipose tissue but not anthropometric markers of health-related variables. J Appl Physiol 2000;89(2):636–43.

[81] Deurenberg P, van der Kooy K, Leenen R, et al. Sex and age specific prediction formulas for estimating body composition from bioelectrical impedance: a cross-validation study. Int J Obes 1991;15(1):17–25.

[82] Schaefer F, Georgi M, Zieger A, et al. Usefulness of bioelectric impedance and skinfold measurements in predicting fat-free mass derived from total body potassium in children. Pediatr Res 1994;35(5):617–24.

[83] Houtkooper LB, Lohman TG, Going SB, et al. Validity of bioelectric impedance for body composition assessment in children. J Appl Physiol 1989;66(2):814–21.

[84] Baumgartner RN, Heymsfield SB, Lichtman S, et al. Body composition in elderly people: effect of criterion estimates on predictive equations. Am J Clin Nutr 1991;53(6):1345–53.

[85] Segal KR, Gutin B, Presta E, et al. Estimation of human body composition by electrical impedance methods: a comparative study. J Appl Physiol 1985;58(5):1565–71.

[86] Segal KR, Van Loan M, Fitzgerald PI, et al. Lean body mass estimation by bioelectrical impedance analysis: a four-site cross-validation study. Am J Clin Nutr 1988;47(1):7–14.

2

The Prevalence of Obesity

Holly R. Wyatt

Most health care providers are seeing more overweight and obese patients than ever before in their practices, which is not surprising, because more than half of the US population is overweight or obese. Health care providers are facing a modern-day public health crisis that is rapidly getting worse and that increasingly negatively affects patient morbidity, mortality, and health care expenditures. This chapter describes the obesity epidemic and explains how it arose.

The definition and classification of obesity in adults—what is the problem?

By definition, *obesity* is an excessive accumulation of body fat. Current methods that accurately measure body fat are impractical and costly for large-scale use, so simple measures of weight for height that correlate with body fat are used to identify overweight and obesity. The body mass index (BMI) has gained widespread acceptance in the scientific community as the tool of choice in assessing overweight and obesity in most adults [1]. *Body mass index* is defined as weight in kilograms divided by height in meters squared. This formula initially was developed to compare weight independent of height, but it is used today to provide a strong, although not always perfect, correlation with body fat.

Because BMI is correlated with body fat, this measure satisfactorily classifies most people into the appropriate weight category [2–5]. Use of BMI results in misclassification of some individuals, however. For example, a very muscular individual such as an elite athlete might have high amounts of lean muscle and might be classified incorrectly as overweight. The same may be true for edematous individuals. Body mass index may underestimate fat in the frail, elderly population that has lost large amounts of lean muscle. Waist circumference measurements, when combined with BMI, further reduce the number of patients who will be misclassified. A normal waist circumference (<35 inches for women and <40 inches for men) alerts the health care practitioner that a high BMI might not be secondary to excessive body fat but instead muscle [6]. Alternatively, a high waist circumference in the face of a normal BMI also alerts the practitioner that the individual could be at risk from an increased body fat level [6,7]. Clinical judgment needs to be used when assessing these rare individuals.

Body mass index has become the standard measure for clinicians to use in classifying patients as overweight or obese because it is highly correlated with percentage of body fat and because morbidity and mortality increase with increasing BMI [1,4]. One must realize, however, that there is substantial variation in the percentage of body fat at each level of BMI, somewhere in the range of 30% to 40% [4]. Men at each BMI level have a lower percentage of body fat than women, and older individuals have more body fat than younger ones at the same BMI [4]. Because the clinical management of obesity is based on preventing or treating the comorbidities and mortality associated with excess fat, BMI works well for identifying patients at risk because of their weight. Body mass index also works well when making decisions about whether on not obesity treatment is indicated in patients.

There is good agreement as to how to classify individuals based on BMI. In 1998, the World Health Organization (WHO) committee and The National Institutes of Health defined overweight as a BMI of 25 to 29.9 kg/m^2 and obesity as a BMI of 30 kg/m^2 or higher [1,8]. This classification has become the worldwide standard and has allowed uniform comparisons of obesity rates within and across populations. A BMI cutoff of approximately 25 kg/m^2 seems to be optimal for detecting individuals whose weight may affect their health negatively, while not erroneously detecting the over-lean [5]. Body mass index cutoffs are based on data showing that health risks increase beginning at a BMI of 25 kg/m^2 and increase even more steeply after a BMI greater than or equal to 30 kg/m^2 [9,10]. There is considerable debate about whether certain ethnic groups, such as Asians, may require different cutoffs based on ethnic-specific health risks [11,12].

Body mass indices greater than 30 kg/m^2 are subdivided into several subcategories: mild obesity (obesity class I, BMI 30.0–34.9 kg/m^2), moderate obesity (obesity class II, BMI 35.0–39.9 kg/m^2), and extreme obesity (obesity class III, BMI $\geq$ 40 kg/m^2) (Table 1) [1]. The higher the obesity subcategory, the higher the risk of morbidity from the excessive weight and the more aggressive treatments are indicated in the management of these individuals. For example, a BMI of 40 kg/m^2 or higher (extreme obesity) is the subcategory of obesity in which surgical procedures are considered as a viable treatment option when other efforts at therapy have failed [1]. Although surgery carries an increased risk as a treatment option, this degree of

Table 1
Classification and current age-adjusted prevalence of overweight and obesity in adults
according to BMI

Classification	BMI	Age-adjusted prevalence (%) NHANES 1999
Overweight	25.0–29.9	34
Obesity	≥30	27
Class 1	30.0–34.9	
Class 2	35.0–39.9	
Extreme (class 3)	≥40	

excessive body fat also carries an increased risk of developing comorbidities
from the excess weight [13]. In this way, appropriate treatment options are
tied to the degree of obesity and associated heath risks.

Current prevalence of obesity—where are we now?

Prevalence refers to the total number of existing cases of a disease
or condition in a given population at a specified time point. Using standard BMI cutoffs, one can divide the population into groups and compare
these groups across geographic boundaries, between genders, among ethnic
groups, and over periods of time. According to the most recent population
study from the 1999 National Health and Nutrition Examination Survey
(NHANES), 61% of individuals in the US population can be classified as
overweight or obese (BMI ≥ 25 kg/m^2; age-adjusted) (Table 1) [14]. More
than one third (34%) are overweight, defined as a BMI of 25 to 29.9 kg/m^2,
and 27% are obese (BMI ≥ 30 kg/m^2) [14].

The distribution of overweight and obesity is not divided equally among
the population. Ethnicity, gender, and age all influence the distribution of
overweight and obesity within the US population. In general, the prevalence
of obesity increases from age 20 to age 60, then decreases [5,15]. Because
of this tendency, most prevalence rates are age-adjusted, which means they
have been adjusted statistically to remove the effect of age differences in the
populations that are being compared. Fig. 1 shows the age-adjusted
prevalence of non-Hispanic whites, non-Hispanic blacks, and Mexican
Americans in the United States with a BMI greater than or equal to 25
kg/m^2 and broken down by overweight (BMI 25.0–29.9 kg/m^2) and obesity
criteria (BMI ≥ 30 kg/m^2). Both overweight and obesity are higher in non-
Hispanic black and Mexican-American ethnic groups than non-Hispanic
white individuals, according to the 1988 to 1994 NHANES III data [15].
Some groups of Native Americans, such as the Pima Indians of Arizona, are
reported to have even higher rates of obesity [16].

In the most recent NHANES, the prevalence of overweight (BMI 25–29.9
kg/m^2) was higher for men than women, the prevalence of BMIs 30 to 34.9
kg/m^2 was similar for men and women, and the prevalence of BMIs greater
than or equal to 35 kg/m^2 was higher for women than men [15]. There were

The Prevalence of Obesity

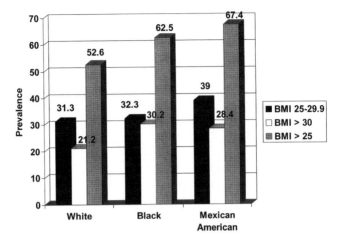

Fig. 1. Age-adjusted prevalence rates of overweight and obesity in the United States for non-Hispanic whites, non-Hispanic blacks, and Mexican Americans. (*Data from* Flegal KM, Carroll MD, Kuczmarski RJ, Johnson CL. Overweight and obesity in the United States: prevalence and trends, 1960–1994. Int J Obes 1998;22:39–47.)

some differences in this general pattern when broken down by gender and ethnic or racial group, however (Fig. 2). More white men than white women tend to be overweight, but not obese. The proportion of black women who were overweight or obese (BMI ≥ 25 kg/m^2) was higher than the proportion of black men (67% versus 58%) [15]. The age-adjusted prevalence of overweight or obesity in Mexican-American women and men tends to be approximately the same (Fig. 2); however, more Mexican-American women than men were classified as obese (BMI ≥ 30 kg/m^2). In addition, the age-adjusted prevalence of overweight or obesity is higher in non-Hispanic black and Mexican-American women than non-Hispanic white women (66.5% and 67.6%, respectively, versus 45.5%) (Fig. 2) [15]. Although an inverse relationship between socioeconomic status and obesity for women has been shown to exist, especially in developed countries [17], these ethnic and racial differences have been shown to persist even after controlling for socioeconomic status [5].

Weight gain is also a serious problem in children and adolescents. The most recent preliminary data from NHANES 1999 estimate that 13% of children aged 6 to 11 and 14% of adolescents aged 12 to 19 are overweight (BMI $\geq$ 95th percentile, revised National Centers for Health Statistics/Centers for Disease Control growth charts) [18]. Data from NHANES III (1988–1994) revealed that approximately 10% to 11% of every age and sex group of children and adolescents was overweight [19]. In boys, the highest percentage of overweight ($\geq$95th percentile, revised National Centers for Health Statistics/Centers for Disease Control growth charts) occurred in non-Hispanic blacks (12.3%), and the lowest percentage of overweight occurred among non-Hispanic white girls (9.8%) [18]. The prevalence

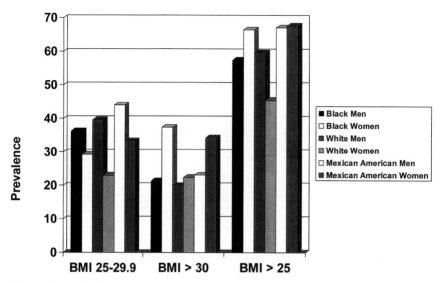

Fig. 2. Age-adjusted prevalence rates of overweight and obesity broken down by race-ethnic group for men and women. (*Data from* Flegal KM, Carroll MD, Kuczmarski RJ, Johnson CL. Overweight and obesity in the United States: prevalence and trends, 1960–1994. Int J Obes 1998;22:39–47.)

figures for adolescents vary from report to report [20,21]. Part of the problem comes from the fact that different percentile cutoffs are used for classifying youth at risk for adverse health consequences because of their weight. The results of all of the reports are consistent in showing that weights of youth in this country have increased dramatically between the 1980s and today [19,20,22]. This increase is of concern, because overweight adolescents are at increased risk for becoming overweight adults [23].

Time trends in the prevalence of obesity—how did we get here?

The prevalence of overweight and obesity in the US population has increased dramatically between the 1970s and the 1990s. The prevalence of individuals with a BMI of 25 kg/m^2 or higher has increased from 46% in the 1970s, to 54.4% in the 1980s and 1990s, to 61% by the latest NHANES 1999 data [14]. This increase in prevalence is almost entirely due to an increase in the prevalence of obesity (BMI $\geq$ 30 kg/m^2). Obesity has increased by almost 11 percentage points from the 1970s to 1999, with most of the rise occurring in the past decade [14].

From the 1970s to 1994, the prevalence of class I obesity (BMI 30–34.9 kg/m^2) increased from 9.6% to 14.4% overall, with men increasing from 9.5% to 14.6% and women from 10.5% to 14.2% [15]. Class II (BMI 35.0–39.9 kg/m^2) and class III obesity (BMI $\geq$ 40 kg/m^2) also increased during this time period (2.8%–5.2% and 1.3%–2.9%, respectively) [15]. In contrast, the prevalence of overweight defined as a BMI of 25 to 29.9 kg/m^2 has remained fairly constant during this same period (Fig. 3) [15].

Obesity has been increasing in every state in the nation. The Behavioral Risk Factor Surveillance Survey (BRFSS), a random-digit, cross-sectional telephone survey conducted in all states, collects self-reported weights and heights along with responses to questions about personal behaviors that increase risk for one or more of the 10 leading causes of death. In 2000, based on 184,450 participants in 50 states, the BRFSS found a 61% increase in obesity (BMI ≥ 30) since 1991 [24,25]. Overweight or obesity (BMI ≥ 25 kg/m^2) increased from 45% to 56.4% [24]. In 1991, four of the participating states in the BRFSS had obesity rates greater than 15%; by 2000, all participating states except Colorado had rates greater than 15% [24]. These data show that the average weight of US adults increased by 0.5 kg from 1999 to 2000 [24]. These estimates are probably conservative and lower than other population-based measurements, because self-reported weights usually are underestimated, and self-reported heights are overestimated.

How much weight are we gaining?

The Coronary Artery Risk Development in Young Adults (CARDIA) study is a population-based prospective study of cardiovascular risk factors that followed up more than 5000 young men and women (aged 18–30

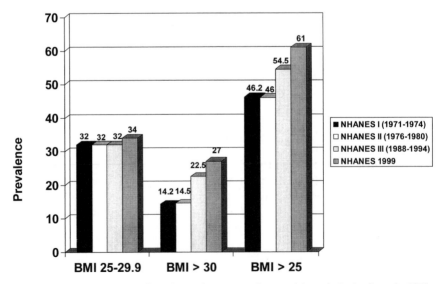

Fig. 3. Time trends for age-adjusted prevalence rates of overweight and obesity from the 1970s to 1999. (*Data from* Flegal KM, Carroll MD, Kuczmarski RJ, Johnson CL. Overweight and obesity in the United States: prevalence and trends, 1960–1994. Int J Obes 1998;22:39–47 and National Centers for Health Statistics, Centers for Disease Control. Prevalence of overweight and obesity among adults: United States, 1999. Available at: http://www.cdc.gov/nchs/products/pubs/pubd/hestats/obese/obse99.htm. Accessed September 1, 2002.)

at baseline) over the course of 10 years. In this cohort, the prevalence of overweight and obesity increased markedly over time in all race-sex groups [26]. The prevalence of overweight increases ranged from 23.7% at baseline to 41.6% at year 10 in white women to 47.8% baseline to 71.6% at year 10 for African-American women. Prevalence of the most severe obesity category, BMI greater than or equal to 40, more than doubled in all groups. The amount of weight gain during the 10-year period was reported to range from 11.9 kg in African-American women to 6.9 kg in white women [26]. The largest increases in weight occurred in the youngest, and the smallest increase occurred in the oldest race-age groups in all race-sex groups. Weight maintenance occurred in only a minority of individuals in all groups except for normal-weight white women, 51% of whom maintained their baseline weight [26]. These results and others show no sign of slowing in the 1990s.

Several studies, including CARDIA, have shown that the early to mid-twenties are periods of particular concern for weight gain among young adults [26–28]. These patterns have implications for targets for obesity-prevention measures. Health care providers should be aware that obesity needs to be addressed in the young adult years, a time possibly preceding the actual development of obesity-related comorbidities, but a time of high risk for weight gain. Additionally, even modest weight gain after age 18 years has been shown to increase the risk of heart disease [29].

Why are we gaining weight as a population?

Smoking cessation has been considered as a contributing factor in the increasing prevalence of overweight and obesity [30]. Many investigators have hypothesized that it is a possible explanation for the increase in obesity because smoking cessation started in the 1960s and 1970s and could result in weight gain, especially in the older-men subgroup [31]. Although it is true that a substantial increase in BMI is associated with smoking cessation [32], data from NHANES suggest that smoking cessation does not explain most of the weight gain the US population is experiencing [33]. In the CARDIA study, similar rates of weight gain were seen in smokers and in those who had never smoked [26]. Other studies have reported similar findings and agree that although smoking cessation may have played a small role, it alone does not account for the dramatic increase in overweight and obesity in the United States [34–36].

In energy balance terms, the increase in the weight of the population is due to energy intake that exceeds energy expenditure [37,38]. The social and environmental causes that facilitate this imbalance are harder to identify. Increased availability of energy-dense foods, large portion sizes, and lower levels of physical activity, both at work and at home, have been proposed as the cause of the increase. The WHO concluded that the fundamental causes of overweight and obesity worldwide are a fall in spontaneous and work-related physical activity and the overconsumption of high-fat, energy-dense diets [8]. In general, there has been a decrease in the percentage of calories of fat in the diet, an increase in total calories, and little change in the absolute amount of fat grams in the diet. In 2000, the BRFSS reported that 27% of US adults did not engage in any leisure-time physical activity, and 28.8% were not regularly active [24]. These rates are similar to rates reported in 1998. Reductions in overall physical activity may be largely attributable to decreases in activities of daily living that are much more difficult to document, however.

Flegal and Troiano [39] investigated the changes in the distribution of BMI using mean-difference plots that allow qualitative visual comparisons among the multiple NHANES data sets. They found an increasing skew with greater shift in the upper part of the weight distribution, which means that the heaviest subgroup of the population is much heavier in the NHANES III than prior surveys. In addition to the skew, they also found a general shift of the distribution upward, indicating an increase in BMI across the whole population, suggesting that the increase in obesity from NHANES II to NHANES III is not caused solely from the heaviest getting heavier. This finding is in opposition to the view that the increase in obesity is seen largely in specific age groups and especially in those at the tail end of the weight distribution [31]. Flegal and Troiano [39] found that the entire BMI distribution for adults had shifted over time, with some parts of the distribution shifting more than others. Older men showed a larger shift than young men, but no part of the distribution was unresponsive. There is an overall increase in obesity across all groups. This general shift points to a population-based cause for the increase in obesity that health care providers are facing, which suggests that the factors that are responsible operate broadly for almost the entire adult population, with a stronger effect on the upper portion of the distribution, possibly representing increased susceptibility in that subgroup. The whole population is susceptible and gaining significant amounts of weight, but some may be more susceptible and gaining more than others.

This analysis is important because it provides information that is useful to those working to stop the increase in weight. It suggests that the causes of obesity should be sought at the population level rather than focusing exclusively on individuals. Changes in energy balance on the individual level are likely secondary to environmental changes that affect the entire population. Interventions need to be considered, not just at the individual level, but also at the population level.

The prevalence of obesity throughout the world

The obesity epidemic is not confined to the United States or even to developed countries. The prevalence of overweight has been reported to be increasing throughout the world—in Canada, Mexico, Europe, Australia, Russia, China, South Africa, Saudi Arabia, Mauritius, and Western Samoa

[34,40–44]. Recent consensus of BMI cutoffs has allowed obesity prevalence rates to be compared among countries and regions of the world. The results are alarming, showing that most countries in the world have a significant obesity problem. Currently, the WHO estimates that there are more than 300 million obese adults (BMI $\geq$ 30 kg/m^2) [45]. This number translates into an 8.2% global prevalence of obesity [46].

The prevalence of overweight and obesity is rising to epidemic proportions in "westernized" developed countries and also is growing in countries that are just starting to develop. Traditionally, excess body weight was a sign of affluence, but now overweight and obesity are being seen in lower socioeconomic classes [47]. This global obesity epidemic is referred to as a "nutrition transition" by several nutrition experts and reflects just how quickly obesity can develop under the right set of economic and environmental conditions [47,48]. Many countries are now facing a double burden of undernutrition for some and an epidemic of obesity and health-related complications for others in the same geographic area. The WHO estimates that the global prevalence of obesity is 4.8% in developing countries, 17.1% in economies in transition, and 20.4% in developed market economy countries [46].

Prevalence of obesity-related comorbidities—what is the problem with gaining weight?

Obesity is a known risk factor for type 2 diabetes, heart disease, stroke, hypertension, osteoarthritis, sleep apnea, and some forms of cancer [1,49]. Gaining weight is not just a cosmetic problem but is correlated directly with the increase in the prevalence of many serious health disorders.

Type 2 diabetes has been associated with increased adiposity in studies worldwide. This serious comorbidity is one of the main reasons increasing weight will have a major impact on the general health and economic burden the United States faces with the obesity epidemic. It is estimated that 15.6 million adults in the United States have diabetes [50]. Approximately 95% of these persons have type 2 diabetes. Of those with type 2 diabetes, almost half (46%) have a BMI greater than or equal to 30 kg/m^2, and 67% have a BMI greater than or equal to 27 kg/m^2 [49]. From 1990 to 2000, the self-reported diagnosis of diabetes increased by 49%, from 4.9% to 7.3% [24]. This increase in diagnosed diabetes was correlated highly with obesity. Must et al [51], using the NHANES III data set, estimated that the prevalence of type 2 diabetes strongly increases in prevalence with increasing weight class among both younger and older participants. Colditz et al [52] found that the relative risk of diabetes increases by approximately 25% for each additional unit of BMI higher than 22 kg/m^2.

The metabolic syndrome, a cluster of coronary heart disease risk factors sharing insulin resistance in common, recently has been getting increased attention from the medical community. The third annual report of the

National Cholesterol Education Program Expert Panel on Detection, Evaluation, and Treatment of High Blood Cholesterol in Adults (Adult Treatment Panel III) emphasized the importance of diagnosing and treating patients with the metabolic syndrome [53]. The diagnosis of the metabolic syndrome is discussed further elsewhere in this book. The prevalence for metabolic syndrome in NHANES III (1988–1994) was approximately 22% (24% age-adjusted) [54]. The prevalence increased from 6.7% in young participants (aged 20–29 years) to 43.5% in participants aged 60 to 69 years [54]. Mexican Americans had the highest age-adjusted prevalence of the metabolic syndrome (31.9%). It is likely that the increase in obesity from 1994 to the present has resulted in an even higher prevalence than the 22% from the NHANES III data. It is estimated that approximately 47 million people living in the United States have the metabolic syndrome [54].

Looking to the future—where will we be tomorrow?

The prevalence of obesity is likely to increase in the years ahead. None of the epidemiologic studies to date has shown any signs that the increase in obesity is slowing. Some investigators have used the obesity trends to project that everyone will be obese by the year 2030 [55]. In all likelihood, a minority of individuals will prove to be genetically resistant to obesity, but these projections are cause for great alarm. The United States is still leading the way in the obesity epidemic, but the rest of the world is following closely behind.

Summary

During the past several decades, obesity has increased substantially, making it a true epidemic and a public health crisis that both health care providers and the public are going to have to face. Currently, 61% of the US population is overweight or obese and therefore at increased risk for a number of diseases that are associated with increased body fat. Indeed, the obesity epidemic already is leading to dramatic increases in type 2 diabetes and the metabolic syndrome. Almost a quarter of the population currently has metabolic syndrome, which places them at high risk for the development of coronary heart disease. The future of the general health of the US population depends on identifying and providing the best treatment and prevention strategies for obesity in the years ahead.

References

[1] National Heart, Lung, and Blood Institute Obesity Education Initiative Expert Panel. Clinical guidelines on the identification, evaluation, and treatment of overweight and obesity in adults: the evidence report. Obes Res 1998;6(Suppl 2):51S–209S.
[2] Hortobagyi T, Israel RG, O'Brien KF. Sensitivity and specificity of the Quetelet index to assess obesity in men and women. Eur J Clin Nutr 1994;48:369–75.

[3] Heymsfield SB, Allison DB, Heshka S, Pierson RN Jr. Assessment of human body composition. In: Allison DB, editor. Handbook of assessment methods for eating behavior and weight related problems: measures, theory, and research. Thousand Oaks (CA): Sage Publications; 1995. p. 515–60.

[4] Gallagher D, Visser M, Sepulveda D, Pierson RN, Harris T, Heymsfield SB. How useful is body mass index for comparison of body fatness across age, sex, and ethnic groups. Am J Epidemiol 1996;143:228–39.

[5] Allison DB, Saunders SE. Obesity in North America: an overview. Med Clin North Am 2000;84:305–32.

[6] National Institutes of Health, National Heart, Lung, and Blood Institute. North American Association for the Study of Obesity. The practical guide: identification, evaluation, and treatment of overweight and obesity in adults. NIH Publication 00–4084. Bethesda (MD): National Institutes of Health, National Heart, Lung, and Blood Institute; 2000.

[7] Lemieux S, Prud'homme D, Brouchard C, Tremblay A, Despres J. A single threshold value of waist girth identifies normal weight and overweight subjects with excess visceral adipose tissue. Am J Clin Nutr 1996;64:685–93.

[8] World Health Organization. Obesity: preventing and managing the global epidemic. Report of a WHO Consultation on Obesity, Geneva, June 3–5, 1997. Geneva: World Health Organization; 1998.

[9] Manson JE, Stampfer MJ, Hennekens CH, Willett WC. Body weight and longevity: a reassessment. JAMA 1987;257:353–8.

[10] Troiano RP, Frongillo EA, Sobal J, Levstsky DA. The relationship between body weight and mortality: a quantitative analysis of combined information from existing studies. Int J Obes Relat Metab Disord 1996;20:63–75.

[11] Wang J, Thorton JC, Russell M, et al. Asians have lower body mass index but higher body fat than whites: comparison of anthropometric measurements. Am J Clin Nutr 1994; 60:23–8.

[12] Wang J, Thorton JC, Burastero S, et al. Comparison of body mass index and body fat percent among Puerto Ricans, blacks, whites and Asians living in New York City area. Obes Res 1996;4:377–84.

[13] Gastrointestinal surgery for severe obesity. National Institutes of Heath Consensus Development Conference Statement. Am J Clin Nutr 1992;55:615S–619S.

[14] National Centers for Health Statistics, Centers for Disease Control. Prevalence of overweight and obesity among adults: United States, 1999. Available at: http://www.cdc.gov/nchs/products/pubs/pubd/hestats/obese/obse99.htm. Accessed September 1, 2002.

[15] Flegal KM, Carroll MD, Kuczmarski RJ, Johnson CL. Overweight and obesity in the United States: prevalence and trends, 1960–1994. Int J Obes 1998;22:39–47.

[16] Price RA, Charles MA, Pettit DJ, et al. Obesity in Pima Indians: large increases among post-World War II birth cohorts. Am J Phys Anthropol 1993;92:473–9.

[17] Sobal J, Stunkard A. Socioeconomic status and obesity: a review of the literature. Psychol Bull 1989;105:260–75.

[18] National Centers for Health Statistics, Centers for Disease Control. Overweight among US children and adolescents, data brief. Available at: http://www.cdc.gov/nchs/nhanes.htm. Accessed September 1, 2002.

[19] Troiano RP, Flegal KM. Overweight children and adolescents: description, epidemiology and demographics. Pediatrics 1998;101(Suppl 3):497–504.

[20] Troiano RP, Flegal KM. Overweight prevalence among youth in the United States: why so many numbers? Int J Obes 1999;23(Suppl 2):S22–7.

[21] Flegal KM, Ogden CL, Wei R, Kuczmarski RL, Johnson CL. Prevalence of overweight in US children: comparison of US growth charts from the Centers of Disease Control and Prevention with other reference values for body mass index. Am J Clin Nutr 2001;73: 1086–93.

[22] Wang Y, Monteiro C, Popkin BM. Trends of obesity and underweight in older children and adolescents in the United States, Brazil, China, and Russia. Am J Clin Nutr 2002;75:971–7.

[23] Serdula MK, Ivery D, Coates JR, Freedman DS, Williamson DF, Byers T. Do obese children become obese adults? A review of the literature. Prev Med 1993;22:167–77.

[24] Mokdad AH, Bowman BA, Ford ES, Vinicor F, Marks JS, Koplan JP. The continuing epidemics of obesity and diabetes in the United States. JAMA 2001;286:1195–200.

[25] Mokdad A, Serdula M, Dietz W, Bowman B, Marks J, Koplan J. The spread of the obesity epidemic in the United States, 1991–1998. JAMA 1999;282:1519–22.

[26] Lewis CE, Jacobs DR, McCreath H, Kiefe CI, Schreiner PJ, Smith DE, et al. Weight gain continues in the 1990s: 10 year trends in weight and overweight from the CARDIA study. Am J Epidemiol 2000;151:1172–81.

[27] Rissanen A, Heliovarra M, Aromaa A. Overweight and anthropometric changes in adulthood: a prospective study of 17,000 Finns. Int J Obes 1988;12:391–401.

[28] Williamson DF, Kahn HS, Remington PL, et al. The 10-year incidence of overweight and major weight gain in US adults. Arch Intern Med 1990;150:665–72.

[29] Willett WC, Manson JE, Stampfer MJ, et al. Weight, weight change, and coronary heart disease in women: risk within the normal weight range. JAMA 1995;273:461–5.

[30] Pi-Sunyer FX. The fattening of America [editorial]. JAMA 1994;272:238–9.

[31] Kuller LH. The epidemiology of obesity in adults in relationship to cardiovascular disease. In: Fletcher GF, Grundy SM, Hayman LL, editors. Obesity: impact on cardiovascular disease. Armonk, (NY): Futura Publishing Company; 1999. p. 3–29.

[32] Molarius A, Seidell JC, Kuulasmaa K, et al. Smoking and relative body weight: an international perspective from the WHO MONICA Project. J Epidemiol Commun Health 1997;51:252–60.

[33] Flegal KM, Troiano RP, Pamuk ER, Kuczmarski RJ, Campbell SM. The influence of smoking cessation on the prevalence of overweight in the United States. N Engl J Med 1995;333:1165–70.

[34] Shah M, Hannan PJ, Jeffery RW. Secular trends in body mass index in the adult population of three communities from the upper mid-western part of the USA: the Minnesota Heart Health Program. Int J Obes 1991;15:499–503.

[35] Boyle CA, Dobson AJ, Egger G, Magnus P. Can the increasing weight of Australians be explained by the decreasing prevalence of cigarette smoking? Int J Obes 1994;18:55–60.

[36] Wolk A, Rossner S. Effects of smoking and physical activity on body weight: development in Sweden between 1980 and 1989. J Int Med 1995;237:287–91.

[37] Hill JO. An overview of the etiology of obesity. In: Fairburn CG, Brownell KD, editors. Eating disorders and obesity: a comprehensive handbook. 2nd edition. New York (NY): The Guilford Press; 2002. p. 460–4.

[38] Peters JC, Wyatt HR, Donahoo WT, Hill JO. From instinct to intellect: the challenge of maintaining healthy weight in the modern world. Obes Rev 2002;3:69–74.

[39] Flegal KM, Troiano RP. Changes in the distribution of the body mass index of adults and children in the US population. Int J Obes 2000;24:807–18.

[40] Kuskowska-Wolk A, Bergstrom R. Trends in body mass index and prevalence of obesity in Swedish men, 1980–89. J Epidemiol Commun Health 1993;47:103–8.

[41] Bennett SA, Magnus P. Trends in cardiovascular risk factors in Australia: results from the National Heart Foundation's Risk Factor Prevalence Study, 1980–1989. Med J Aust 1994;161:519–27.

[42] Popkin BM, Paeratakul S, Ge K, Zhai F. Body weight patterns among the Chinese: results from the 1989 and 1991 China Health and Nutrition Surveys. Am J Public Health 1995;85:690–4.

[43] Hodge AM, Dowse GK, Gareeboo H, Tuomilehto J, Alberti KG, Zimmet PZ. Incidence, increasing prevalence, and predictors of change in obesity and fat distribution over 5 years in the rapidly developing population of Mauritius. Int J Obes 1996;20:137–46.

[44] Prentice AM, Jebb SA. Obesity in Britain: gluttony or sloth? BMJ 1995;19:924–7.

[45] World Health Organization (WHO). Controlling the global obesity epidemic. Available at: http://www.who.int/nut/obs.htm. Accessed August 30, 2002.

[46] World Health Organization (WHO). Global database on obesity and body mass index (BMI) in adults. Available at: http://www.who.int/nut/db_bmi.htm. Accessed August 30, 2002.

[47] James WPT. A world view of the obesity problem. In: Fairburn CG, Brownell KD, editors. Eating disorders and obesity: a comprehensive handbook. 2nd edition. New York (NY): The Guilford Press; 2002. p. 411–6.

[48] McLellan F. Obesity rising to alarming levels around the world. Lancet 2002;359:1412.

[49] National Task Force on the Prevention and Treatment of Obesity. Overweight, obesity and health risk. Arch Intern Med 2000;160:898–904.

[50] Harris MI, Flegal KM, Cowie CC, et al. Prevalence of diabetes impaired fasting glucose and impaired glucose tolerance in US adults: the Third National Heath and Education Survey, 1988–1994. Diabetes Care 1998;21:518–24.

[51] Must A, Spadano J, Coakley E, Field A, Colditz G, Dietz W. The disease burden associated with overweight and obesity. JAMA 1999;282:1523–9.

[52] Colditz GA, Willett WC, Rotnitzky A, Manson JE. Weight gain as a risk factor for clinical diabetes mellitus in women. Ann Intern Med 1995;122:481–6.

[53] National Institutes of Health. Third Report of the National Cholesterol Education Program Expert Panel on Detection, Evaluation, and Treatment of High Blood Cholesterol in Adults (Adult Treatment Panel III). NIH publication 01–3670. Bethesda (MD): National Institutes of Health; 2001.

[54] Ford ES, Giles WH, Dietz WH. Prevalence of the metabolic syndrome among US adults: findings from the Third National Health and Nutrition Examination Survey. JAMA 2002;287:356–9.

[55] Foreyt JP, Goodrick GK. The ultimate triumph of obesity. Lancet 1995;15:134–5.

3

Etiology of Obesity

Catherine M. Kotz

Allen S. Levine

Charles J. Billington

As the prevalence of obesity rapidly increases, it is apparent that something is very wrong with the way humans—children and adults, males and females alike—manage body weight. This "mismanagement" of body weight has resulted in obesity becoming one of the most important issues on the national health agenda. The causes of obesity, like other complex phenotypes, are generally understood as a combination of genetic tendency and environmental challenge. Recent obesity science has begun to more thoroughly identify the details of both contributions to the problem, but whether or not understanding will progress fast enough to blunt the remarkable increase in obesity prevalence is very much in doubt.

Genes

For the laboratory scientist, the best-known part of the story derives from the recent power of biomedical genetics. Several decades of searching has identified a number of animal models in which obesity appears as a result of a single gene mutation. The most famous of these is probably the ob/ob mouse, which is afflicted with an early onset obesity characterized by increased eating and decreased energy expenditure via metabolic rate. The investigation of this mouse strain led to the identification of leptin, a hormone secreted by fat tissue in amounts roughly comparable to total fat mass [1]. The *ob* gene is a recessive gene located on human chromosome 6 that codes for leptin, a 145 amino acid peptide produced in adipose and secreted into the bloodstream. Leptin binds to a receptor in the arcuate nucleus of the hypothalamus to decrease feeding behavior [2]. Both mouse and human homologs have been cloned, and when injected into obese mice or rats (peripherally and centrally), the animals decrease feeding [3–6]. Leptin administration also results in increased metabolic rate, and chronic administration results in loss of body weight when given to experimental animals [3–6]. Similar abnormalities occur when the leptin receptor, crucially expressed in the hypothalamus, is seriously mutated as it is in the db/db mouse and the Fa/Fa rat [7–9]. The significance of these findings was made apparent when it was found that some humans suffer from the same type of genetic abnormality in leptin or its receptor [10,11]. These people also had early onset obesity as a prominent manifestation of their condition, and their plight makes real the possibility of single gene obesities in humans. At this point, it appears that only a very few people will be found with this particular genetic defect. Nonetheless, the "proving" of human genetic obesity has greatly impacted the thinking of both the lay public, who now may be inclined to blame their obesity problem on their genes, and the thinking of scientists and science policy makers, who have focused considerable resources on further search for obesity genes and means to understand their effects.

Research encouraged by the interest in leptin has led to additional discoveries about the brain mechanisms that normally respond to leptin, and about the genes that partially define these mechanisms. Leptin is currently thought to interact with two groups of neurons in the hypothalamus. One group of hypothalamic neurons normally makes neuropeptide Y, which acts as a neuromodulator promoting food intake and positive energy balance, and leptin interaction with its receptor suppresses the positive energy balance function of these neurons [8]. Another group of neurons also responds to leptin binding to its receptor, but in this case the action of leptin is to enhance the formation of the prohormone/proneuromodulator, pro-opiomelanocortin (POMC), and its product melanocyte-stimulating hormone (MSH) [12]. This neural influence normally suppresses food intake and through additional means promotes negative energy balance. The action of α-MSH takes place at melanocortin receptors, and this system of POMC/MSH/melanocortin receptor is an additional important site of single gene defects, both in animals and in humans [11,13–16]. Recent data suggests that more people may be affected by genetic abnormalities in this system than have been found to be affected by leptin abnormalities, but even so the contribution of abnormalities in this system is likely to explain a small minority of human obesity.

Several other genes contribute to obesity in rodents, and the biology of these genes provides additional clues to potential obesity genetics in humans. The *fat* gene is a recessive gene on chromosome 8 that encodes carboxypeptidase E, which cleaves proinsulin and prepro neuropeptide Y (NPY), both peptides involved in feeding behavior [7,17,18]. Mice with a mutation in this gene develop adult onset obesity associated with type II diabetes. *Tub* is a recessive gene on chromosome 7 and mice with this mutation also develop adult onset obesity associated with type II diabetes

[7]. Finally, a defect in the gene that encodes β_3-adrenergic receptors is also associated with obesity. Stimulation of the β_3-adrenergic receptors increases metabolism, and a replacement mutation at position 64 of the amino acid arginine for tryptophan is associated with a slower metabolism and propensity to gain weight [19–21].

Among those people whose obesity is at least partly the result of their genes, most have polygenic obesity. Estimates of the number of genes that might contribute to the obesity phenotype have varied, but many would agree that the number of potential contributors is around 40. The obesity phenotype in polygenic obesity is seen as a result of interaction, in any given individual, between some smaller number of these traits. Most of these genes are yet to be identified, and the manner of their interactions is currently unknown. Accordingly, solid statements about the proportion of an individual's obesity attributable to genetic cause will be a long time coming.

Ecology

A century ago, the more pressing issue was one of food availability, or how to ensure that there was sufficient food supply. Agricultural and engineering advances have solved food production problems and the question of how to ensure adequate food supply is now one of food distribution. This is exemplified by the fact that just as the prevalence of obesity is increasing worldwide, so does hunger remain a problem on all continents. What has changed is the ratio of hungry to obese and the pattern of distribution. In almost all countries, the number of hungry has lessened, whereas obesity has increased dramatically. Further, in developed countries, small and rare pockets of hunger exist within a society that has available an excessive and readily accessible food supply, whereas in underdeveloped countries, the pattern is reversed, with small pockets of profound obesity existing in sharp contrast to surrounding areas of famine.

They are many indications that the Western lifestyle, particularly the American version of that lifestyle, promotes obesity in a broad spectrum of its citizens. Studies have shown that members of specific ethnic groups gain weight during the geographical transition over generations from one part of the world to the United States. In addition, it is now quite clear that obesity appears in those parts of any country with sufficient resources to adopt an American lifestyle [22–25]. In many cases, even a partial adoption of the American way, in the form of fast food or automobile oriented transportation patterns, can result in an increase in average body weight for height.

The profound obesity promoting effect of the Western lifestyle has been labeled "the toxic environment." The concept is emerging that the environment is so dangerous that it is likely that essentially all Americans will become obese in the next 50 years. Obesity scholars and activists generally support some attempts to change the environment, and this desire for change has also been manifest in government and governmental agencies.

While the recognition of this danger has become widespread, however, a full understanding of why the environment is so dangerous has not yet fully emerged.

With respect to basic energy balance, some reasons for the environmental toxicity are apparent. On average the typical American consumes more calories than a citizen of any other country, and from a historical perspective that same American consumed significantly more calories than did his or her ancestors 50, 100, or 200 years ago. At the same time, the physical intensity of activity associated with work has diminished for the average American, particularly in the last 25 years. The popular versions of these concepts are that we can blame the success of fast food, television, and computers for many of the obesity problems that Americans suffer. These concepts are clearly correct in a limited way but likely do not provide a full explanation for what has happened in the United States.

Additional explanations for obesity based on macronutrient consumption have also been offered. Dietary fat is currently the most accepted nutritional feature associated with obesity. For most of the last 20 years, probably in part related to a concern about fat relationship to cholesterol, dietary fat has been the component of the diet, which was thought to be the biggest problem. The most straightforward version of this argument is that fat is naturally more energy-dense then carbohydrate or protein, so extra consumption of fat is more likely to create a calorie imbalance. Additional features of fat that may further contribute to its mischief are that it is highly palatable in many forms and routinely sought after by animals and humans. A current addition to the argument is that fat may actually be directly toxic to body weight regulatory mechanisms (and may thus create leptin resistance). Skeptics of the dietary fat explanation for obesity have noted that obesity prevalence has skyrocketed during a time when the percentage of dietary fat reported by Americans has diminished. This critique is weakened by the fact that the percentage of fat in American diets has only diminished because total calorie levels have been increased by additional consumption of carbohydrates. The absolute amount of fat calories in the American diet probably has not changed for a few decades. From an energy balance point of view, the persistence of fat consumption may itself be a problem [26].

Currently, carbohydrates are the popular malefactor implicated in the genesis of obesity. While some of the explanations for why carbohydrates might be a problem rely on various forms of physiologic magic, there are nonetheless biologically plausible reasons to be concerned about the amount of carbohydrates eaten by the typical American. The most important of these reasons, as suggested above, is that an increase in total calories has been quickly and easily achieved by introduction of additional carbohydrates. One factor that might be particularly germane is the consumption of sugared beverages, particularly soda pop. There is clear evidence that pop consumption has nearly doubled over the last 25 years [27]. Even though a portion of that extra consumption has been of diet beverages, the consumption of energy in this form has increased greatly. During the period of obesity prevalence explosion, this extra energy has mainly been in the form of high fructose corn syrup. In addition to contribution of calorie-sweetened beverages to energy balance, there are current theories suggesting that fructose may be a more important problem than other forms of carbohydrate for metabolic reasons.

Beyond these issues, there are also strong suggestions that certain forms of carbohydrates, fats, or combinations of these macronutrients in the diet are particularly rewarding when consumed and may actually increase intake based on biological drive for that type of reward. Although it would not be accurate to refer to these highly palatable foods and drinks as addictive, there is some indication that a form of dependence on these substances can occur for biological reasons as evidenced by the finding that chronic ingestion of palatable solutions can lead to changes in neurochemical systems involved in drug dependence [28]. For example, in rats exposed to glucose solution, daily dopamine D_1-receptor binding increased significantly in the nucleus accumbens core and shell, a region importantly implicated in reward-based feeding [29]. Also, opioid μ_1-receptor binding increased significantly in the cingulate cortex, hippocampus, locus coeruleus, and accumbens shell [29]. Other investigators have shown that food reward can affect drug-taking behavior. For example, the replacement of water with a bottle of a saccharin solution will decrease self-administration of reinforcing drugs in primates [30]. Also, it has been found that animals that prefer sweet-tastants will self-administer more cocaine than those that demonstrate no sweet preference [31]. If these notions continue to gain additional evidentiary support, then there may be reason to more carefully evaluate the rewarding qualities of foods in the etiology of obesity.

Energy expended has also been undergoing change in the American environment. Most obviously, much of the physically strenuous work has been transformed into knowledge and service work, which depends more on offices and computers than on the traditional understanding of the word labor. Limited measurements of the quantitative impact of this change are available, but few scholars doubt the significance. More controversial is the role of voluntary exercise associated with activities like sport. While most poll data indicate that Americans do less exercise, there is nonetheless a successful business in fitness. One way to understand these disparate trends is to note that some people, probably a minority, respond to exercise positively, while others, probably a majority, will only exercise when the incentive to do so becomes very strong.

One phenotypic behavior of obese individuals is extreme efficiency of movement, and very little spontaneous movement. Although this sparing of energy expenditure may be the result of becoming obese, there is also evidence to suggest that low levels of activity play a causative role. In one study that followed children from infancy to late childhood, it was demonstrated that energy expenditure at 3 months of age in children who later became obese was 20% less than that in those who remained lean [32]. In studies of families with varying levels of physical activity, it was shown that children in families with low activity levels were more likely to be obese [33,34]. These studies demonstrate that low levels of spontaneous physical activity may be a very important determinant of obesity. Recent work by Levine and Jensen have demonstrated that individuals vary dramatically in the amount of body weight gained in response to overeating and that much of this variation is due to thermogenesis from nonvolitional or "spontaneous" exercise [35]. The source of this activity is incompletely defined but has been attributed to fidgeting [36]. The term coined for the energy expended by nonvolitional activity is *nonexercise activity thermogenesis* (NEAT). Those with enhanced capacity for NEAT are less susceptible to weight gain [35]. Recent work has demonstrated that fidgeting-like activities have significant thermogenic potential and may have important implications for energy balance [36,37]. In a very recent study in rats, Levine et al [38] investigated whether enhanced energy expenditure observed in hyperthyroidism could be attributed to increases in NEAT. In this study, rats given injections of triiodothyronine (T3) for 14 days were shown to have increased spontaneous physical activity and NEAT, and the energy expenditure associated with hyperthyroidism appears to be related to these changes in activity. However, the mechanism behind NEAT is still unknown. Leptin does not appear to be involved in activation of NEAT, as leptin changes in response to overfeeding do not correlate with changes in NEAT [35,39]. A recent study of the response to overfeeding in self-reported restrained and unrestrained eaters indicates that restrained eaters have reduced NEAT, which may contribute to enhanced susceptibility to weight gain in restrained eaters [40].

Another important incentive to which humans are known to respond is economic. Studies of the economic contributions to obesity are in a relatively early phase, but the evidence tends to support some common-sense notions. In a dynamic and competitive marketplace, the value of time rises for nearly all individuals. One consequence of the high value of time is that eating that can take place quickly may be very desirable [41]. Economic data suggests that obesity increases in those communities with more restaurants, and that obesity further increases when the price of fast food falls [42,43]. Furthermore, competition between restaurants is in good part based on perceived value, so that portion sizes have greatly increased over the past 25 years. Restaurant advocates would argue that people can exert both will and satiety to stop their consumption at appropriate levels, but biological studies from food labs shows the expected finding that an increase in portion size will produce increased consumption [44,45].

Economic values have also driven some of the changes in physical activity that have occurred. The best example of this change occurs in the traditionally nonbusiness setting of the public school. Budgetary pressures have led to the downsizing or elimination of physical education and sports in schools, and evidence indicates that this change is associated with the decline in the degree to which children and adolescents are physically active. There are indications that programs like community centers can partially address this difficulty, but these programs are also under budgetary pressures [44]. Furthermore, schools, which are forced to be entrepreneurial, have sought additional resources from business in return for the placement of products such as vending machines purveying calorie-sweetened beverages and cafeterias selling popular fast foods [46]. Attempts to educate students about healthy body weight must now compete with the attention given these popular nuisances. More broadly, the increased value of individual time referred to above provides a disincentive for individuals of all ages to exercise, or even to choose a mode of transportation that is more active but slower.

The concept of ecology indicates that crucial components of individual energy balance are only partially under individual control. Food and activity choices can also be determined by surrounding individuals and by the culture, resources, and circumstances that are present. Still, these choices have a biological context and it is useful to recognize that humans have the capacity to change their ecology. We can further recognize that the technological ability to change our ecology, as well as the efficiency with which this change can take place, have been greatly increased by our industry and economy. When we find that there are many restaurants selling large portions cheaply, we know that this is a change in our ecology that we have collectively created. Motivations for making these changes are rooted in our own biology. Although cynics would conclude that the human ability to efficiently change ecology so as to maximize obesity poses an insurmountable barrier to combating the problem, a hopeful conclusion is that problems that we have created can be fixed by us. The caveat is that solutions at the individual level would be difficult to achieve until we collectively make decisions to change our ecology in favorable ways.

There is some evidence that obesity may have a viral link. The possibility that a viral infection could contribute to obesity is based on data indicating that in chickens, an adenovirus is associated with central adiposity [47,48]. Furthermore, the presence of serum antibodies to this adenovirus in humans has been associated with obesity [49]. However, the contribution of a viral mechanism to human obesity is likely a small fraction of affected individuals because in all of the cases where the virus has been able to produce obesity in rats or monkeys it was associated with low cholesterol, which is in contrast to the obese phenotype in humans [48,50].

Role of the brain

The brain plays a central role in the effect of gene-environment interactions on obesity. All of the above-mentioned genetic and viral abnormalities associated with obesity impact important energy regulatory processes in the brain. Conditions in our environment also affect the brain, and our cognition dictates the foods we choose and whether we exercise. The majority of drugs that have been used to treat obesity act on brain mechanisms to reduce appetite. Furthermore, the success of drugs or treatments that target a nonbrain mechanism (eg, the use of dietary lipase inhibitors or stomach stapling procedures), ultimately resides in changes that occur in the brain, because the success of these weight-loss strategies is due to learned avoidance of unpleasant consequences of eating too much food or fat.

Studies by Tataranni and colleagues indicate that brain activity as measured by glucose uptake within specific cortical and limbic regions during hunger and satiation is different between the obese and the lean, in both men and women [51,52]. Whether these differences precede the obese state or occur as a result of obesity is an active area of investigation. Preliminary studies of postobese individuals suggest that most of these differences disappear as a result of weight loss, with the exception of persistent differences in hippocampal activity [53]. The hippocampus has a primary role in learning and forming memories, and as such may contribute to the learning of food preferences [54]. Current techniques do not allow for measurement of brain plasticity in humans, but basic science studies suggest that new connections can be formed in a relatively rapid time-frame [55,56], and that learning involves forming new connections or remodeling of old connections. This plasticity can be both disadvantageous and advantageous for body weight regulation, since it allows for the development of preferences for perhaps "unhealthy" foods and practices, but also allows for unlearning of unhealthy practices through cognitive and behavioral training.

In addition to leptin, NPY, and POMC circuits mentioned above, there are a variety of other important neurotransmitters, including peptides, monoamines, and amino acids that participate in determining feeding behavior. Some of these compounds may regulate spontaneous activity levels, which would result in alterations in energy expenditure, and as Bray [57,58] has studied in detail, many of these neurotransmitters have more direct effects on energy expenditure. Bray demonstrated an inverse relationship between energy intake and energy expenditure for many neuroregulatory compounds. One example of this is the finding that neuropeptide Y and opioids, both of which increase feeding, in turn decrease sympathetic nervous system firing to and activity of brown adipose tissue, which would result in decreased energy expenditure [59–63]. Conversely, serotonin, corticotrophin releasing hormone (CRH), and urocortin, all of which decrease feeding, result in activation of the sympathetic nervous system [64,65]. This dual effect on food intake and expenditure can lead to powerful effects on body weight. Urocortin is a peptide related to CRH that binds to CRH receptors more avidly than

CRH [66] and may be more potent that CRH in decreasing feeding [67,68]. Recent studies in our laboratory have demonstrated that urocortin in the paraventricular nucleus decreases nocturnal feeding, deprivation-induced feeding, and feeding induced by neuropeptide Y [65]. Another putative satiety signal is cocaine- and amphetamine-regulated transcript (CART), which also inhibits the feeding response to neuropeptide Y and both normal and deprivation-induced feeding. Furthermore, endogenous levels of CART in the arcuate nucleus is decreased following food deprivation and antisera against CART increases feeding in normal rats [69]. In animals with defective leptin signaling, CART mRNA is absent, and leptin administration in obese mice up-regulates CART mRNA [69], indicating that CART may interact with leptin in feeding regulation. Orexins A and B (also known as hypocretins 1 and 2) are two recently characterized peptides that not only play a role in the stimulation of feeding but also induce activity and energy expenditure when given centrally [70,71]. Prepro-orexin mRNA levels are increased following food deprivation [71], which is consistent with what would be expected for an orexigenic compound. However, mice with specific depletion of orexin-containing neurons do not become lean as one might expect; rather, they become obese [72]. Importantly, the activity levels of these mice were also decreased dramatically. Thus, although the mice were eating less, they were also expending less energy with the net effect being weight gain.

The above examples illustrate the complexity of brain mechanism operating to maintain appropriate feeding behavior and activity levels. It is clear that there are many opportunities for overlap, and plasticity ensures adaptability. Finally, this is a small sampling of some of the data linking the brain with the regulation of feeding and energy expenditure. There are numerous other equally relevant neuropeptides and other compounds not discussed here, and ongoing research efforts are rapidly uncovering previously unidentifed mechanisms influencing energy balance.

Summary

It is evident that both genes and environment contribute to obesity. There are some important challenges in defining the gene–environment interaction, because these concepts in current form do not mix well. The conceptions underlying current views about genetic mechanisms focus on an adipostat, in which body fat content would be homeostatically maintained at fixed levels. Biological stability of body weight is inconsistent with the burgeoning numbers of obese people and with the toxic environment invoked by many to explain this phenomenon. Attempts to reconcile the inconsistencies between genetic and environmental understandings have pursued a few lines. This interaction would commonly be seen as environmental challenges working on sensitive, gene-defined mechanisms, in which some are more sensitive than others. Another concept holds that the genetic constitution has defined an obese genotype, which has not been fully expressed in phenotype until the last 25 years because of limited calorie availability or the need for expended energy. The mechanisms of brain regulation may provide a more detailed answer, as suggested above, in which genetically defined components interact with each other and with the environment, then regulate appetite and activity in accord with contributions of both genes and environment.

One potentially useful perspective is to consider energy intake and energy expenditure as sums of several individual contributions. In the case of intake, some eating is to provide for current energy and glucose needs and some other intake sustains a basal level of fat storage and leptin signaling, while additional intake is for purposes of pleasure, mood, or social purposes. Although these individual motivations to eat can be separated conceptually in this way, each of these motivations is also represented by a mechanism in the brain. Further, these individual brain-based motivations likely interact and support one another. For example, we obviously eat more when hungry, but we eat even more when we are hungry and the food is very good and in great variety. In this case the biological mechanisms that signal short-term energy need work along with the biological mechanisms that respond to the desirability of presented food. A similar, differentiated but interacting set of biological phenomena is found on the energy expenditure side. Much more work needs to be done to better understand these interacting motivations and biological mechanisms, and this work represents a significant challenge.

When seen in this way, the beginnings of an explanation for obesity etiology can be glimpsed. Although it is clear that defects in mechanisms related to leptin signaling and like phenomena can produce obesity in a fraction of the population, it is not necessary to invoke widespread leptin signaling defects to explain the general appearance of obesity. It is more likely that our success in providing good food and a comfortable lifestyle feeds into biological mechanisms that encourage us to pursue more food and greater comfort. We are able to change our environment, or our ecology, so as to enrich the environment with the features that we like. It is therefore likely that it is the power and efficiency to change our own environment, which poses the greatest challenge, but mercifully opens the possibility of redress. Humans collectively decided to change their ecology in this way, generally for reasons that had nothing to do with health. Once we understand the threat, we can change it for the better.

References

[1] Caro JF, et al. Leptin: the tale of an obesity gene. Diabetes 1996;45:1455–62.
[2] Elmquist JK. Hypothalamic pathways underlying the endocrine, autonomic, and behavioral effects of leptin. Int J Obes Relat Metab Disord 2001;25(Suppl 5):S78–82.

[3] Weigle DS, et al. Recombinant ob protein reduces feeding and body weight in the ob/ob mouse. J Clin Invest 1995;96:2065–70.

[4] Halaas JL, et al. Weight-reducing effects of the plasma protein encoded by the obese gene. Science 1995;269:543–6.

[5] Campfield LA, et al. Recombinant mouse OB protein: evidence for a peripheral signal linking adiposity and central neural networks. Science 1995;269:546–9.

[6] Pelleymounter MA, et al. Effects of the obese gene product on body weight regulation in ob/ob mice. Science 1995;269:540–3.

[7] Coleman DL, Eicher EM. Fat (fat) and tubby (tub): two autosomal recessive mutations causing obesity syndromes in the mouse. J Hered 1990;81:424–7.

[8] Williams G, et al. The hypothalamus and the control of energy homeostasis: different circuits, different purposes. Physiol Behav 2001;74:683–701.

[9] Williams G, Harrold JA, Cutler DJ. The hypothalamus and the regulation of energy homeostasis: lifting the lid on a black box. Proc Nutr Soc 2000;59:385–96.

[10] Montague CT, et al. Congenital leptin deficiency is associated with severe early-onset obesity in humans. Nature 1997;387:903–8.

[11] Clement K. Monogenic forms of obesity: from mice to human. Ann Endocrinol (Paris) 2000;61(Suppl 6):39–49.

[12] Cone RD, et al. The arcuate nucleus as a conduit for diverse signals relevant to energy homeostasis. Int J Obes Relat Metab Disord 2001;25(Suppl 5):S63–7.

[13] Pritchard LE, Turnbull AV, White A. Pro-opiomelanocortin processing in the hypothalamus: impact on melanocortin signalling and obesity. J Endocrinol 2002;172:411–21.

[14] Shintani M, Ogawa Y, Nakao K. Obesity induced by abnormality in leptin receptor and melanocortin-4 receptor. Nippon Rinsho 2002;60:404–9.

[15] Benoit S, et al. CNS melanocortin system involvement in the regulation of food intake. Horm Behav 2000;37:299–305.

[16] Krude H, et al. Severe early-onset obesity, adrenal insufficiency and red hair pigmentation caused by POMC mutations in humans. Nat Genet 1998;19:155–7.

[17] Weigle DS, Kuijper JL. Obesity genes and the regulation of body fat content. Bioessays 1996;18:867–74.

[18] Naggert JK, et al. Hyperproinsulinaemia in obese fat/fat mice associated with a carboxypeptidase E mutation which reduces enzyme activity. Nat Genet 1995;10: 135–42.

[19] Lamont LS. Beta-blockers and their effects on protein metabolism and resting energy expenditure. J Cardiopulm Rehabil 1995;15:183–5.

[20] Yen TT. Beta-agonists as antiobesity, antidiabetic and nutrient partitioning agents. Obes Res 1995;3(Suppl 4):531S–6S.

[21] Astrup A. The sympathetic nervous system as a target for intervention in obesity. Int J Obes Relat Metab Disord 1995;19(Suppl 7):S24–8.

[22] Popkin BM, Doak CM. The obesity epidemic is a worldwide phenomenon. Nutr Rev 1998;56:106–14.

[23] Popkin BM. The nutrition transition and obesity in the developing world. J Nutr 2001;131:871S–3S.

[24] Bell AC, Ge K, Popkin BM. The road to obesity or the path to prevention: motorized transportation and obesity in China. Obes Res 2002;10:277–83.

[25] Popkin BM. Nutrition in transition: the changing global nutrition challenge. Asia Pac J Clin Nutr 2001;10:S13–8.

[26] Bray GA, Popkin BM. Dietary fat intake does affect obesity. Am J Clin Nutr 1998;68: 1157–73.

[27] USDA. What and where our children eat—1994 nationwide survey results. Food and Nutrition Research Briefs April 1996. p. 1–7.

[28] Levine AS, Kotz CM, Gosnell BA. Sugars: hedonic aspects, neuroregulation, and energy balance. Am J Clin Nutr, in press.

[29] Colantuoni C, et al. Excessive sugar intake alters binding to dopamine and mu-opioid receptors in the brain. Neuroreport 2001;12:3549–52.

[30] Gosnell BA. Sucrose intake predicts rate of acquisition of cocaine self-administration. Psychopharmacology (Berl) 2000;149:286–92.

[31] Carroll ME, Carmona GG, May SA. Modifying drug-reinforced behavior by altering the economic conditions of the drug and a nondrug reinforcer. J Exp Anal Behav 1991;56:361–76.

[32] Schutz Y. The role of physical inactivity in the etiology of obesity. Ther Umsch 1989;46:281–90.

[33] Birch LL, Davison KK. Family environmental factors influencing the developing behavioral controls of food intake and childhood overweight. Pediatr Clin North Am 2001;48:893–907.

[34] Davison KK, Birch LL. Child and parent characteristics as predictors of change in girls' body mass index. Int J Obes Relat Metab Disord 2001;25:1834–42.

[35] Levine JA, Eberhardt NL, Jensen MD. Role of nonexercise activity thermogenesis in resistance to fat gain in humans. Science 1999;283:212–4.

[36] Levine J, et al. Measurement of the components of nonexercise activity thermogenesis. Am J Physiol Endocrinol Metab 2001;281:E670–5.

[37] Levine JA, Schleusner SJ, Jensen MD. Energy expenditure of nonexercise activity. Am J Clin Nutr 2000;72:1451–4.

[38] Levine JA, et al. Effect of hyperthyroidism on spontaneous physical activity and energy expenditure in rats. J Appl Physiol 2003;94:165–70.

[39] Levine JA, Eberhardt NL, Jensen MD. Leptin responses to overfeeding: relationship with body fat and nonexercise activity thermogenesis. J Clin Endocrinol Metab 1999;84:2751–54.

[40] Bathalon GP, et al. The energy expenditure of postmenopausal women classified as restrained or unrestrained eaters. Eur J Clin Nutr 2001;55:1059–67.

[41] DeMaria AN. Of fast food and franchises. J Am Coll Cardiol 2003;41:1227–8.

[42] Drewnowski A. Fat and sugar: an economic analysis. J Nutr 2003;133:838S–40S.

[43] French SA. Pricing effects on food choices. J Nutr 2003;133:841S–3S.

[44] Mitka M. Economist takes aim at "big fat" US lifestyle. JAMA 2003;289:33–4.

[45] Kottke TE, Wu LA, Hoffman RS. Economic and psychological implications of the obesity epidemic. Mayo Clin Proc 2003;78:92–4.

[46] Stitzel K. School nutrition programs: a legislative perspective. J Am Diet Assoc 2003;103:439–40.

[47] Dhurandhar NV, et al. Transmissibility of adenovirus-induced adiposity in a chicken model. Int J Obes Relat Metab Disord 2001;25:990–6.

[48] Dhurandhar NV, et al. Increased adiposity in animals due to a human virus. Int J Obes Relat Metab Disord 2000;24:989–96.

[49] Dhurandhar NV, et al. Association of adenovirus infection with human obesity. Obes Res 1997;5:464–9.

[50] Dhurandhar NV, et al. Human adenovirus Ad-36 promotes weight gain in male rhesus and marmoset monkeys. J Nutr 2002;132:3155–60.

[51] Gautier JF, et al. Differential brain responses to satiation in obese and lean men. Diabetes 2000;49:838–46.

[52] Gautier JF, et al. Effect of satiation on brain activity in obese and lean women. Obes Res 2001;9:676–84.

[53] Gautier JF, et al. Differences in the brain response to satiation in lean, obese and post-obese individuals. Obes Res 2001;9(Suppl 3):56S.

[54] Tracy AL, Jarrard LE, Davidson TL. The hippocampus and motivation revisited: appetite and activity. Behav Brain Res 2001;127:13–23.

[55] Vautrin J, Barker JL. Presynaptic quantal plasticity: Katz's original hypothesis revisited. Synapse 2003;47:184–99.

[56] Murphy TH. Activity-dependent synapse development: changing the rules. Nat Neurosci 2003;6:9–11.

[57] Bray GA. Reciprocal relation of food intake and sympathetic activity: experimental observations and clinical implications. Int J Obes Relat Metab Disord 2000;24(Suppl 2): S8–17.

[58] Bray GA. The nutrient balance hypothesis: peptides, sympathetic activity, and food intake. Ann N Y Acad Sci 1993;676:223–41.

[59] Billington CJ, et al. Neuropeptide Y in hypothalamic paraventricular nucleus: a center coordinating energy metabolism. Am J Physiol 1994;266:R1765–70.

[60] Billington CJ, Levine AS. Hypothalamic neuropeptide Y regulation of feeding and energy metabolism. Curr Opin Neurobiol 1992;2:847–51.

[61] Egawa M, Yoshimatsu H, Bray GA. Neuropeptide Y suppresses sympathetic activity to interscapular brown adipose tissue in rats. Am J Physiol 1991;260:R328–34.

[62] Egawa M, Yoshimatsu H, Bray GA. Effect of beta-endorphin on sympathetic nerve activity to interscapular brown adipose tissue. Am J Physiol 1993;264:R109–15.

[63] Kotz CM, et al. Effects of opioid antagonists naloxone and naltrexone on neuropeptide Y-induced feeding and brown fat thermogenesis in the rat. Neural site of action. J Clin Invest 1995;96:163–70.

[64] Egawa M, Yoshimatsu H, Bray GA. Effect of corticotropin releasing hormone and neuropeptide Y on electrophysiological activity of sympathetic nerves to interscapular brown adipose tissue. Neuroscience 1990;34:771–5.

[65] Wang CF, et al. Feeding inhibition by urocortin in the rat hypothalamic paraventricular nucleus. Am J Physiol 2001;280:R473.

[66] Vaughan J, et al. Urocortin, a mammalian neuropeptide related to fish urotensin I and to corticotropin-releasing factor. Nature 1995;378:287–92.

[67] Jones DN, et al. The behavioural effects of corticotropin-releasing factor-related peptides in rats. 1988;138:124–32.

[68] Spina M, et al. Appetite-suppressing effects of urocortin, a CRF-related neuropeptide. Science 1996;273:1561–4.

[69] Kristensen P, et al. Hypothalamic CART is a new anorectic peptide regulated by leptin. Nature 1998;393:72–6.

[70] de Lecea L, et al. The hypocretins: hypothalamus-specific peptides with neuroexcitatory activity. Proc Natl Acad Sci U S A 1998;95:322–7.

[71] Sakurai T, et al. Orexins and orexin receptors: a family of hypothalamic neuropeptides and G protein-coupled receptors that regulate feeding behavior. Cell 1998;92:573–85.

[72] Hara J, et al. Genetic ablation of orexin neurons in mice results in narcolepsy, hypophagia, and obesity. Neuron 2001;30:345–54.

4

Metabolic Syndrome

Maria L. Collazo-Clavell

Michael D. Jensen

Metabolic syndrome describes a cluster of metabolic and cardiovascular risk factors [1]. The constellation of truncal obesity, glucose intolerance, dyslipidemia (high triglycerides, low high-density lipoprotein [HDL] cholesterol, small low-density lipoprotein [LDL] cholesterol), and hypertension has been recognized relatively recently and has been referred to by different names [2–4]. *Syndrome X, metabolic syndrome X, insulin-resistance syndrome,* and, more recently, *metabolic syndrome* are terms used to describe this cohort of patients recognized to be at increased risk for cardiovascular heart disease (CHD) and mortality [5]. Although frequently referred to, it was not until 1998 that a working definition for metabolic syndrome was proposed by the World Health Organization (WHO) [6]. Most recently, the Third Report of the National Cholesterol Education Program (NCEP III) recognized metabolic syndrome as a clinical entity and proposed a set of clinical criteria for diagnosis [1].

The NCEP criteria for a diagnosis of metabolic syndrome include the presence of three or more risk determinants as outlined in Table 1. This differs from the WHO criteria in that it proposes lower values for blood pressure and serum triglycerides for a diagnosis. Although insulin resistance and proinflammatory and prothrombotic states are thought to be important components of metabolic syndrome, measures of these components are not included in the NCEP criteria because they are not easily identified during routine clinical evaluation [1].

Ford et al [7] reported the prevalence of metabolic syndrome among adults in the United States using the NCEP III diagnostic criteria. The results of the NHANES III survey, which was conducted in 1994, indicated that 22% of adults in the United States met the criteria for metabolic syndrome. Today, the prevalence of metabolic syndrome is likely higher, considering the rise in the prevalence of obesity since the NHANES III survey.

Table 1
Clinical identification of metabolic syndrome

Risk factor	Defining level
Abdominal obesity (waist circumference)	
Men	> 102 cm (> 40 in)
Women	> 88 cm (> 35 in)
Triglycerides	≥150 mg/dL
HDL cholesterol	
Men	<40 mg/dL
Women	<50 mg/d/L
Blood pressure	≥130/85 mm Hg
Fasting glucose	≥110 mg/dL

Abbreviation: HDL, high-density lipoprotein.
From Third Report of the National Cholesterol Education Program (NCEP) expert panel on detection, evaluation, and treatment of high blood cholesterol in adults (Adult Treatment Panel III): final report. Circulation 2001;106:3143–421.

The health implications of metabolic syndrome are worrisome, both for the individual patient and for the population at large. The presence of metabolic syndrome increases the risks for CHD at any given LDL cholesterol level [1]. Unless reversed, the rising prevalence of metabolic syndrome threatens the recent improvements in CHD risks that have been achieved by lowering of the average LDL cholesterol in the population. Metabolic syndrome is now considered a risk factor for premature CHD equal to cigarette smoking [1].

Metabolic syndrome and insulin resistance

Multiple cross-sectional studies have identified insulin resistance as a common finding in persons with metabolic syndrome [4,8,9]. However, the role of insulin resistance as the cause for the clustering of clinical abnormalities that define metabolic syndrome remains actively debated. The San Antonio Heart Study first reported that individuals with higher plasma insulin concentrations, at their baseline exam, were more likely to develop hypertension, type 2 diabetes mellitus, hypertriglyceridemia, and low HDL after 8 years of follow-up [4]. As a result of this and multiple other studies, insulin resistance is considered to be an active contributor to the pathophysiological processes increasing an individual's risk for CHD [1].

Pathophysiology of metabolic syndrome: insulin resistance and related complications

The properties of excess adipose tissue, which contribute to the metabolic complications of obesity, are now somewhat better understood. The fact that a central or upper body fat distribution is predictive of the metabolic complications of obesity was an important clue [10]. The most important function of adipose tissue is to store lipid fuel (fatty acids in the form of triglycerides) and release free fatty acids (FFAs) and glycerol into the circulation via lipolysis. FFAs provide the majority of circulating lipid fuel. Lipolysis is capable of providing 50% to 100% of daily energy needs. Adipose tissue lipolysis is regulated primarily by insulin (inhibition) [11] and catecholamines (stimulation) [12]. Upper body obesity is associated with several abnormalities of adipose tissue lipolysis, most notably with higher FFA concentrations, due to excess release in the postabsorptive [13] and postprandial [14] periods. Abnormally high FFA concentrations can contribute to or account for a number of the metabolic complications of central obesity [15].

Insulin resistance

The term *insulin resistance* is typically used when referring to the inability of insulin to promote glucose uptake, oxidation, and storage, as well as to inhibit the release of glucose into the circulation. The primary site of insulin-stimulated glucose uptake, oxidation, and storage is skeletal muscle. The principal site of glucose production is the liver. Insulin resistance initially leads to hyperinsulinemia, a possible independent cardiovascular risk factor, and may eventually lead to the development of type 2 diabetes mellitus.

The ability of insulin to stimulate glucose disposal in muscle (and thus maintain normal glucose tolerance) and suppress plasma FFA concentrations is reduced in upper body obesity. Creating high plasma FFA concentrations via experimental manipulations can induce a state of insulin resistance both in the muscle (glucose uptake) [16] and in the liver (glucose release) [17], independent of obesity. Thus, abnormal regulation of adipose tissue FFA export can potentially explain much of the insulin resistance with respect to glucose metabolism.

It has been suggested that abnormalities in the production of adipose tissue hormones and peptides also contribute to metabolic syndrome. These compounds include adiponectin, resistin, tumor necrosis factor α (TNF-α), interleukin 6 (IL-6), plasminogen activator inhibitor 1 (PAI-1), and angiotensinogen. Adiponectin is a protein with structural similarity to collagen expressed in high concentration by adipocytes. Adiponectin concentrations are inversely related to body fat mass and are also especially low in adults with type 2 diabetes mellitus and coronary heart disease. Serum concentrations of adiponectin are negatively correlated with fasting plasma insulin concentrations and positively correlated with insulin sensitivity independent of body fat. Because of these findings, it has been suggested that adiponectin has a cardioprotective effect. No direct data are available to support or refute this hypothesis. Resistin is also a protein produced by adipocytes. In rodents, administration of resistin produces insulin resistance, whereas neutralizing resistin with specific antibodies improves insulin sensitivity. In humans, however, resistin was inconsistently found in muscle and fat, and there were no differences between patients with type 2 diabetes mellitus or insulin resistance when compared with healthy controls. The findings thus far do not support a primary role for resistin in the relationship between insulin resistance and obesity in humans. TNF-α and IL-6 are cytokines that can be produced by adipocytes and are variably increased in obesity and insulin resistance. Adipose tissue is not the sole source of these cytokines, and any evidence that they play a direct role in the insulin resistance of metabolic syndrome is currently lacking. PAI-1 is produced by many cell types, including adipocytes. Serum PAI-1 concentrations are also elevated in obesity and may contribute to the prothrombotic tendencies.

Islet-cell failure/type 2 diabetes mellitus

The risk of developing type 2 diabetes is high in persons with metabolic syndrome. Type 2 diabetes requires defects in both insulin secretion and insulin action. Many obese individuals are insulin resistant, yet only a portion will develop diabetes mellitus; therefore, it follows that those who develop type 2 diabetes develop pancreatic beta cell decompensation. FFAs have been shown to modulate insulin secretion, but it has not yet been demonstrated that they have a long-term adverse effect on islet β-cell function in humans. A potential explanation for the development of β-cell failure in obesity is the overproduction of islet amyloid polypeptide. This protein is cosecreted with insulin, and because of its tertiary structure (which is different in humans and rodents) can form toxic amyloid deposits in β-cells. Amyloid deposits have been found in the pancreatic islets obtained at autopsy from patients with type 2 diabetes mellitus.

Hypertension

Blood pressure can be increased by a number of mechanisms. Increased circulating blood volume, abnormal vasoconstriction, decreased vascular relaxation, and increased cardiac output may all contribute to hypertension in obesity. It has been proposed that the ability of hyperinsulinemia to increase renal sodium absorption contributes to hypertension via increased circulating blood volume. Abnormalities of vascular resistance may also contribute to the pathophysiology of obesity-related hypertension. Under some experimental conditions, elevated FFAs have been found to cause increased vasoconstriction [18] and reduced nitric oxide–mediated vasorelaxation, similar to that seen in metabolic syndrome. It has also been suggested that there is an increased activity of the sympathetic nervous system [19] in some obesity phenotypes and that this contributes to obesity-associated hypertension. Angiotensinogen (also produced by adipocytes), a precursor of the vasoconstrictor angiotensin II, is positively correlated with blood pressure in some studies [20].

Dyslipidemia

Upper body obesity and type 2 diabetes mellitus are associated with increased triglycerides, decreased HDL cholesterol, and a high proportion of small, dense LDL particles. This dyslipidemia contributes to the increased cardiovascular risk observed in metabolic syndrome. Fasting hypertriglyceridemia is caused by increased hepatic secretion of very low-density lipoprotein (VLDL). The elevated VLDL secretory rate may well be driven by increased delivery of FFA to the liver, which increases triglyceride synthesis and subsequently VLDL apoB-100 secretion [21]. Low HDL cholesterol and the increase in small, dense LDL particles are likely an indirect consequence of elevated, triglyceride-rich VLDL mediated via increased cholesterol ester transfer protein (CETP) and hepatic lipase activity.

Therapy

The incidence of CHD increases with each component of metabolic syndrome present [5]. As a result, treatment and control of all components is imperative. A comprehensive approach should have two goals in mind: improve modifiable risk factors contributing to insulin resistance and, when indicated, the institution of pharmacotherapy to achieve the clinical goals desired.

Weight loss

Weight loss as modest as 5% to 10% has been shown to lead to improvements in all components of the metabolic syndrome [22–32]. The most recent study to corroborate this claim is the Diabetes Prevention Program. In this study, lifestyle change with dietary modification, regular physical activity, and 7% weight loss was shown to decrease the incidence of developing type 2 diabetes mellitus by over 50% over 4 years compared with the control cohort. The dietary changes emphasized included caloric restriction, with <30% of total calories as fat, <7% of total calories as saturated fat, and increased fiber (15g/1000 kcal) [33].

Unfortunately, weight loss remains a challenging prescription. There is significant confusion regarding effective dietary changes to achieve weight loss, as well as a wealth of unproven claims that misguide patients. The Adult Treatment Panel (ATP) proposes the Therapeutic Lifestyle Changes Diet (Table 2). It encourages a hypocaloric diet with decreased intake of dietary fat, with specific guidelines for saturated, monounsaturated, and polyunsaturated fat intake while promoting increased intake of dietary fiber [1]. Simply said, it promotes increased intake of fruits and vegetables, whole

Table 2
Macronutrient recommendations for the Therapeutic Lifestyle Changes Diet

Component	Recommendation
Polyunsaturated fat	Up to 10% of total calories
Monounsaturated fat	Up to 20% of total calories
Total fat	25–35% of total calories[a]
Carbohydrate[b]	50–60% of total calories[a]
Dietary fiber	20–30 grams/day
Protein	Approximately 15% of total calories

[a] The ATP III allows an increase of total fat to 35% of total calories and a reduction in carbohydrate to 50% for persons with metabolic syndrome. Any increase in fat intake should be in the form of either polyunsaturated or monounsaturated fat.

[b] Carbohydrate should derive predominately from foods rich in complex carbohydrates including grains (especially whole grains), fruits, and vegetables.

grain carbohydrates, and legumes while limiting the intake of meat, whole-fat dairy products, simple sugars, refined carbohydrates, and salt. Similar dietary guidelines have been shown to be effective in the prevention and treatment of hypertension [34].

Long-term adherence to dietary modification is difficult; however, behavioral treatment and regular follow-up with a health professional can improve long-term compliance [35–37]. Physical activity can enhance weight loss, and regular physical activity plays a major role in the prevention of weight regain [38–41].

Medications for the treatment of obesity should be considered for individuals who meet the recommended criteria. Agents currently available for the chronic treatment (>1 year) of obesity will be discussed in detail later in this chapter.

Physical activity

Physical activity is frequently advised as part of a weight loss program. Although physical activity increases energy expenditure, thereby facilitating weight loss [23,25,42], regular physical activity provides health benefits even in the absence of weight loss. Regular physical activity is known to improve insulin resistance and glucose control [43–47]. The Nurses Health Study, a prospective cohort survey of over 70,000 nurses, evaluated the risk for type 2 diabetes mellitus according to physical activity level. Physical activity was defined by quintile of metabolic equivalent task score based on time spent per week on each of eight common activities. The relative risk for rype 2 diabetes mellitus was lower with higher activity scores [48]. Regular physical activity is associated with favorable lipid changes [25,49], lower blood pressure [50,51], and decreased fibrinogen [7,52]. These changes may be responsible for the lower mortality rates (including cardiovascular disease mortality rates) observed in fit individuals regardless of weight [53–57].

The current recommendation for physical activity by the Surgeon General includes 30 minutes of physical activity most days of the week [58]. More recently, a complete review of available studies has suggested that 45 to 60 minutes per day of physical activity is needed to prevent unhealthy weight gain [59]. This amount of physical activity can be achieved in a flexible manner. Studies have shown that both aerobic and strengthening exercises provide health benefits [60–62]. The time of physical activity can be accrued in a continuous or intermittent manner [63,64]. For example, three exercise bouts of 10 minutes in duration offer benefits similar to a single 30-minute session. This information can be helpful to those individuals who are unable to perform prolonged bouts of activity as a result of time or physical limitations. Informal exercise programs, such as those completed at home, have equal benefits to more structured programs performed at a gym [64,65]. Nonexercise activity also provides benefits. Levine et al [66] demonstrated that activities throughout the day, such as walking and climbing stairs, can provide substantial contributions to energy metabolism and weight management. Essentially, any type of physical activity is worth doing.

Individual recommendations for physical activity must take into consideration multiple factors. Fitness level, limitations to exercise (eg, musculoskeletal symptoms, time), and socioeconomic circumstances can impair an individual's ability to comply with recommendations outlined. As a result, activities advised should be SMART: Specific, Measurable, Attainable, Realistic, and Trackable. For individuals who are able to walk, the use of pedometers are recommended for tracking daily activity. A total of 10,000 steps per day are recommended for cardiovascular fitness [67].

Pharmacotherapy

Therapeutic lifestyle changes should be the foundation targeting modifiable risk factors promoting insulin resistance. However, in many circumstances lifestyle changes may not be sufficient to achieve the clinical goals desired, warranting the initiation of pharmacotherapy. Historically, the components of metabolic syndrome have been targeted independently; as a result, multiple pharmacological agents are available that have been proven effective at controlling hyperglycemia, hypertension, and hyperlipidemia. In the past decade, agents that target insulin resistance and the chronic management of obesity have been added to the armamentarium.

Obesity

The pharmacological treatment of obesity has been marked by multiple challenges. Available therapeutic agents have been used as single or combination therapy, despite the absence of clinical trials proving their long-term safety and efficacy [68–70]. The complications that resulted left many physicians apprehensive toward the new obesity drugs available [71].

Medical therapy should be considered for the obese individual (body mass index > 30 kg/m^2) or the overweight individual (body mass index >27 kg/m^2), with weight-related morbidity. It is most effective as a component of a weight management regimen, including dietary advice, regular physical activity, behavioral therapy, and routine medical follow-up [72]. Two agents, currently approved for the long-term treatment of obesity, are sibutramine and orlistat.

Sibutramine is a selective serotonin and adrenergic reuptake inhibitor first released in 1997 [73]. It enhances satiety, thereby limiting caloric intake. Several randomized, placebo-controlled clinical trials have shown the efficacy of sibutramine (doses 10–15 mg/day) at promoting weight loss after 6 to 12 months of therapy [74,75]. The weight loss observed is modest, 5% to 10%, but associated with improvements in metabolic parameters [75]. The most common side effects include dryness of the mouth, insomnia, constipation, and headaches. The most worrisome complication is the potential for significant elevations in blood pressure [73]. As a result, routine medical follow-up is imperative. There are several contraindications to the use of sibutramine therapy, a frequently encountered one being active treatment with selective serotonin reuptake inhibitors (because of the risk of serotonin syndrome) [76].

Response to sibutramine can be assessed early in the course of therapy. Clinical trials suggests that nonresponders—individuals who failed to lose 1% of their initial body weight after 4 weeks of treatment—experienced no additional weight loss, despite continued therapy for 12 months [73]. Weight loss plateaus 6 months into therapy; however, when compared with placebo, improved rates of weight maintenance are reported after 24 months [75].

Orlistat is a pancreatic lipase inhibitor that reduces the absorption of dietary fat [77]. Compared with placebo, 120 mg of orlistat administered three times a day is more effective at promoting weight loss after 12 months [78,79]. Weight loss of 5% to 10% was associated with statistically significant improvements in metabolic parameters decreasing cardiovascular risk factors and the risk for development of type 2 diabetes mellitus [78–81]. At the end of the 12-month weight loss arm, subjects were randomized to either continued therapy with orlistat or placebo. Orlistat was superior to placebo at promoting weight maintenance for up to 12 months. Of interest, subjects randomized to placebo during the weight loss arm and later randomized to orlistat experienced continued weight loss. The cohort of subjects randomized to orlistat for both the weight loss and weight maintenance arms experienced some weight regain. At the end of the 24-month trial, weights between these two cohorts were not statistically different. This supports a role for orlistat at promoting continued weight loss after initial lifestyle changes [79].

Gastrointestinal side effects are common but tend to improve with decreased intake of dietary fat [77]. As a result, orlistat is best initiated when the individual has instituted some dietary changes. This decreases the risk for gastrointestinal side effects that can interfere with long-term compliance and, hence, efficacy. Decreases in fat-soluble vitamin concentrations have been observed, but no fat-soluble vitamin deficiencies have been reported. However, intake of a daily multivitamin is recommended. Orlistat does not interfere with the intestinal absorption and efficacy of most medications. Caution must be exercised with medications influenced by fat absorption (eg, warfarin, cyclosporine) [77].

To date, no long-term clinical trials have studied the efficacy of combination therapy with sibutramine and orlistat.

Insulin resistance

Metformin was one of the first insulin sensitizers available. It improves insulin resistance, mainly at the liver, by decreasing hepatic gluconeogenesis, lowering hepatic glucose output, and improving glycemia [82,83]. In addition to its antihyperglycemic effects, metformin has appetite suppressant properties, leading to decreased caloric intake and promoting a modest amount of weight loss. Metformin therapy is associated with improvements in serum lipids with lowering of serum triglycerides, LDL cholesterol, and rise in HDL cholesterol [84–86]. In individuals with impaired glucose tolerance, metformin (1500 mg daily) was shown to decrease the risk for progression to Type 2 diabetes mellitus compared with placebo, but was less effective than lifestyle changes in preventing progression to Type 2 diabetes mellitus [87].

At present, metformin is not approved by the US Food and Drug Administration for the treatment of metabolic syndrome or its components, with the exception of type 2 diabetes mellitus. As a result, caution must be exercised with regard to potential side effects and contraindications to therapy.

Another class of insulin sensitizers are the thiazolidinediones. Agents in this category that are currently available are rosiglitazone and pioglitazone. Neither has been associated with the high incidence of liver toxicity, in contrast to their predecessor, troglitazone. Both compounds improve insulin resistance, likely via their activation of the peroxisome proliferator-activated receptor (PPAR)-γ receptor in various tissues. Adipose tissue is thought to be an important site of action of thiazolidinediones; perhaps improvement in adipose handling of fatty acids mediates some of the benefits with regard to insulin resistance, glycemia, and lipids. Unlike metformin, thiazolidinediones are associated with weight gain, gain of fat mass, and fluid retention. Fortunately, the beneficial effects of metabolic parameters appear to overshadow the weight gain on metabolic abnormalities [88]. Thiazolidinediones are not currently approved for the treatment of metabolic syndrome in the absence of type 2 diabetes.

Diabetes mellitus

With the exception of metformin and alpha reductase inhibitors (acarbose, miglitol), most pharmacologic agents in the treatment of type 2 diabetes mellitus (eg, thiazolidinediones, sulfonylureas, and insulin) are associated with weight gain [89]. As a result, in the absence of contra-indications, metformin should be the first line agent for the treatment of type 2 diabetes mellitus in patients with metabolic syndrome. Beneficial effects of metformin on weight have also been observed, when used in combination with sulfonylureas, thiazolidinediones, and insulin [89].

However, combination therapy is often required to achieve more aggressive glycemic goals. In the United Kingdom Prospective Diabetes Study, subjects in the intensive treatment arm were more frequently taking more than one oral agent or insulin. Improved glycemic control was associated with a trend toward decreased cardiovascular events, barely missing statistical significance [90,91]. This is the first study to support a beneficial effect of improved glycemic control on cardiovascular outcomes.

Dyslipidemia

The dyslipidemia defining the metabolic syndrome (high triglycerides, low HDL, small LDL) has long been recognized to promote premature CHD [92,93]. The contribution by each component of this triad to the development of CHD has been difficult to dissect [1].

The current ATP III guidelines identify LDL cholesterol as the primary target in lipid-lowering therapy [1]. 3-hydroxy-3-methylglutaryl coenzyme A inhibitors are by far the most potent agents available to lower LDL choles-terol and have been shown to be effective in lowering the risk for cardiovas-cular events both in primary and secondary prevention studies [94–98].

Yet improving atherogenic dyslipidemia leads to benefits beyond LDL lowering by lowering the risk for cardiovascular events. Nicotinic acid and fibrates have been shown to improve all elements of this triad in both primary and secondary intervention studies [99–101]. They are particularly effective at lowering serum triglycerides and have been shown to decrease risks for CHD [100,102].

Moderate elevations of serum triglycerides (150–199 mg/dL) should be managed with therapeutic lifestyle changes. For triglyceride values between 200 and 499 mg/dL, non-HDL cholesterol should be determined (total cholesterol – HDL cholesterol). Non-HDL cholesterol reflects the presence of remnant triglyceride-rich lipoproteins that are known to be atherogenic. The target non-HDL cholesterol should be 30 points higher than the target LDL cholesterol. When triglycerides are above 500 mg/dL, triglyceride lowering becomes the primary target of therapy [1].

Hypertension

A detailed discussion of all pharmacologic agents available for the treatment of hypertension is beyond the scope of this publication. However, in the individual with metabolic syndrome, the choice of an antihypertensive agent must be made with careful consideration.

Angiotensin-converting enzyme inhibitors (ACE) are effective in the treatment of hypertension and provide beneficial effects to other components of metabolic syndrome [103]. Clinical studies suggest ACE inhibitors may provide insulin-sensitizing effects and decrease the risk for the development of type 2 diabetes mellitus [104] and cardiovascular events. ACE inhibitors are generally well tolerated, although careful consideration to contraindications to their use and potential side effects must be considered [103].

Calcium channel blockers and angiotensin receptor blockers are also effective in controlling hypertension without aggravating other components of the metabolic syndrome [103]. Beta-blockers may promote weight gain and thiazide diuretics can impair insulin sensitivity, contributing to the development of hyperglycemia. In the absence of clinical indications requiring the specific use of these agents, they are generally avoided as first-line therapy in the individual with metabolic syndrome [103].

Inflammation/hypercoagulability

Thrombosis, platelet hyperaggregability, and inflammation are increasingly being recognized as factors that increase the risk for acute coronary syndromes [105]. Aspirin and other antiplatelet therapies have been shown to decrease the risk of acute coronary events, mostly in secondary prevention studies [106,107]. These processes are commonly present in individuals with metabolic syndrome. However, guidelines for the use of aspirin therapy as a primary prevention have not been firmly established.

Summary

In conclusion, metabolic syndrome describes a cluster of metabolic and cardiovascular risk factors known to increase an individual's risk for the development of cardiovascular heart disease. As defined by the NCEP III, the prevalence of metabolic syndrome is rising and threatens the recent advances at lowering cardiovascular risks achieved by lowering LDL cholesterol. Hence, it is important to determine whether or not an individual meets the criteria for metabolic syndrome. Insulin resistance has been recognized as an active contributor to the pathophysiological processes increasing the risk for CHD. As a result, management of metabolic syndrome mandates a new treatment paradigm: the first step is to target modifiable risk factors contributing to insulin resistance (eg, obesity, inactivity), followed by careful consideration of the pharmacotherapy used to achieve clinical goals desired for improving glycemia, hypertension, and dyslipidemia.

References

[1] Third Report of the National Cholesterol Education Program (NCEP) expert panel on detection, evaluation, and treatment of high blood cholesterol in adults (Adult Treatment Panel III): final report. Circulation 2001;106:3143–421.

[2] Reaven G. Pathophysiology of insulin resistance in human disease. Physiol Rev 1995;75:473–86.

[3] Lopez-Candales A. Metabolic syndrome X: a comprehensive review of the pathophysiology and recommended therapy. J Med 2001;32:283–300.

[4] Haffner S, Valdez R, Hazuda H, et al. Prospective analysis of the insulin-resistance syndrome (syndrome X). Diabetes 1992;41:715–22.

[5] Isomaa B, Almgren P, Tuomi T, et al. Cardiovascular morbidity and mortality associated with the metabolic syndrome. Diabetes Care 2001;24:683–9.

[6] Alberti KG, Zimmet PZ. Definition, diagnosis and classification of diabetes mellitus and its complications. Part 1: diagnosis and classification of diabetes mellitus provisional report of a WHO consultation. Diabet Med 1998;15:539–53.

[7] Ford E, Giles W, Dietz W. Prevalence of the metabolic syndrome among US adults: findings from the third National Health and Nutrition Examination Survey. JAMA 2002;287:356–9.

[8] Kolaczynski J, Caro J. Insulin resistance: site of the primary defect or how the current and the emerging therapies work. J Basic Clin Physiol Pharmacol 1998;9:281–94.

[9] Zimmet P, Boyko EJ, Collier G, et al. Etiology of the metabolic syndrome: potential role of insulin resistance, leptin resistance, and other players. Ann N Y Acad Sci 1999;892:25–44.

[10] Kissebah A, Vydelingum N, Murray R, et al. Relation of body fat distribution to metabolic complications of obesity. J Clin Endocrinol Metab 1982;54:254–60.

[11] Jensen M, Caruso M, Heiling V, et al. Insulin regulation of lipolysis in nondiabetic and IDDM subjects. Diabetes 1989;38:1595–601.

[12] Divertie G, Jensen M, Cryer P, et al. Lipolytic responsiveness to epinephrine in nondiabetic and diabetic humans. Am J Physiol 1997;272:E1130–5.

[13] Jensen M, Haymond M, Rizza R, et al. Influence of body fat distribution on free fatty acid metabolism in obesity. J Clin Invest 1989;83:1168–73.

[14] Roust L, Jensen M. Postprandial free fatty acid kinetics are abnormal in upper body obesity. Diabetes 1993;42:1567–73.

[15] Sheehan M, Jensen M. Metabolic complications of obesity. In: Cullen J, editor. Obesity. Philadelphia: WB Saunders; 2000. p. 363–85.

[16] Kelley D, Mokan M, Simoneau J, et al. Interaction between glucose and free fatty acid metabolism in human skeletal muscle. J Clin Invest 1993;92:91–8.

[17] Ferrannini E, Barrett E, Bevilacqva S, et al. Effect of fatty acids on glucose production and utilization man. J Clin Invest 1983;72:1737–47.

[18] Goodfriend T, Egan B. Nonesterified fatty acids in the pathogenesis of hypertension: theory and evidence. Prostaglandins Leukot Essent Fatty Acids 1997;57:57–63.

[19] Reaven G, Lithell H, Landsberg L. Hypertension and associated metabolic abnormalities—the role of insulin resistance and the sympathoadrenal system. N Engl J Med 1996;334:374–81.

[20] Schorr U, Blaschke K, Turan S, et al. Relationship betweeen angiotensinogen, leptin, and blood pressure levels in young normotensive men. J Hypertens 1998;16:1475–80.

[21] Lewis G, Uffelman K, Szeto L, et al. Interaction between free fatty acids and insulin in the acute control of very low density lipoprotein production in humans. J Clin Invest 1995;95:158–66.

[22] Hellenius M, de Faire U, Berglund B, et al. Diet and exercise are equally effective in reducing risk for cardiovascular disease. Results of a randomized controlled study in men with slightly to moderately raised cardiovascular risk factors. Atherosclerosis 1993;103: 81–91.

[23] Katzel L, Bleecker E, Colman E, et al. Effects of weight loss vs aerobic exercise training on risk factors for coronary disease in healthy, obese, middle-aged and older men. A randomized controlled trial. JAMA 1995;274:1915–21.

[24] Simkin-Silverman L, Wing R, Hansen D, et al. Prevention of cardiovascular risk factor elevations in healthy premenopausal women. Prev Med 1995;24:509–17.

[25] Stefanick M, Mackey S, Sheehan M, et al. Effects of diet and exercise in men and postmenopausal women with low levels of HDL cholesterol and high levels of LDL cholesterol. N Engl J Med 1998;339:12–20.

[26] Svendsen O, Hassager C, Christiansen C. Effect of an energy-restrictive diet, with or without exercise, on lean tissue mass, resting metabolic rate, cardiovascular risk factors, and bone in overweight postmenopausal women. Am J Med 1993;95:131–40.

[27] Wood P, Stefanick M, Williams P, et al. The effects on plasma lipoproteins of a prudent weight-reducing diet, with or without exercise, in overweight men and women. N Engl J Med 1991;325:461–6.

[28] Dengel J, Katzel L, Goldberg A. Effect of an American Heart Association diet, with or without weight loss, on lipids in obese middle-aged and older men. Am J Clin Nutr 1995;62:715–21.

[29] Jalkanen L. The effect of a weight reduction program on cardiovascular risk factors among overweight hypertensives in primary health care. Scand J Soc Med 1991;19:66–71.

[30] Wood P, Stefanick M, Dreon D, et al. Changes in plasma lipids and lipoproteins in overweight men during weight loss through dieting as compared with exercise. N Engl J Med 1988;319:1173–9.

[31] Pan X, Li G, Hu Y, et al. Effects of diet and exercise in preventing NIDDM in people with impaired glucose tolerance. The Da Qing IGT and Diabetes Study. Diabetes Care 1997;20:537–44.

[32] Manning R, Jung R, Leese G, et al. The comparison of four weight reduction strategies aimed at overweight diabetic patients. Diabet Med 1995;12:409–15.

[33] Tuomilehto J, Lindstrom J, Eriksson J, et al. Prevention of type 2 diabetes mellitus by changes in lifestyle among subjects with impaired glucose tolerance. N Engl J Med 2001;344:1343–50.

[34] Sacks F, Svetkey L, Vollmer W, et al. Effects on blood pressure of reduced dietary sodium and the Dietary Approaches to Stop Hypertension (DASH) diet. DASH-Sodium Collaborative Research Group. N Engl J Med 2001;344:3–10.

[35] Wadden T, Foster G, Letizia K. One-year behavioral treatment of obesity: comparison of moderate and severe caloric restriction and the effects of weight maintenance therapy. J Consult Clin Psychol 1994;62:165–71.

[36] Long C, Simpson C, Allott E. Psychological and dietetic counselling combined in the treatment of obesity: a comparative study in a hospital outpatient clinic. Hum Nutr Appl Nutr 1983;37:94–102.

[37] Wadden T, Stunkard A. Controlled trial of very low calorie diet, behavior therapy, and their combination in the treatment of obesity. J Consult Clin Psychol 1986;54:482–8.

[38] Ewbank P, Darga L, Lucas C. Physical activity as a predictor of weight maintenance in previously obese subjects. Obes Res 1995;3:257–63.

[39] Klesges R, Klesges L, Haddock C, et al. A longitudinal analysis of the impact of dietary intake and physical activity on weight change in adults. Am J Clin Nutr 1992;55:818–22.

[40] Ching P, Willett W, Rimm E, et al. Activity level and risk of overweight in male health professionals. Am J Public Health 1996;86:25–30.

[41] Williamson D, Madans J, Anda R, et al. Recreational physical activity and ten-year weight change in a US national cohort. Int J Obes Relat Metab Disord 1993;17:279–86.

[42] Garrow J, Summerbell C. Meta-analysis: effect of exercise, with or without dieting, on the body composition of overweight subjects. Eur J Clin Nutr 1995;49:1–10.

[43] Burstein R, Epstein Y, Shapiro Y, et al. Effect of an acute bout of exercise on glucose disposal in human obesity. J Appl Physiol 1990;69:299–304.

[44] Devlin J, Hirshman M, Horton E, et al. Enhanced peripheral and splanchnic insulin sensitivity in NIDDM men after single bout of exercise. Diabetes 1987;36:434–9.

[45] DeFronzo R, Sherwin R, Kraemer N. Effect of physical training on insulin action in obesity. Diabetes 1987;36:1379–85.

[46] Reitman J, Vasquez B, Klimes I, et al. Improvement of glucose homeostasis after exercise training in non-insulin-dependent diabetes. Diabetes Care 1984;7:434–41.

[47] Trovati M, Carta Q, Cavalot F, et al. Influence of physical training on blood glucose control, glucose tolerance, insulin secretion, and insulin action in non-insulin- dependent diabetic patients. Diabetes Care 1984;7:416–20.

[48] Hu F, Sigal R, Rich-Edwards J, et al. Walking compared with vigorous physical activity and risk of type 2 diabetes in women: a prospective study. JAMA 1999;282: 1433–9.

[49] Leon A, Connett J, Jacobs D Jr., Rauramaa R. Leisure-time physical activity levels and risk of coronary heart disease and death. The Multiple Risk Factor Intervention Trial. JAMA 1987;258:2388–95.

[50] Blair S, Goodyear N, Gibbons L, et al. Physical fitness and incidence of hypertension in healthy normotensive men and women. JAMA 1984;252:487–90.

[51] Martin J, Dubbert P, Cushman W. Controlled trial of aerobic exercise in hypertension. Circulation 1990;81:1560–7.

[52] King D, Carek P, Mainous A 3rd, et al. Inflammatory markers and exercise: differences related to exercise type. Med Sci Sports Exerc 2003;35:575–81.

[53] Ekelund L, Haskell W, Johnson J, et al. Physical fitness as a predictor of cardiovascular mortality in asymptomatic North American men. The Lipid Research Clinics Mortality Follow-up Study. N Engl J Med 1988;319:1379–84.

[54] Blair S, Kohl H 3rd, Paffenbarger R Jr, et al. Physical fitness and all-cause mortality. A prospective study of healthy men and women. JAMA 1989;262:2395–401.

[55] Blair S, Kampert J, Kohl H 3rd, et al. Influences of cardiorespiratory fitness and other precursors on cardiovascular disease and all-cause mortality in men and women. JAMA 1996;276:205–10.

[56] Lee C, Blair S, Jackson A. Cardiorespiratory fitness, body composition, and all-cause and cardiovascular disease mortality in men. Am J Clin Nutr 1999;69:373–80.

[57] Blair S, Brodney S. Effects of physical inactivity and obesity on morbidity and mortality: current evidence and research issues. Med Sci Sports Exerc 1999;31:S646–62.

[58] Howell J. The 1996 Surgeon General's report on physical activity and health. Nurse Pract Forum 1996;7:104.

[59] Saris WH, Blair SN, van Baak MA, et al. How much physical activity is enough to prevent unhealthy weight gain? Outcome of the IASO 1st Stock Conference and consensus statement. Obes Rev 2003;4:101–14.

[60] Ballor D, Harvey-Berino J, Ades P, et al. Contrasting effects of resistance and aerobic training on body composition and metabolism after diet-induced weight loss. Metabolism 1996;45:179–83.

[61] Ades P, Ballor D, Ashikaga T, et al. Weight training improves walking endurance in healthy elderly persons. Ann Intern Med 1996;124:568–72.

[62] Wadden T, Vogt R, Andersen R, et al. Exercise in the treatment of obesity: effects of four interventions on body composition, resting energy expenditure, appetite, and mood. J Consult Clin Psychol 1997;65:269–77.

[63] Donnelly J, Jacobsen D, Heelan K, et al. The effects of 18 months of intermittent vs. continuous exercise on aerobic capacity, body weight and composition, and metabolic fitness in previously sedentary, moderately obese females. Int J Obes Relat Metab Disord 2000;24:566–72.

[64] Jakicic J, Winters C, Lang W, et al. Effects of intermittent exercise and use of home exercise equipment on adherence, weight loss, and fitness in overweight women: a random- ized trial. JAMA 1999;282:1554–60.

[65] Andersen R, Wadden T, Bartlett S, et al. Effects of lifestyle activity vs structured aerobic exercise in obese women: a randomized trial. JAMA 1999;281:335–40.

[66] Levine J, Eberhardt N, Jensen M. Role of nonexercise activity thermogenesis in resistance to fat gain in humans. Science 1999;283:212–4.

[67] Leermakers E, Dunn A, Blair S. Exercise management of obesity. Med Clin North Am 2000;84:419–40.

[68] Bray G. Use and abuse of appetite-suppressant drugs in the treatment of obesity. Ann Intern Med 1993;119:707–13.

[69] Guy-Grand B, Apfelbaum M, Crepaldi G, et al. International trial of long-term dexfenfluramine in obesity. Lancet 1989;2:1142–5.

[70] Weintraub M. Long-term weight control study: conclusions. Clin Pharmacol Ther 1992;51:642–6.

[71] Connolly H, Crary J, McGoon M, et al. Valvular heart disease associated with fenfluramine-phentermine. N Engl J Med 1997;337:581–8.

[72] Clinical guidelines on the identification. Evaluation, and treatment of overweight and obesity in adults—the evidence report. National Institutes of Health. Obes Res 1998; 6(Supp 2):51S–209S.

[73] Lean M. Sibutramine—a review of clinical efficacy. Int J Obes Relat Metab Disord 1997;21(Suppl 1):S30–6 [discussion: 37–9].

[74] Wirth A, Krause J. Long-term weight loss with sibutramine: a randomized controlled trial. JAMA 2001;286:1331–9.

[75] James W, Astrup A, Finer N, et al. Effect of sibutramine on weight maintenance after weight loss: a randomised trial. STORM Study Group. Sibutramine Trial of Obesity Reduction and Maintenance. Lancet 2000;356:2119–25.

[76] Lantz M. Serotonin syndrome. A common but often unrecognized psychiatric condition. Geriatrics 2001;56:52–3.

[77] Guerciolini R. Mode of action of orlistat. Int J Obes Relat Metab Disord 1997;21(Suppl 3):S12–23.

[78] Davidson M, Hauptman J, DiGirolamo M, et al. Weight control and risk factor reduction in obese subjects treated for 2 years with orlistat: a randomized controlled trial. JAMA 1999;281:235–42.

[79] Sjostrom L, Rissanen A, Andersen T, et al. Randomised placebo-controlled trial of orlistat for weight loss and prevention of weight regain in obese patients. European Multicentre Orlistat Study Group. Lancet 1998;352:167–72.

[80] Lindgarde F. The effect of orlistat on body weight and coronary heart disease risk profile in obese patients: the Swedish Multimorbidity Study. J Intern Med 2000;248: 245–54.

[81] Heymsfield S, Segal K, Hauptman J, et al. Effects of weight loss with orlistat on glucose tolerance and progression to type 2 diabetes in obese adults. Arch Intern Med 2000;160:1321–6.

[82] Sirtori CR, Pasik C. Re-evaluation of a biguanide, metformin: mechanism of action and tolerability. Pharmacol Res 1994;30:187–228.

[83] Bailey CJ, Turner RC. Metformin. N Engl J Med 1996;334:574–9.

[84] Giugliano D, Quatraro A, Consoli G, et al. Metformin for obese, insulin-treated diabetic patients: improvement in glycaemic control and reduction of metabolic risk factors. Eur J Clin Pharmacol 1993;44:107–12.

[85] DeFronzo RA, Goodman AM. Efficacy of metformin in patients with non-insulin-dependent diabetes mellitus. The Multicenter Metformin Study Group. N Engl J Med 1995;333:541–9.

[86] Stumvoll M, Nurjhan N, Perriello G, et al. Metabolic effects of metformin in non-insulin-dependent diabetes mellitus. N Engl J Med 1995;333:550–4.

[87] Knowler WC, Barrett-Connor E, Fowler SE, et al. Reduction in the incidence of type 2 diabetes with lifestyle intervention or metformin. N Engl J Med 2002;346:393–403.

[88] Mudaliar S, Henry RR. New oral therapies for type 2 diabetes mellitus: the glitazones or insulin sensitizers. Annu Rev Med 2001;52:239–57.

[89] DeFronzo RA. Pharmacologic therapy for type 2 diabetes mellitus. Ann Intern Med 1999;131:281–303.

[90] Effect of intensive blood-glucose control with metformin on complications in overweight patients with type 2 diabetes (UKPDS 34). UK Prospective Diabetes Study (UKPDS) Group. Lancet 1998;352:854–65.

[91] Intensive blood-glucose control with sulphonylureas or insulin compared with conventional treatment and risk of complications in patients with type 2 diabetes (UKPDS 33). UK Prospective Diabetes Study (UKPDS) Group. Lancet 1998;352:837–53.

[92] Austin M, Breslow J, Hennekens C, et al. Low-density lipoprotein subclass patterns and risk of myocardial infarction. JAMA 1988;260:1917–21.

[93] Austin M, King M, Vranizan K, et al. Atherogenic lipoprotein phenotype. A proposed genetic marker for coronary heart disease risk. Circulation 1990;82:495–506.

[94] Prevention of cardiovascular events and death with pravastatin in patients with coronary heart disease and a broad range of initial cholesterol levels. The Long-Term Intervention with Pravastatin in Ischaemic Disease (LIPID) Study Group. N Engl J Med 1998;339: 1349–57.

[95] Downs J, Clearfield M, Weis S, et al. Primary prevention of acute coronary events with lovastatin in men and women with average cholesterol levels: results of AFCAPS/ TexCAPS. Air Force/Texas Coronary Atherosclerosis Prevention Study. JAMA 1998;279:1615–22.

[96] Shepherd J, Cobbe S, Ford I, et al. Prevention of coronary heart disease with pravastatin in men with hypercholesterolemia. West of Scotland Coronary Prevention Study Group. N Engl J Med 1995;333:1301–7.

[97] Randomised trial of cholesterol lowering in 4444 patients with coronary heart disease: the Scandinavian Simvastatin Survival Study (4S). Lancet 1994;344:1383–9.

[98] Sacks F, Pfeffer M, Moye L, et al. The effect of pravastatin on coronary events after myocardial infarction in patients with average cholesterol levels. Cholesterol and Recurrent Events Trial investigators. N Engl J Med 1996;335:1001–9.

[99] Vega G, Grundy S. Lipoprotein responses to treatment with lovastatin, gemfibrozil, and nicotinic acid in normolipidemic patients with hypoalphalipoproteinemia. Arch Intern Med 1994;154:73–82.

[100] Frick M, Elo O, Haapa K, et al. Helsinki Heart Study: primary-prevention trial with gemfibrozil in middle-aged men with dyslipidemia. Safety of treatment, changes in risk factors, and incidence of coronary heart disease. N Engl J Med 1987;317:1237–45.

[101] Guyton J, Blazing M, Hagar J, et al. Extended-release niacin vs gemfibrozil for the treatment of low levels of high-density lipoprotein cholesterol. Niaspan-Gemfibrozil Study Group. Arch Intern Med 2000;160:1177–84.

[102] Secondary prevention by raising HDL cholesterol and reducing triglycerides in patients with coronary artery disease: the Bezafibrate Infarction Prevention (BIP) study. Circulation 2000;102:21–7.

[103] Blackshear JL, Schwartz GL. Step care therapy for hypertension in diabetic patients. Mayo Clin Proc 2001;76:1266–74.

[104] Vermes E, Ducharme A, Bourassa MG, et al. Enalapril reduces the incidence of diabetes in patients with chronic heart failure: insight from the Studies Of Left Ventricular Dysfunction (SOLVD). Circulation 2003;107:1291–6.

[105] Fuster V, Lewis A. Conner Memorial Lecture. Mechanisms leading to myocardial infarction: insights from studies of vascular biology. Circulation 1994;90:2126–46.

[106] Hennekens C, Dyken M, Fuster V. Aspirin as a therapeutic agent in cardiovascular disease: a statement for healthcare professionals from the American Heart Association. Circulation 1997;96:2751–3.

[107] Hansson L, Zanchetti A, Carruthers S, et al. Effects of intensive blood-pressure lowering and low-dose aspirin in patients with hypertension: principal results of the Hypertension Optimal Treatment (HOT) randomised trial. HOT Study Group. Lancet 1998;351:1755–62.

5

The Menopause and Obesity

Jennifer C. Lovejoy

Obesity is a major health problem in the United States. It is estimated that 61% of the U.S. population is either overweight or obese (Body Mass Index $\geq$ 25 kg/m^2) [1]. According to the most recent National Health and Nutrition Examination Survey (NHANES III, 1988–1994), the prevalence of obesity is substantially higher in women (24.9%) than in men (19.9%) [1]. Additionally, 8.4% of women and 3.9% of men aged 25 to 34 years experience a major weight gain (greater than 10 kg) [2]. For women in the early menopausal years (aged 50 to 59 years), the prevalence of obesity increased by 47% between 1991 and 1998 [3].

Obesity is particularly common among minority women. In NHANES III, nearly 40% of black women and 34% of Mexican-American women had a BMI that was greater than 30 kg/m^2 [1]. Among some Native American groups, more than 50% to 80% of the adult women are obese [4] (p. 142S). Furthermore, among women but not men, poverty or low socioeconomic status is a risk factor for obesity. The prevalence of obesity in women at, or below, the poverty level is approximately 50%, regardless of ethnic group; women in higher income groups have significantly lower prevalence rates [4] (p. 146S).

At any level of BMI, women have a greater percentage of body fat than men, so a woman's risk of being "overfat" is higher, even at BMIs that are within the normal range. For example, Blew et al [5] recently assessed the relationship between BMI and percentage of fat in 317 postmenopausal women aged 40 to 66 years. Using 38% fat as a criterion for obesity, the cutoff BMI in this population was 24.9 kg/m^2. Wellens et al [6] similarly suggested that a BMI of 23 kg/m^2 might provide a better cutoff for defining obesity in premenopausal white women, based on their percentage of body fat.

The reasons for the excess rates of obesity in women are not entirely clear; however, it has been shown that hormonal fluctuations during pregnancy and menopause increase the obesity risk. The role of menopause in the development of obesity may be particularly important as women's life spans increase, with the result that women in most developed countries live substantial portions of their life in the postmenopausal state.

Weight and total body fat changes at menopause

Several studies addressed the issue of weight changes at menopause. Wing et al [9] reported data from the Healthy Women Study, a longitudinal study of cardiovascular risk changes in middle-aged women. The average weight gain in this population of perimenopausal women was 2.25 kg, although 20% of the population gained 4.5 kg or more. Although this study suggested that weight gain is a significant issue for middle-aged women, there was no difference in mean weight gain of women who remained pre-menopausal compared with those who underwent menopause.

In contrast, several studies reported that menopause is specifically associated with an increase in body weight that is independent of aging. Pasquali et al [9] reported that BMI was significantly higher among peri-menopausal and postmenopausal women compared with premenopausal women in a population study in Italy. The differences remained significant after adjusting for age, diet, activity, and smoking habits. Aloia et al [9] applied a four-compartment model of body composition analysis to 155 white women aged 51.4 years ± 13.5 years. They found that menopause is associated with a gain in body fat; the rate of change in body fat differed in pre- and postmenopausal women. Toth et al [10] studied 53 pre- and postmenopausal women of similar age (47 years versus 51 years). They reported that body weight was 6% higher and body fat was 17% higher in the postmenopausal women. The menopause-related increase in fat mass remained significant, even after adjusting statistically for age and body weight.

The question of changes in body weight at menopause has been examined in epidemiologic studies. The recent Study of Women's Health Across the Nation (SWAN) surveyed approximately 13,000 women of different ethnic backgrounds who lived in various areas of the United States [11]. BMI was significantly higher in perimenopausal women and women who had surgical menopause compared with premenopausal women. BMI in women who had undergone natural menopause was not significantly different from pre-menopausal women, however.

Weight gain at menopause is not without adverse health consequences. In the longitudinal study by Wing et al [7] women who gained weight at menopause had significant increases in total cholesterol, LDL-cholesterol, and insulin levels, whereas women who were weight stable during the menopause transition had no change in any cardiovascular or metabolic variable at follow-up. This study suggested that weight gain is common during the perimenopausal years and some of the increased health risk that is typically associated with the hormonal changes of menopause, may, in fact, be caused by weight gain. Prevention of excess weight gain at the time of menopause should thus be both a clinical and public health goal.

Changes in fat distribution at menopause

Changes in fat distribution at menopause resulting in increased abdominal fat in postmenopausal women have been observed. Using anthropometric measures of abdominal fat (waist-to-hip ratio, WHR) in a cross-sectional analysis of age-matched cohorts, Wing et al [12] found that postmenopausal women in the Healthy Women Study had a higher WHR than premenopausal women. Conversely, Den Tonkelaar et al [13] and Pasquali et al [8] reported that postmenopausal women did not have an increased WHR compared with premenopausal women after statistically adjusting for BMI and age. WHR is a poor measure of intra-abdominal fat distribution, however, and more sensitive indicators are likely needed to detect changes in fat distribution at menopause.

In support of this idea, several studies that used radiograph imaging techniques suggested that there may be a shift in abdominal fat distribution at menopause, even if there is no change in the WHR. Several studies with body composition analysis by dual-energy X-ray absorptiometry (DEXA) reported increased upper body or trunk fat in postmenopausal women; however, age-matched controls were not used in these studies so it is difficult to separate the effects of menopause from those of aging [14,15]. Conversely, Svendsen et al [16] statistically controlled for the effects of aging and observed a significant independent effect of menopausal status on total and abdominal fat percentage.

Studies that used CT scan as a direct measure of intra-abdominal fat in pre- and postmenopausal women have consistently found an increase in visceral abdominal fat with menopause. In one study, Enzi et al [17] reported that postmenopausal women have a decreased subcutaneous-to-visceral fat ratio by CT scan compared with age-matched premenopausal women; this pattern is typically associated with worsened health risk factors. Findings of increased visceral fat in postmenopausal women independent of aging were also reported in several other studies [18–21]. Thus, existing studies of regional fat distribution changes at menopause that use sophisticated measures of intra-abdominal fat consistently suggested that menopause accelerates the accumulation of abdominal visceral fat.

Effects of hormone replacement therapy on body weight and fat distribution

Although it is not uncommon for patients to believe that hormone replacement therapy (HRT) increases body weight, most studies suggested that HRT use is associated with lower body weight. The Postmenopausal Estrogen/Progestin Intervention trial was one of the largest studies to prospectively examine the effects of HRT on body weight. This randomized, placebo-controlled, clinical trial of 875 women found that women who were assigned to estrogen replacement (with or without progestin) had a significantly lower weight gain at the end of 3 years than women who were given placebo [22]. Similarly, in the Rancho Bernardo population study in southern California, women who used HRT, either continuously or intermittently over a 15 year follow-up, had significantly lower BMI than women who had never used HRT [23].

The SWAN study also examined the question of HRT use and body weight in their large population of U.S. women [11]. HRT use was associated with lower BMI independent of ethnicity (26.5 versus 27.3 kg/m^2). Furthermore, HRT users were less likely to be obese (BMI greater than 30 kg/m^2) than non-HRT users (22.6% versus 27.2%). The data on HRT and body weight are somewhat contradictory, however, because Davies et al [24] examined body weight trajectories over time in postmenopausal women who used or did not use HRT and found that both groups gained similar amounts of weight over time.

The existing literature consistently suggests that exogenous HRT influences abdominal fat accumulation. Several studies reported that HRT is associated with significantly lower WHR in postmenopausal women [22,25–28]. Using DEXA, Haarbo et al [29] reported that HRT prevented the increase in intra-abdominal fat that was seen in placebo-treated postmenopausal women over a 2-year period. Even in a short-term study, women who were treated with HRT for 12 weeks had decreased total fat mass and abdominal fat mass by DEXA compared with a placebo control group [30]. These studies confirmed that intra-abdominal fat distribution is strongly influenced by female reproductive steroids.

Factors influencing weight gain and fat distribution at menopause

It is not clear why women may be especially vulnerable to rapid weight gain at the time of menopause. It was reported that physical activity during leisure time is decreased in menopausal women [31] and that women with the lowest physical activity have the greatest weight gains during the perimenopause [7]. It was also suggested that menopausal women have a slightly decreased resting metabolic rate (RMR) [31]. Decreases in metabolic rate might be expected in postmenopausal women because of their loss of lean tissue mass and loss of the luteal-phase increase in energy expenditure [32]. A decrease in physical activity and even a small decrease in RMR could contribute to a positive energy balance and weight gain in menopausal women.

Eating behavior may play a role in the development of obesity at menopause. In one longitudinal study, food intake was increased as a result of menopause [31]. Furthermore, Hays et al [33] recently reported that increased dietary disinhibition scores on the Eating Inventory significantly predicted weight gain and current BMI in 638 healthy, postmenopausal women aged 55 to 65 years.

There is strong evidence that reproductive steroids influence body fat distribution in women. In particular, estrogens seem to promote lower body (gluteo-femoral) fat accumulation, whereas androgens have been associated with an upper body fat distribution in premenopausal [34] and postmenopausal white women [25]. At menopause, there is a shift in the ratio of androgens to estrogens. Ovarian estrogen production ceases whereas adrenal androgen production continues; this may relate to changes in fat distribution occurring at this time. The mechanism for this effect was proposed by Rebuffe-Scrive and colleagues [35] to relate to alterations in lipoprotein lipase activity in different fat depots in premenopausal compared with postmenopausal women. Specifically, after menopause, there is decreased lipoprotein lipase activity in femoral adipocytes combined with a loss of the high lipolytic responsiveness of abdominal and mammary adipocytes observed in premenopausal women, both of which would tend to predispose toward accumulation of central, abdominal body fat.

Genetic factors may also play a role in the accumulation of body fat at menopause. In one study that compared abdominal fat accumulation in postmenopausal monozygotic versus dizygotic twins, genetic factors contributed 60% of the variance in total and central body fat [36]. The heritability of abdominal body fat measured by DEXA was independent of the heritability of total body fat; the genetic effects were not affected by estrogen use.

Treatment of the obese, postmenopausal woman

In general, recommendations for treating overweight or obese postmenopausal women are similar to recommendations for treating overweight premenopausal women. Because menopause seems to be associated with decreased energy expenditure (metabolic rate and physical activity) and possibly increased energy intake, most, if not all, women who enter the perimenopausal period should be counseled in behavioral strategies to increase activity and decrease caloric intake.

Several studies examined weight loss therapy in postmenopausal women. There is no evidence that behavioral therapies (ie, diet and exercise treatment) are any less effective in postmenopausal women than they are in younger women [37,38]. Specifically, weight loss treatment may be particularly beneficial to reduce visceral adiposity and cardiovascular health risk factors in postmenopausal women [39].

There has been some concern about undertaking intentional weight loss in older women (and the elderly, in general) because aging and menopause are associated with reductions in lean body mass, particularly skeletal muscle, which weight loss could exacerbate. Gallagher et al [38] performed a 16-week dietary weight loss program in obese, postmenopausal women with detailed measures of body composition to determine the degree of change in fat-free components. Subjects lost 9.6 ± 3.0 kg of body weight, of which 19.5% was fat-free mass, an amount that was similar to that observed in premenopausal women during weight loss. The relative losses of body cell mass, skeletal muscle, and appendicular lean soft tissue were appropriate and consistent with the reductions in total body weight. Of importance, follow-up measures in these subjects 2 years after the weight loss study showed that body weight and fat mass remained below baseline values, whereas fat-free mass was not significantly different from baseline. This suggested that weight loss in postmenopausal women, even in the absence of vigorous exercise training, does not have adverse effects on lean body mass.

Conversely, bone loss may be a significant issue of concern during weight loss in postmenopausal women, a population that is at risk for osteoporosis. Weight loss can be associated with decreased bone mineral density or increased bone turnover. Ricci et al [40] reported that moderate calorie restriction for 6 months in postmenopausal women resulted in a decrease in total-body bone mineral density of 1.2%, with increased rates of bone resorption. Because of the potential for bone loss during obesity treatment, weight-bearing exercise should be considered an important component of any postmenopausal weight loss program. Additionally, consideration may be given to performing periodic assessments of bone mineral density during weight loss programs in postmenopausal women.

Several studies examined the impact of genetics on the ability of postmenopausal women to lose weight. Tchernof et al [41] studied the effect of weight loss in postmenopausal women with or without the Trp64Arg β3-adrenoceptor gene variant. There were similar losses in body weight and body fat during a dietary weight loss program, but carriers of the Trp64Arg allele lost 43% less visceral abdominal fat during weight loss than non-carriers. Another recent study by this group found that carriers and non-carriers of the Trp64Arg allele had similar declines in resting metabolic rate after a weight loss program; this suggested that this particular genotype should not be a hindrance to weight reduction in postmenopausal women [42].

Summary

In summary, menopause tends to be associated with an increased risk of obesity and a shift to an abdominal fat distribution with associated increase in health risks. Changes in body composition at menopause may be caused by the decrease in circulating estrogen, and, for fat distribution shifts, the relative increase in the androgen-estrogen ratio is likely to be important. Clinicians need to be aware of the likelihood of weight gain during the perimenopausal and postmenopausal years because behavioral strategies for weight loss can be effectively used in this population. Weight loss or prevention of weight gain is likely to have significant health benefits for older women.

References

[1] Flegal KM, Carroll MD, Ogden CL, et al. Prevalence and trends in obesity among US adults, 1999–2000. JAMA 2002;288:1723–7.
[2] Williamson DF, Kahn HS, Byers T. The 10-yr incidence of obesity and major weight gain in black and white US women aged 30–55 y. Am J Clin Nutr 1991;53:1515S–8S.
[3] Mokdad AH, Serdula MK, Dietz WH, et al. The spread of the obesity epidemic in the United States, 1991–1998. JAMA 1999;282:1519–22.
[4] National Heart Lung and Blood Institute. Clinical guidelines on the identification, evaluation and treatment of overweight and obesity in adults - the evidence report. Obes Res 1998;6(Suppl. 2):146S.
[5] Blew RM, Sardinha LB, Milliken LA, et al. Assessing the validity of body mass index standards in early postmenopausal women. Obes Res 2002;10(8):799–808.
[6] Wellens RI, Roche AF, Khamis HJ, et al. Relationships between the body mass index and body composition. Obes Res 1996;4:35–44.
[7] Wing RR, Matthews KA, Kuller LH, et al. Weight gain at the time of menopause. Arch Intern Med 1991;151:97–102.
[8] Pasquali R, Casimirri F, Labate AMM, et al. Body weight, fat distribution and the menopausal status in women. Int J Obes 1994;18:614–21.
[9] Aloia JF, Vaswani A, Ma R, et al. Aging in women - the four-compartment model of body composition. Metabolism 1996;45:43–8.
[10] Toth MJ, Tchernof A, Sites CK, et al. Effect of menopausal status on body composition and abdominal fat distribution. Int J Obes 2000;24:226–31.
[11] Matthews KA, Abrams B, Crawford S, et al. Body mass index in mid-life women: relative influence of menopause, hormone use, and ethnicity. Int J Obes 2001;25:863–73.
[12] Wing RR, Matthews KA, Kuller LH, et al. Waist to hip ratio in middle-aged women: associations with behavioral and psychosocial factors and with changes in cardiovascular risk factors. Arterio Thromb 1991;11:1250–7.
[13] Den Tonkelaar I, Seidell JC, van Noord PAH, et al. Fat distribution in relation to age, degree of obesity, smoking habits, parity and estrogen use: a cross-sectional study in 11825 Dutch women participating in the DOM-project. Int J Obes 1990;14:753–61.
[14] Dawson-Hughes B, Harris S. Regional changes in body composition by time of year in healthy postmenopausal women. Am J Clin Nutr 1992;56:307–13.
[15] Ley CJ, Lees B, Stevenson JC. Sex- and menopause-associated changes in body-fat distribution. Am J Clin Nutr 1992;55:950–4.
[16] Svendsen OL, Hassager C, Christiansen C. Age- and menopause-associated variations in body composition and fat distribution in healthy women as measured by dual-energy X-ray absorptiometry. Metabolism 1995;44:369–73.
[17] Enzi G, Gasparo M, Biondetti PR, et al. Subcutaneous and visceral fat distribution according to sex, age, and overweight, evaluated by computed tomography. Am J Clin Nutr 1986;44:739–46.
[18] Hunter GR, Kekes-Szabo T, Trueth MJ, et al. Intra-abdominal adipose tissue, physical activity and cardiovascular risk in pre- and postmenopausal women. Int J Obes 1996;20:860–5.
[19] Kotani K, Tokunaga K, Fujioka S, et al. Sexual dimorphism of age-related changes in whole-body fat distribution in the obese. Int J Obes 1994;18:207–12.

[20] Zamboni M, Armellini G, Milani MP, et al. Body fat distribution in pre- and postmenopausal women: metabolic and anthropometric variables and their inter-relationships. Int J Obes 1992;16:495–504.

[21] Zamboni M, Armellini F, Harris T, et al. Effects of age on body fat distribution and cardiovascular risk factors in women. Am J Clin Nutr 1997;66:111.

[22] Espeland MA, Stefanick ML, Kritz-Silverstein D, et al. Effect of postmenopausal hormone therapy on body weight and waist and hip girths. J Clin Endocrinol Metab 1997; 82:1549–56.

[23] Kritz-Silverstein D, Barrett-Connor E. Long-term postmenopausal hormone use, obesity and fat distribution in older women. JAMA 1996;275:46–9.

[24] Davies KM, Heaney RP, Recker RR, et al. Hormones, weight change and menopause. Int J Obes 2001;25:874–9.

[25] Kaye SA, Folsom AR, Prineas RJ, et al. The association of body fat distribution with lifestyle and reproductive factors in a population study of postmenopausal women. Int J Obes 1990;14:583–91.

[26] Perry AC, Allison M, Applegate EB, et al. The relationship between fat distribution and coronary risk factors in sedentary postmenopausal women on and off hormone replacement therapy. Obes Res 1998;61:40–6.

[27] Reubinoff BE, Wurtman J, Rojansky N, et al. Effects of hormone replacement therapy on weight, body composition, fat distribution and food intake in early postmenopausal women: a prospective study. Fertil Steril 1995;64:963.

[28] Troisi RJ, Wolf AM, Manson JE, et al. Relation of body fat distribution to reproductive factors in pre- and postmenopausal women. Obes Res 1995;3:143–51.

[29] Haarbo J, Marslew U, Gotfredsen A, et al. Postmenopausal hormone replacement therapy prevents central distribution of body fat after menopause. Metabolism 1991;40: 1323–6.

[30] Sorensen MB, Rosenfalck AM, Hojgaard L, et al. Obesity and sarcopenia after menopause are reversed by sex hormone replacement therapy. Obes Res 2001;9:622–6.

[31] Poehlman ET, Toth MJ, Gardner AW. Changes in energy balance and body composition at menopause: a controlled, longitudinal study. Ann Int Med 1995;123:673–5.

[32] Heymsfield SB, Gallagher D, Poehlman ET, et al. Menopausal changes in body composition and energy expenditure. Exp Gerontol 1994;29:377–89.

[33] Hays NP, Bathalon GP, McCrory MA, et al. Eating behavior correlates of adult weight gain and obesity in health women aged 55–65 y. Am J Clin Nutr 2002;75:476–83.

[34] Pasquali R, Casimirri F, Cantobelli S, et al. Insulin and androgen relationships with abdominal body fat distribution in women with and without hyperandrogenism. Horm Res 1993;39:179–87.

[35] Rebuffe-Scrive M, Eldh J, Hafstrom L-O, et al. Metabolism of mammary, abdominal and femoral adipocytes in women before and after menopause. Metabolism 1986;35: 792–7.

[36] Samaras K, Spector TD, Nguyen TV, et al. Independent genetic factors determine the amount and distribution of fat in women after the menopause. J Clin Endocrinol Metab 1997;82:781–5.

[37] Cordero-MacIntyre ZR, Peters W, Libanati CR, et al. Effect of a weight-reduction program on total and regional body composition in obese postmenopausal women. Ann N Y Acad Sci 2000;904:526–35.

[38] Gallagher D, Kovera AJ, Clay-Williams G, et al. Weight loss in postmenopausal obesity: no adverse alterations in body composition or protein metabolism. Am J Physiol 2000;279:E124–31.

[39] Kuller LH, Simkin-Silverman LR, Wing RR, et al. Women's Healthy Lifestyle Project: a randomized clinical trial: results at 54 months. Circulation 2001;103:32–7.

[40] Ricci TA, Heymsfield SB, Pierson RN Jr, et al. Moderate energy restriction increases bone resorption in obese postmenopausal women. Am J Clin Nutr 2001;73:347–52.

[41] Tchernof A, Starling RD, Turner A, et al. Impaired capacity to lose visceral adipose tissue during weight reduction in obese postmenopausal women with the Trp64Arg β_3-adrenoceptor gene variant. Diabetes 2000;49:1709–13.

[42] Rawson ES, Nolan A, Silver K, et al. No effect of the Trp64Arg β_3-adrenoceptor gene variant on weight loss, body composition, or energy expenditure in obese, Caucasian postmenopausal women. Metabolism 2002;51:801–5.

6

Problems in Childhood Obesity

Sandra Hassink

Childhood obesity is reaching epidemic proportions. Data from the National Longitudinal Study of Youth show that by 1998, 21.5% of black children, 21.8% of Hispanic children, and 12.3% of white children had a body mass index that was greater than the 95th percentile for age and sex [1]. Obesity is a chronic disease with a multifactorial cause and a strong gene-environment interaction. Obesity has been linked to increased morbidity from cardiovascular disease [2,3], dyslipidemia [4], diabetes [5], hypertension [6], and cancer [7]. These morbidities are not confined to adults; risks of high BMI values in adulthood and the prevalence of cardiovascular and other diseases increase markedly for children aged 8 years and older with BMI values higher than the 85th percentile for age [8]. Complications of childhood obesity that require immediate evaluation and treatment include upper airway obstruction, slipped capital femoral epiphysis, pseudotumor cerebri, and nonalcoholic steatohepatitis.

Physicians and health care practitioners are faced with increasing numbers of obese children in their care. These obese children with morbidity require immediate evaluation and treatment to prevent progression of disease and long-term disability. The following descriptions of commonly encountered problems in the obese child represent those that are encountered in clinical practice. An expanded list of obesity-related morbidity by system is found in Table 1.

Evaluation of the obese pediatric patient

Obesity is defined as excess fat mass for age and sex. Adipose tissue stores change as children grow and differ between boys and girls, particularly

Table 1
Obesity-related morbidity in the pediatric population

Morbidity	Associated findings
Neurologic	
Pseudotumor cerebri	Headache, vomiting, visual changes
Pulmonary	
Upper airway obstruction	Sleep apnea, enuresis, orthopnea, daytime tiredness, napping, poor school performance
Asthma	Occult exercise-induced asthma, shortness of breath on exercise
Cardiovascular	
Cardiomyopathy of obesity	Dyspnea on activity, cardiac enlargement, poor ventricular function
Hypertension	Proteinuria, left ventricular enlargement
Dyslipidemia	Elevated cholesterol, triglycerides, low high-density lipoprotein cholesterol
Orthopedic	
Slipped capital femoral epiphysis	Limp, limitation of motion of hip, hip and/or knee pain
Blount disease	Tibia vara, knee pain
Gastrointestinal	
Nonalcoholic fatty liver disease	Elevated transaminases, enlarged liver, progression to fibrosis, cirrhosis
Gastroesophageal reflux	Abdominal discomfort, vomiting
Endocrine	
Type 2 diabetes	May present with polyuria, polydipsia, or ketoacidosis. Also may be associated with infection or discovered on routine urinalysis.
Polycystic ovary syndrome	Irregular menses, hirsutism, acanthosis nigricans
Psychological	
Depression	Depressed affect, poor school performance, suicidal ideation
Anxiety	Excessive worry, emotional eating pattern
Poor self-esteem	Decreased participation in social/school activities

during puberty. Direct measurements of body fat such as hydrodensitometry, bioelectrical impedance, or dual energy x-ray absorptiometry are used in research studies. Body mass index, defined as weight in kilograms divided by the square of the height in meters, is correlated with direct measures of adiposity [9] and is the commonly used clinical measure of obesity.

In contrast with the adult measure, BMI changes with age, paralleling a child's increases in height and weight. The Centers for Disease Control (CDC) recently published new growth charts for children that include charts for BMI (Fig. 1). A child with a BMI that is higher than the 85th percentile but lower than the 97th percentile is considered overweight; and a child with a BMI that is greater than the 97th percentile is classified as obese [10].

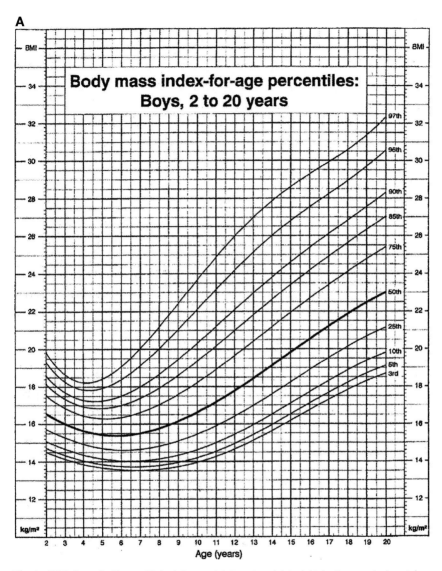

Fig. 1. CSC Growth Charts: United States. (A) Boys' and (B) girls' body mass index charts. Body mass index equals weight in kilograms divided by the square of the height in meters or weight in pounds times 703 and divided by the square of the height in inches.

In addition to its association with an increased risk of adult obesity, childhood obesity is linked with a wide range of other disorders (Table 2) that should be included in the evaluation of an obese pediatric patient. Obesity in childhood and adolescence is associated with increased adult obesity and its attendant health consequences and is responsible for significant, often unrecognized, morbidity in childhood and adolescence.

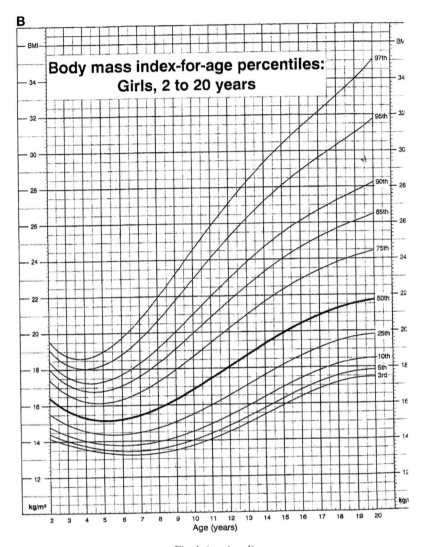

Fig. 1 (*continued*)

Nonalcoholic steatohepatitis

Example: A 16-year-old boy comes to you for help with his weight. He wants to increase his exercise tolerance and "look better." His parents are concerned because there is a family history of obesity and diabetes. His height of 179.2 cm (>95%) and weight of 152 kg (>95%) give him a BMI of 47.5 kg/m² (>97%).

On his initial metabolic screen, his fasting insulin is 35.8 μU/L, glucose is 87 mg/dL, and hemoglobin (Hgb) A_1C is 5.7%. His cholesterol is mildly elevated at 189 mg/dL with high-density lipoprotein cholesterol of 36 mg/dL,

Table 2
Disorders associated with obesity in childhood

Disorder	Associated findings
Genetic	
Prader-Willi syndrome	Infantile hypotonia, cognitive delay, short stature, behavioral/psychological problems
Bardet-Biedl syndrome	Short stature, cognitive delay, retinitis pigmentosa, renal disease
Alstrom syndrome	Nerve deafness, diabetes, pigmentary retinal degeneration, cataracts
Hypothalamic obesity	
Head injury	Associated neurological deficits
CNS Malignancy/radiation/surgery	Associated neurological deficits
Endocrine disorders	
Cushing's syndrome	Hypertension, centripetal obesity, stria, hypercortisolemia
Hypothyroidism	Constipation, myxedema, lethargy
Growth hormone deficiency	Short stature
Psychosocial	
Physical or sexual abuse	Obesity may follow episode of abuse
Depression/anxiety	Associated with pharmacotherapy or changes in eating and activity behavior

low-density lipoprotein cholesterol of 191 mg/dL, and triglycerides of 170 mg/dL. His aspartate aminotransferase is 85 μ/L, alanine aminotransferase is 148 μ/L, and gamma-glutamyltransferase (GGT) is 105 μ/L. His physical examination is normal, but you note a liver edge at 1 cm below the right costal margin. You are surprised and evaluate him for other causes of liver disease, including alpha-1 anti-trypsin deficiency, Wilson's disease, hemachromatosis, infectious hepatitis, hypopituitarism, and autoimmune diseases, which are negative. An ultrasound of his liver demonstrates echogenicity with an estimated 35% fat.

This patient has nonalcoholic fatty liver disease (NAFLD). Nonalcoholic fatty liver disease describes a continuum of conditions that range from simple steatosis at the most clinically benign end of the spectrum, through nonalcoholic steatohepatitis (NASH), to cirrhosis and end-stage liver disease (Fig. 2) [11]. NAFLD was originally described in adults [12] and the progression from fatty liver to cirrhosis is not well understood. Fibrosis may be extensive with relatively moderate elevations in transaminases (see Fig. 2). One theory is that an individual may have a genetic predisposition for hepatic fibrosis and then experience a "second hit," that causes chronic oxidative stress [13], which results in fibrotic changes in the liver. Leptin deficient ob/ob mice did not develop hepatic fibrosis despite obesity, fatty liver, and diabetes [14], which led to speculation that leptin may play a role in hepatic fibrosis because all but a few, obese individuals have high circulating levels of leptin. Obesity and type 2 diabetes are the strongest predictors of progression of fibrosis [15]. Age is also a risk factor for cirrhosis [15], which may reflect increased duration of risk for the "second

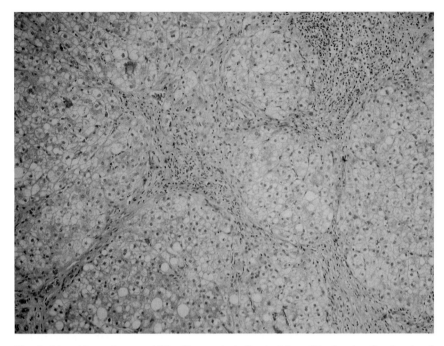

Fig. 2. Liver biopsy from a child with nonalcoholic steatohepatitis showing fine bands of bridging fibrosis that divide the hepatic parenchyma. Hepatocytes show accumulation of microvesicular fat with inflammatory foci within the lobule.

hit" that is believed to initiate fibrosis. Baldridge et al [16] reviewed liver biopsies of 14 obese children aged 10 to 18 years with steatosis without a known cause. Mild to marked steatosis and portal fibrosis with mild inflammatory infiltrate was found in all biopsies. Children with NAFLD may be at increased risk for cirrhosis if obesity is not reversed and other risk factors, such as alcohol consumption, are not avoided.

Weight loss will reverse elevations in aminotransferases and reduce hepatic steatosis, and it may decrease fibrosis. In a small series of pediatric patients with elevated aminotransferases and fatty liver on ultrasound, those who lost at least 10% of their excess weight normalized ALT and AST values and decreased ultrasound evidence of fatty infiltration [17]. When liver biopsies were performed in adults after weight loss, all had reduced steatosis, but only 50% had a reduction in fibrosis. Rapid weight loss may actually increase fibrosis because of an increase of free fatty acids to the liver and increased lipid peroxidation with resultant increased oxidative stress. This led to the conclusion that rapid weight loss should be avoided in these patients [18].

In adults, the management of diabetes with metformin was shown to reduce ALT and decrease liver volume, but follow-up liver biopsies were not performed [19]. 3-hydroxy-3-methylglutaryl coenzyme A (HMG-CoA) reductase inhibitors were shown to decrease growth of human hepatic stellate cells independent of their effect on cholesterol synthesis [20]. Studies are underway to evaluate HMG-CoA reductase inhibitors as a potential therapy for NASH. Ursodeoxycholic acid and vitamin E therapy have been tried but are as yet unproven therapeutically in reducing inflammatory activity and fibrosis.

Points to remember

Obesity is a risk factor for NAFLD, and even mild obesity may be associated with elevation of liver enzymes and hepatic steatosis. Metabolic evaluation of the obese child should include evaluation of liver function.

Nonalcoholic fatty liver disease is a diagnosis of exclusion; other causes of liver disease should be ruled out before a diagnosis is made.

Weight loss was shown to reverse the elevation of liver enzymes and to reduce steatosis and the histopathological changes that are associated with NASH but may not completely reverse fibrotic changes.

Upper airway obstructions/sleep apnea

Example: A mother in your practice brings her 8-year-old son in for his yearly physical. She tells you that he is doing "okay" in school but is being teased about his weight and often seems tired when he comes home from school. She does not have any other concerns about him at the time of the visit.

You note that his height of 134 cm (90%) and weight of 54.8 kg (>95%) give him a BMI of 30.6 kg/m^2, which is greater than the 97th percentile for age and sex. His blood pressure is 112/62 mm Hg. In your review of systems, you note that he snores at night; his mother does not know if there are any pauses in his breathing but says that he is sleeping on three to four pillows and it is hard to wake him up in the morning. You request a sleep study, which shows significant apnea and oxygen desaturation.

Obstructive sleep apnea syndrome (OSAS) in children is defined as a disorder of breathing during sleep that is characterized by prolonged, partial upper airway obstruction or intermittent complete obstruction (obstructive apnea) that disrupts normal ventilation during sleep and normal sleep patterns [21]. Sleep apnea is a frequent and significant comorbidity of obesity. Parents may not comment on snoring or sleep disturbance unless specifically asked. Often there is a family history of sleep apnea, and the parents often feel that this breathing pattern is "normal" for the child. Obstructive sleep apnea was noted in obese infants as young as 5 months of age [22].

A combination of increased fat mass, increased muscle relaxation during sleep, and enlarged tonsils and adenoids are frequently cited as etiologic factors for sleep apnea. The prevalence of OSAS in obese children is not known, but in one study [23], 59% of obese children with positive sleep histories had sleep apnea. A recent study found a significant correlation between fasting insulin levels and sleep apnea in a group of obese children [24].

Symptoms of sleep apnea can include nighttime awakening, restless sleep, difficulty awaking in the morning, daytime somnolence, napping, enuresis, decreased concentration, and poor school performance [25]. Significant deficits on measure of attention motor efficiency and graphomotor ability were documented in patients with sleep apnea [26].

Pulmonary hypertension [27], systemic hypertension [28], cor pulmonale, and right heart failure [29] are complications of OSAS. Untreated OSAS may result in cardiorespiratory failure and death [30].

History, audio and video taping, and overnight oximetry and daytime nap polysomnography are poor predictors of OSAS. The definitive diagnosis of OSAS is made by nighttime polysomnography [31].

Treatment includes weight loss, tonsilladenoidectomy, if indicated, and continuous positive airway pressure (CPAP) or bilevel positive airway pressure (BPAP). In adults, weight loss significantly improves symptoms of OSAS with a reduction in the apnea/hypopnea index and increase in nocturnal oxygen saturation. Functional residual capacity and expiratory reserve volume increase, and pharyngeal function improves [32]. Weight loss also reduced apneic episodes, hypoxemia, and daytime sleepiness in a group of obese children [33].

Tonsillectomy and adenoidectomy may provide relief of the obstruction [34]. Postoperative pulmonary edema occurs in some children, so close monitoring is imperative. Obstructive symptoms may remain even after surgery; children may need to be maintained on CPAP or BPAP support until weight loss is achieved.

Continuous positive airway pressure delivers constant air pressure by way of a mask, which leads to mechanical stenting of the airway and improved functional residual capacity. Bilevel positive airway pressure is similar, but delivers airway pressure that varies with inspiration and expiration. Both are an effective treatment for symptomatic children who can tolerate wearing the mask at night. Children who use this mode of therapy report an increased energy level, improved concentration, and increased activity level. CPAP and BPAP must be individually adjusted in the sleep laboratory for each patient, and compliance must be regularly monitored.

Points to remember

Ask specifically about sleep disturbances, snoring, and sleep position. Families will often disregard these symptoms.

Obstructive sleep apnea syndrome should be especially considered in obese children with poor school performance and concentration difficulties.

Sleep symptoms can evolve over time. Keep asking about sleep disturbance as you follow these children. Weight gain, intercurrent upper respiratory infections, and tonsillar enlargement can provoke symptoms.

Slipped capital femoral epiphysis

Example: A 12-year-old boy comes to your office complaining of knee pain. His parents have noticed that he has been limping intermittently, which interferes with his activity. His height of 159 cm and weight of 96.1 kg give him a BMI of 38.1 kg/m^2. He has no other specific complaints. On examination, you note marked limitation of rotation of his left hip and send him for an immediate radiograph.

This young man has a slipped capital femoral epiphysis (SCFE) of the left hip. This condition is an orthopedic emergency that requires immediate treatment. The cause remains unknown, but there is an increased association with obesity [35], puberty [36], and rapid growth [1]. Slipped capital femoral epiphysis refers to the medial and posterior displacement of the femoral epiphysis through the growth plate relative to the femoral neck [37]. The preferential site of slipping within the epiphysis is a zone of hypertrophic cartilage cells under the influence of gonadal hormones and growth hormone [38]. This condition was reported in a child as young as 5 years [39].

Slipped capital femoral epiphysis should be suspected and immediately evaluated in a patient who presents with limp, as did this patient. The condition can also present with complaints of groin, thigh, or knee pain that is referred by sensory cutaneous nerves that pass close to the hip capsule. Motion of the hip in abduction and internal rotation is limited on examination. The initial radiographic examination includes an anteroposterior view of the pelvis that includes both hips. This allows for comparison of the hips and helps diagnose bilateral disease, which occurs in up to 20% of patients. The findings are a widened growth plate with the epiphysis slipping posteriorly. A line that is drawn along the anterior femoral neck should intersect the epiphysis in a normal hip. Ultrasound has also been used in the diagnosis of SCFE, with the major finding that the quadriceps muscle is significantly atrophied compared with the asymptomatic hip [40]. Magnetic resonance imaging can detect a widened growth plate and can be used to diagnose preslip conditions [40]. All studies have a small rate of false negative results, and so they can confirm, but not completely rule out, a slipped epiphysis when one is suspected clinically.

Slips in the contralateral hip are common, especially if weight gain continues. Slipped capital femoral epiphysis can also be associated with renal failure, a history of radiation therapy, or primary hypothyroidism [41]. Small series of patients with SCFE were reported to have received gonadotropin-releasing hormone agonists [38] and growth hormone therapy [42].

The goal of treatment in patients with SCFE is to prevent the further slipping of the epiphysis. Stabilization of the hip is accomplished surgically by pinning the affected hip through the epiphysis. Complications of SCFE include avascular necrosis, which results from disruption of the vessels that supply the femoral head causing necrosis and destruction of the hip joint.

Points to remember

A careful hip and knee examination should be a routine part of the evaluation and follow-up of every obese child.

An obese child that complains of, or presents with, hip, knee, groin, or thigh pain should have a complete and thorough examination of his/her hips, including radiological studies.

In an obese child, an unusual or abnormal gait should not be attributed to "excess weight" but should be thoroughly investigated with a careful hip and knee examination.

Prader-Willi syndrome

Example: A 5-year-old girl comes to your office for the first time with pharyngitis and noisy breathing at night. Her parents state that she was a small baby who was difficult to feed, and they were pleased when she began to gain weight at around 18 months of age.

Her BMI is 32.8 kg/m^2 with weight of 33.3 kg, (95%) but her height is 101 cm (3%). Her tonsils are enlarged; she has clear nasal discharge. You notice that her development seems somewhat delayed. In addition to treating her respiratory symptoms, you order genetic testing for Prader-Willi syndrome (PWS).

Single gene defects are a rare but important cause of childhood obesity. Short stature and developmental delay are often associated findings. Prader-Willi syndrome is the most common single gene defect that causes obesity with an incidence of 1 in 10,000 to 1 in 15,000 live births [43]. Prader-Willi syndrome is caused by the absence of the paternally-derived portion of chromosome 15, either a deletion in the region of 15q11-q13 in 70% of the cases, or absence of the paternal chromosome in maternal disomy [44]. The critical region of chromosome 15 is active only in the paternally-inherited chromosome, therefore, PWS is an example of genomic imprinting [45].

The onset of obesity can be between 6 months and 5 to 6 years. The average age of onset of weight gain is 2 years with children suddenly beginning to cross weight percentiles and continues with relentless weight gain through adolescence into adulthood [43]. Obesity is believed to be a result of hypothalamic dysregulation that causes hyperphagia, food obsession, and a decrease in caloric requirement.

Primary features of PWS include infantile hypotonia, a poor sucking reflex, developmental delay, and hypogonadism followed by development of obesity, short stature, and behavioral and psychiatric difficulties that include a greater than average incidence of obsessive compulsive disorder, depression, and mood disorders [43]. Many features of PWS suggest hypothalamic dysfunction; there is a growing body of evidence that supports a relative or absolute growth hormone deficiency. Body composition in children with PWS, even in infancy, is characterized by a marked reduction in lean body mass associated with increased fat mass [46], thereby reducing resting energy expenditure.

Growth hormone therapy is now approved for PWS and has resulted in increases in lean body mass, energy expenditure, and linear growth. Response to growth hormone therapy is greatest in the first 12 months with a reduction in response thereafter [46]. Ongoing studies are underway to assess longterm outcome and risks.

Despite advances in therapy using growth hormone, control of the nutritional environment and access to food are the only current treatments for the obesity secondary to PWS. Children have a driven appetite with a complete inability to control their intake. Families often must lock cabinets and refrigerators because children with PWS will hoard and sneak food to evade nutritional restriction. In addition, because of decreased calorie burning, additional restrictions on daily intake are needed to avoid excessive weight gain. This treatment can place a considerable burden on families and caregivers [43].

Points to remember

Prader-Willi syndrome should be suspected in infants with hypotonia and a poor suck reflex. Because PWS is most often a sporadic, and not familial, genetic disorder, family history is not usually helpful.

In an obese child, short stature with developmental delay and learning disabilities should prompt consideration of a genetic syndrome.

At first, families may feel that locking up food and maintaining nutritional control of their child's diet may be more than they can tolerate; this is the most effective treatment, and, with support and encouragement, it can result in control of the child's obesity.

Pseudotumor cerebri

Example: An obese 15-year-old girl comes to your office complaining of headaches that have been bothering her for the past several weeks. She has a history of sinus disease and allergies and is taking a nonprescription decongestant. She denies any other medication or drug use.

On her funduscopic examination, you are startled to see papilledema. Further investigation reveals peripheral visual field cuts. Magnetic resonance imaging is normal, but the neurologist finds an increased cerebrospinal fluid pressure on lumbar puncture with a diagnosis of pseudotumor cerebri.

Pseudotumor cerebri is defined as raised intracranial pressure with papilledema and a normal cerebrospinal fluid in the absence of ventricular enlargement. The cause of pseudotumor cerebri is unknown. In a series of case-controlled studies in adolescents and adults, obesity and recent weight gain were the only factors that were found significantly more often in patients with pseudotumor cerebri than control patients [47]. In childhood, pseudo-tumor cerebri has been associated with mastoiditis, lateral sinus thrombosis [48], hypoparathyroidism [49], steroid treatment [50,51] and withdrawal [52], thyroid replacement [53], and systemic lupus [54]. Nalidixic acid, ciproflox-acin, and tetracycline therapy have been associated with pseudotumor cerebri in children but without a clear dose-response relationship [47]. Vitamin A [55] and isoretinoin [56] therapy are established causes of pseudotumor cerebri.

Pseudotumor cerebri can present with headache, with or without vomiting. Neck, shoulder, and back pain have also been reported [47]. Papilledema is the hallmark of this diagnosis but may not be present initially. Occasionally, papilledema is found asymptomatically on physical examination. Loss of peripheral visual fields and reduction in visual acuity may be present at diagnosis [57]. Treatment with acetazolamide [57], lumboperitoneal shunt (in severe cases), and weight loss lead to remission of symptoms [58]. Pseudotumor cerebri is a rare but serious complication of obesity that can occur in the pediatric patient.

Points to remember

A funduscopic examination should be a routine part of the examination of the obese child.

Children may not complain of visual field disturbances. When suspicious, testing for visual field deficits should be performed.

Pseudotumor cerebri is essentially a diagnosis of exclusion after other causes of increased intracranial pressure are eliminated.

Dysmetabolic syndrome

Example: An 11-year-old girl comes in for her yearly physical. Her height of 158.3 cm and weight of 102.8 kg give her a calculated BMI of 41.1 kg/m^2. Her blood pressure is 122/82 mm Hg (greater than 95%).

Her family history is strongly positive for cardiovascular disease, her mother has type 2 diabetes, and her father has hypertension and elevated lipid levels. Her paternal grandfather has a history of a stroke. Based on her presentation, you obtain fasting insulin of 88 μU/L [normal (nl) > 25 μU/L] and fasting glucose of 110 mg/dL (nl < 110 mg/dL). Her total cholesterol is 192 mg/dL (nl < 170 mg/dl), HDL cholesterol of 33 mg/dl (nl 40–59 mg/dL), and triglyceride level of 199 mg/dL (nl < 149 mg/dL).

Her HDL is low, and she has an elevated serum triglyceride, which is a pattern that is consistent with obesity-associated combined dyslipidemia. Urinalysis, including microscopic sediment examination, is normal. An echocardiogram reports her left ventricular mass to be at the upper limit of normal. This young adolescent has hypertension, obesity, and impaired glucose tolerance with marked hyperinsulinemia, borderline left ventricular hypertrophy, and dyslipidemia, which are the hallmarks of the dysmetabolic syndrome [59].

In adults, the dysmetabolic syndrome is defined as the presence of three or more of the following criteria: (1) abdominal obesity, (2) hypertriglyceridemia (higher than 150 mg/dL), (3) low HDL (HDL cholesterol <40 μg/dL in men and <50 mg/dL in women), (4) high blood pressure (higher than 130/85 mm Hg in adults), and (5) elevated fasting glucose higher than 110 μg/dL [60]. This pattern has also been found in young children and adolescents [61,62] and includes three or more of the following: (1) obesity (BMI > 95% for age and sex), (2) elevated blood pressure (systolic or diastolic pressure >90% for age and sex), (3) abnormal blood lipids (HDL cholesterol <40 mg/dL or triglycerides >150 mg/dL LDL >130 mg/dL), and (4) impaired glucose tolerance (fasting glucose >110 mg/dL, random glucose >200 mg/dL) [63].

A thorough medical evaluation in a child with one identified cardiovascular risk factor and obesity often reveals significant abnormalities in family history, lipid levels, glucose metabolism, and metabolic profile. In these children, the development of diabetes mellitus and arteriosclerosis is imminent [59]. The treatment approach should attend to the range of medical conditions identified.

Obesity

Obesity is either the origin or trigger of this condition and should be addressed vigorously with the family and child. Emphasis should be on increases in physical activity, decreases in inactivity, with particular focus on decreasing television and computer time, and improved nutrition. Best results have been obtained with using a family-based approach with education and behavior modification as major components [64–67]. Emphasis on the familial nature of obesity can often help the family see the need for change; and motivation to change often increases when families become aware of obesity-associated medical conditions.

Prioritizing the needed changes in the context of a particular nutritional and activity environment created by the family can help to identify specific measurable steps toward change. Specific parenting skills that are appropriate to the developmental stage of the child may need to be emphasized to help the family shift nutritional and activity patterns.

Hypertension

Underlying or secondary causes of hypertension should be ruled out in a thorough evaluation. A normal urinalysis and normal plasma creatinine make it unlikely that there is underlying renal disease. Patients with renal dysplasia or renal vascular lesions can have a normal urinalysis and normal plasma creatinine; however, these lesions usually cause severe blood pressure elevations in the range of 20 mm Hg above the 95th percentile [59].

Nonpharmacological approaches to achieve lifestyle change are the first steps to treating essential hypertension in children. A diet that is rich in fruits and vegetables and low-fat dairy products is effective in lowering blood pressure in adults [64]. If lifestyle modification is not effective, then drug therapy may be necessary. Angiotensin-converting enzyme inhibitors are a reasonable choice because they have been clinically studied in children [59].

Impaired glucose tolerance

Hyperinsulinemia and insulin resistance are associated with, and may precede, impaired glucose tolerance [68,69]. Impaired glucose tolerance has been found in up to 25% of obese children and adolescents [70]. Individuals with impaired glucose tolerance are at increased risk for developing type 2 diabetes. Impaired glucose tolerance is defined as a fasting plasma glucose level of less than 126 mg/dL and a 2-hour plasma glucose level of 140 to 200 mg/dL [71]. Type 2 diabetes accounts for between 8% and 45% of diabetes diagnoses in pediatric patients [71].

Evaluation for polycystic ovary syndrome should be included in patients with hyperinsulinemia and impaired glucose tolerance. This syndrome presents in adolescence with hirsutism, acne, obesity, menstrual irregularities, and hyperandrogenemia.

Treatment of impaired glucose tolerance is aimed at preventing further progression of glucose intolerance and onset of type 2 diabetes. Data from adult studies document that changes in lifestyle and exercise in patients with impaired glucose tolerance can improve glucose tolerance [72]. In a pilot study of pediatric patients with obesity, fasting hyperinsulinemia, and family history of type 2 diabetes, metformin reduced fasting blood glucose and insulin levels but did not change insulin sensitivity [73]. Risks of metformin therapy include lactic acidosis, decreased intestinal absorption of Vitamin B_{12} and folate, abdominal discomfort, and diarrhea. Further clinical trials are needed to determine the appropriate use and risks of these medications in children [74].

Dyslipidemia

The pattern of low HDL cholesterol and elevated triglyceride levels is typically associated with obesity. An HDL cholesterol of less than 40 µg/dL is considered a major coronary risk factor in adults [75]. The primary approach in treating the low HDL cholesterol, high triglyceride phenotype is controlling obesity by using the Step I American Heart Association diet and increasing physical activity. Improvement in the lipid profile can occur with even modest reduction in weight [76]. Current guidelines for children focus on lowering LDL cholesterol and do not recommend pharmacological treatment unless the patient is older than 10 years of age and the LDL cholesterol is higher than 190 µg/dL (or above 160 µg/dL with two additional risk factors) [59]. Niacin can lower triglycerides and raise HDL cholesterol but is poorly tolerated. The fibrates have not been used in children and may have unacceptable long-term toxicity. Atorvastatin has positive effects on HDL cholesterol and lowers triglycerides but has been used primarily to lower LDL cholesterol. Drugs that affect bile acid reabsorption tend to raise triglyceride levels and occasionally lower HDL cholesterol. Thus, current pharmacologic options for improving obesity-associated dyslipidemia in children are not yet adequate [59].

Points to remember

Obese children and adolescents are at risk for cardiovascular disease and presence of additional cardiovascular risk factors. Evaluation of obese, pediatric patients should include examination for hypertension, dyslipidemia, hyperinsulinemia, and glucose intolerance.

Obese children with insulin resistance and a family history of diabetes are at risk for type 2 diabetes, the fastest-growing endocrine problem in the pediatric age group.

Moderate weight loss will often correct metabolic abnormalities.

Summary

Clearly, obesity prevention should be at the forefront of our approach to this epidemic problem and the goal of health care providers, public health officials, community, and families. The problems of the obese child are no longer solely those of increased risk for disease, but of disease itself. Health care providers are increasingly challenged to provide evaluation and treatment for the serious comorbidities and complications of obesity in childhood. Many of these comorbidities and complications are "invisible" and require careful and focused history and laboratory evaluation to elicit. Treatment of the complication and comorbidity should be focused on preventing progression, reversing the disease process, and, ultimately, achieving control of obesity with family-based lifestyle changes that will allow the child to maintain a healthy balance between his or her genetic predisposition and the environment.

References

[1] Strauss RS, Pollack HA. Epidemic increase in childhood overweight, 1986–1998. JAMA 2001;286(22):2845–8.
[2] Freedman DS, Dietz WH, Srinivasan SR, et al. The relation of overweight to cardiovascular risk factors among children and adolescents: the Bogalusa Heart Study. Pediatrics 1999;103(6 Pt 1):1175–82.
[3] Lauer RM, Connor WE, Leaverton PE, et al. Coronary heart disease risk factors in school children: the Muscatine study. J Pediatr 1975;86(5):697–706.

[4] Guo S, Beckett L, Chumlea WC, et al. Serial analysis of plasma lipids and lipoproteins from individuals 9–21 y of age. Am J Clin Nutr 1993;58(1):61–7.
[5] Maffeis C, Tato L. Long-term effects of childhood obesity on morbidity and mortality. Horm Res 2001;55(Suppl 1):42–5.
[6] Guo SS, Chi E, Wiemandle W, et al. Serial changes in blood pressure from childhood into young adulthood for females in relation to body mass index and maturational age. Am J Hum Biol 1998;10:589–99.
[7] Pi-Sunyer FX. Medical hazards of obesity. Ann Intern Med 1993;119(7 Pt 2):655–60.
[8] Kuczmarski RJ, Ogden CL, Grummer-Strawn LM, et al. CDC growth charts: United States. Adv Data 2000;314:1–27.
[9] Cole TJ, Bellizzi MC, Flegal KM, et al. Establishing a standard definition for child overweight and obesity worldwide: international survey. BMJ 2000;320(7244):1240–3.
[10] Kiess W, Galler A, Reich A, et al. Clinical aspects of obesity in childhood and adolescence. Obes Rev 2001;2(1):29–36.
[11] Harrison SA, Diehl AM. Fat and the liver—a molecular overview. Semin Gastrointest Dis 2002;13(1):3–16.
[12] Ludwig J, Viggiano TR, McGill DB, et al. Nonalcoholic steatohepatitis: Mayo Clinic experiences with a hitherto unnamed disease. Mayo Clin Proc 1980;55(7):434–8.
[13] Day CP, James OF. Steatohepatitis: a tale of two "hits"? [Editorial]. Gastroenterology 1998;114(4):842–5.
[14] Koteish A, Diehl AM. Animal models of steatosis. Semin Liver Dis 2001;21(1):89–104.
[15] Angulo P, Keach JC, Batts KP, et al. Independent predictors of liver fibrosis in patients with nonalcoholic steatohepatitis. Hepatology 1999;30(6):1356–62.
[16] Baldridge AD, Perez-Atayde AR, Graeme-Cook F, et al. Idiopathic steatohepatitis in childhood: a multicenter retrospective study. J Pediatr 1995;127(5):700–4.
[17] Vajro P, Fontanella A, Perna C, et al. Persistent hyperaminotransferasemia resolving after weight reduction in obese children. J Pediatr 1994;125(2):239–41.
[18] Youssef W, McCullough AJ. Diabetes mellitus, obesity, and hepatic steatosis. Semin Gastrointest Dis 2002;13(1):17–30.
[19] Marchesini G, Brizi M, Bianchi G, et al. Metformin in non-alcoholic steatohepatitis. Lancet 2001;358(9285):893–4.
[20] Mallat A, Preaux AM, Blazejewski S, et al. Effect of simvastatin, an inhibitor of hydroxy-methylglutaryl coenzyme A reductase, on the growth of human Ito cells. Hepatology 1994;20(6):1589–94.
[21] Schechter MS. Technical report: diagnosis and management of childhood obstructive sleep apnea syndrome. Pediatrics 2002;109(4):e69–79.
[22] Kahn A, Mozin MJ, Rebuffat E, et al. Sleep pattern alterations and brief airway obstructions in overweight infants. Sleep 1989;12(5):430–8.
[23] Silvestri JM, Weese-Mayer DE, Bass MT, et al. Polysomnography in obese children with a history of sleep-associated breathing disorders. Pediatr Pulmonol 1993;16(2):124–9.
[24] de la Eva RC, Baur LA, Donaghue KC, et al. Metabolic correlates with obstructive sleep apnea in obese subjects. J Pediatr 2002;140(6):654–9.
[25] Gozal D. Sleep-disordered breathing and school performance in children. Pediatrics 1998;102(3 Pt 1):616–20.
[26] Greenberg GD, Watson RK, Deptula D. Neuropsychological dysfunction in sleep apnea. Sleep 1987;10(3):254–62.
[27] Tal A, Leiberman A, Margulis G, et al. Ventricular dysfunction in children with obstructive sleep apnea: radionuclide assessment. Pediatr Pulmonol 1988;4(3):139–43.
[28] Marcus CL, Greene MG, Carroll JL. Blood pressure in children with obstructive sleep apnea. Am J Respir Crit Care Med 1998;157(4 Pt 1):1098–103.
[29] Massumi RA, Sarin RK, Pooya M, et al. Tonsillar hypertrophy, airway obstruction, alveolar hypoventilation, and cor pulmonale in twin brothers. Dis Chest 1969;55(2):110–4.

[30] Kravath RE, Pollak CP, Borowiecki B, et al. Obstructive sleep apnea and death associated with surgical correction of velopharyngeal incompetence. J Pediatr 1980;96(4):645–8.

[31] Clinical practice guideline: diagnosis and management of childhood obstructive sleep apnea syndrome. Pediatrics 2002;109(4):704–12.

[32] Rubinstein I, Colapinto N, Rotstein LE, et al. Improvement in upper airway function after weight loss in patients with obstructive sleep apnea. Am Rev Respir Dis 1988;138(5): 1192–5.

[33] Willi SM, Oexmann MJ, Wright NM, et al. The effects of a high-protein, low-fat, ketogenic diet on adolescents with morbid obesity: body composition, blood chemistries, and sleep abnormalities. Pediatrics 1998;101(1 Pt 1):61–7.

[34] Kudoh F, Sanai A. Effect of tonsillectomy and adenoidectomy on obese children with sleep-associated breathing disorders. Acta Otolaryngol Suppl 1996;523:216–8.

[35] Kelsey JL, Acheson RM, Keggi KJ. The body build of patients with slipped capital femoral epiphysis. Am J Dis Child 1972;124(2):276–81.

[36] Schlesinger I, Waugh T. Slipped capital femoral epiphysis, unsolved adolescent hip disorder. Orthop Rev 1987;16(1):2–17.

[37] Busch MT, Morrissy RT. Slipped capital femoral epiphysis. Orthop Clin North Am 1987;18(4):637–47.

[38] Kempers MJ, Noordam C, Rouwe CW, et al. Can GnRH-agonist treatment cause slipped capital femoral epiphysis? J Pediatr Endocrinol Metab 2001;14(6):729–34.

[39] Bandyopadhyay S, Teach SJ. Slipped capital femoral epiphysis in a 5 1/2-year-old obese male. Pediatr Emerg Care 1999;15(2):104–5.

[40] Reynolds RA. Diagnosis and treatment of slipped capital femoral epiphysis. Curr Opin Pediatr 1999;11(1):80–3.

[41] Loder RT, Greenfield ML. Clinical characteristics of children with atypical and idiopathic slipped capital femoral epiphysis: description of the age-weight test and implications for further diagnostic investigation. J Pediatr Orthop 2001;21(4):481–7.

[42] Grumbach MM, Bin-Abbas BS, Kaplan SL. The growth hormone cascade: progress and long-term results of growth hormone treatment in growth hormone deficiency. Horm Res 1998;49(Suppl 2):41–57.

[43] Cassidy SB. Prader-Willi syndrome. Curr Probl Pediatr 1984;14(1):1–55.

[44] State MW, Dykens EM. Genetics of childhood disorders: XV. Prader-Willi syndrome: genes, brain, and behavior. J Am Acad Child Adolesc Psychiatry 2000;39(6):797–800.

[45] Lee S, Kozlov S, Hernandez L, et al. Expression and imprinting of MAGEL2 suggest a role in Prader-Willi syndrome and the homologous murine imprinting phenotype. Hum Mol Genet 2000;9(12):1813–9.

[46] Carrel AL, Myers SE, Whitman BY, et al. Sustained benefits of growth hormone on body composition, fat utilization, physical strength and agility, and growth in Prader-Willi syndrome are dose-dependent. J Pediatr Endocrinol Metab 2001;14(8):1097–105.

[47] Lessell S. Pediatric pseudotumor cerebri (idiopathic intracranial hypertension). Surv Ophthalmol 1992;37(3):155–66.

[48] Green M. Benign intracranial hypertension (pseudotumor cerebri). Pediatr Clin North Am 1967;14(4):819–30.

[49] Palmer RF, Searles HH, Boldrey EB. Papilledema and hypoparathyroidism simulating brain tumor. J Neurosurg 1959;16(4):378–84.

[50] Baker RS, Baumann RJ, Buncic JR. Idiopathic intracranial hypertension (pseudotumor cerebri) in pediatric patients. Pediatr Neurol 1989;5(1):5–11.

[51] Walker AE, Adamkiewicz JJ. Pseudotumor cerebri associated with prolonged cortico-steroid therapy. Reports of four cases. JAMA 1964;188:779–84.

[52] Neville BG, Wilson J. Benign intracranial hypertension following corticosteroid with-drawal in childhood. BMJ 1970;3(722):554–6.

[53] Huseman CA, Torkelson RD. Pseudotumor cerebri following treatment of hypothalamic and primary hypothyroidism. Am J Dis Child 1984;138(10):927–31.

[54] DelGiudice GC, Scher CA, Athreya BH, et al. Pseudotumor cerebri and childhood systemic lupus erythematosus. J Rheumatol 1986;13(4):748–52.

[55] Morrice G Jr, Havener WH, Kapetansky F. Vitamin A intoxication as a cause of pseudotumor cerebri. JAMA 1960;173:1802–5.

[56] Roytman M, Frumkin A, Bohn TG. Pseudotumor cerebri caused by isotretinoin. Cutis 1988;42(5):399–400.

[57] Baker RS, Carter D, Hendrick EB, et al. Visual loss in pseudotumor cerebri of childhood. A follow-up study. Arch Ophthalmol 1985;103(11):1681–6.

[58] Newborg B. Pseudotumor cerebri treated by rice reduction diet. Arch Intern Med 1974; 133(5):802–7.

[59] Falkner B, Hassink S, Ross J, et al. Dysmetabolic syndrome: multiple risk factors for premature adult disease in an adolescent girl. Pediatrics 2002;110(1 Pt 1):e1–e5.

[60] National Institutes of Health. National Heart, Lung, and Blood Institute. National Cholesterol Education Program. Third report of the expert panel on detection, evaluation, and treatment of high blood cholesterol in adults (Adult Treatment Panel III). Bethesda (MD): National Institutes of Health; 2002. NIH Publications 01–3670.

[61] Falkner B, Michel S. Obesity and other risk factors in children. Ethn Dis 1999;9(2):284–9.

[62] Sinaiko AR, Donahue RP, Jacobs DR, et al. Relation of weight and rate of increase in weight during childhood and adolescent to body size, blood pressure, fasting insulin, and lipids in young adults. The Minneapolis Children's Blood Pressure Study. Circulation 1999;99(11):1471–6.

[63] Epstein LH, McCurley J, Wing RR, et al. Five-year follow-up of family-based behavioral treatments for childhood obesity. J Consult Clin Psychol 1990;58(5):661–4.

[64] Appel LJ, Moore TJ, Obarzanek E, et al. A clinical trial of the effects of dietary patterns on blood pressure. DASH Collaborative Research Group. N Engl J Med 1997;336(16):1117–24.

[65] Epstein LH, Valoski A, Wing RR, et al. Ten-year follow-up of behavioral, family-based treatment for obese children. JAMA 1990;264(19):2519–23.

[66] Golan M, Fainaru M, Weizman A. Role of behaviour modification in the treatment of childhood obesity with the parents as the exclusive agents of change. Int J Obes Relat Metab Disord 1998;22(12):1217–24.

[67] Jelalian E, Saelens BE. Empirically supported treatments in pediatric psychology: pediatric obesity. J Pediatr Psychol 1999;24(3):223–48.

[68] Sinha R, Fisch G, Teague B, et al. Prevalence of impaired glucose tolerance among children and adolescents with marked obesity. N Engl J Med 2002;346(11):802–10.

[69] Zimmet PZ, Collins VR, Dowse GK, et al. Hyperinsulinaemia in youth is a predictor of type 2 (non-insulin-dependent) diabetes mellitus. Diabetologia 1992;35(6):534–41.

[70] The Expert Committee on the Diagnosis and Classification of Diabetes Mellitus. Report of the Expert Committee on the Diagnosis and Classification of Diabetes Mellitus. Diabetes Care 1999;22(Suppl 1):S5–19.

[71] American Diabetes Association. Type 2 diabetes in children and adolescents. Pediatrics 2000;105(3)(Pt 1):671–80.

[72] Tuomilehto J, Lindstrom J, Eriksson JG, et al. Prevention of type 2 diabetes mellitus by changes in lifestyle among subjects with impaired glucose tolerance. N Engl J Med 2001;344(18):1343–50.

[73] Freemark M, Bursey D. The effects of metformin on body mass index and glucose tolerance in obese adolescents with fasting hyperinsulinemia and a family history of type 2 diabetes. Pediatrics 2001;107(4):e55.

[74] Gidding SS, Bao W, Srinivasan SR, et al. Effects of secular trends in obesity on coronary risk factors in children: the Bogalusa Heart Study. J Pediatr 1995;127(6):868–74.

[75] Rocchini AP. Adolescent obesity and hypertension. Pediatr Clin North Am 1993;40(1):81–92.

[76] American Academy of Pediatrics. National Cholesterol Education Program. Report of the Expert Panel on Blood Cholesterol Levels in Children and Adolescents. Pediatrics 1992;89(3 Pt 2):525–84.

7

Obesity: Food Intake

Alexandra Kazaks

Judith S. Stern

When we lose, I eat. When we win, I eat. I also eat when we're rained out.
Tommy Lasorda, L.A. Dodgers baseball team manager.

This chapter is about the key role that food plays in the cause and treatment of obesity. In our society, food is an integral part of our social structure. We eat to satisfy hunger. We eat when we celebrate. We eat for comfort and entertainment. We share food to show love, hospitality, and social status. Energy intake is a major element in determining whether weight is gained, lost, or maintained. Food is a key player in the successful treatment of obesity and maintenance of lost weight. If your patient is like Tommy Lasorda, your challenge is to help that individual make a special effort to balance energy intake (food) with energy expenditure. To lose weight, energy intake must be less than energy expended.

This chapter discusses some of the changes in our food environment that have encouraged overeating and some research that underlies successful weight loss and maintenance of weight loss. The information will help in the guidance of patients to develop personalized eating plans and reduce energy intake, in part by recognizing the contributions of fat, concentrated carbohydrates, and large portion sizes.

Changes in our food environment

Portion distortion

We are victims of "portion distortion." The increase in portion size has occurred in a number of venues. Consider, for example, eating outside of the home. The average restaurant plate has increased from 10 inches to 12 inches. The maximum serving size of French fries that is available at McDonald's increased from 210 kilocalories in 1955 to 610 kilocalories in 2002 (Fig. 1) [1,2].

Similar increases are seen in the size of soft drinks. At many convenience stores, you can buy a 64-ounce soft drink; the smallest fast food restaurant size is now 10 ounces (Fig. 2). Muffins, bagels, and croissants also suffer from portion distortion. One serving of a cinnamon breakfast roll called a Cinnabon Pecanbon tips the scales at 890 calories. Even the mini Cinnabons are excessive at 430 calories per serving [3]. We have also increased portion sizes when we cook. The traditional *Joy of Cooking* cookbook has modified identical recipes from older editions of the cookbook to yield fewer servings. Portion size began to increase in the 1970s and has been growing ever since [2].

What is the effect of larger portion sizes on food intake? According to research done by Wansink and Park [4], "People use more from larger packages—typically between 9% and 36% more." In a study done for CBS television, the same investigators conducted a "popcorn test." When people were given larger containers of popcorn, they ate an average of 44% more (equal to about 120 kilocalories) than those who got small containers. Movie theater-sized extra large popcorn is 170 ounces or more than 5 quarts. With such large sizes being offered, consumers eat more and get a distorted impression of what is a reasonable serving size.

Portion control is not easy. Many Americans are unaware that standardized portions that are used to develop labeling laws and the Food Guide

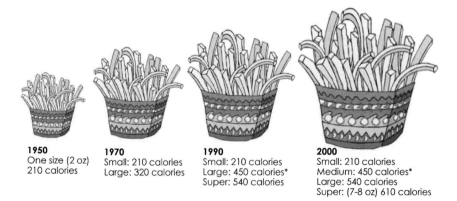

1950	1970	1990	2000
One size (2 oz) 210 calories	Small: 210 calories Large: 320 calories	Small: 210 calories Large: 450 calories* Super: 540 calories	Small: 210 calories Medium: 450 calories* Large: 540 calories Super: (7-8 oz) 610 calories

Fig. 1. Pictorial history of portion sizes of McDonald's French fries. Between 1990 and 2000 large became medium (*From* Stern JS; with permission).

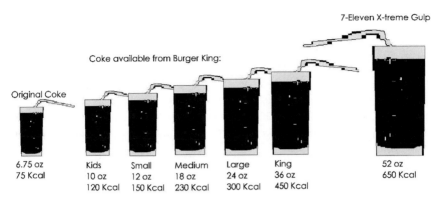

Fig. 2. Beverage portion sizes. Calories per serving without ice. Colas have about 12.5 Kcalories per ounce (*From* Stern JS; with permission).

Pyramid are much smaller than the portions that arecommonly consumed [2]. A standardized serving of cooked meat is 2 to 3 ounces, a serving of fruit juice is 6 ounces, and a serving of soft drink is 8 ounces. Compare the United States Department of Agriculture (USDA) standardized serving of French fries that is 1 ounce or 80 calories with the "medium" serving of McDonald's fries (450 kilocalories) (see Fig. 1). Furthermore, serving sizes on food labels are not always the same as those on the USDA Food Guide Pyramid. The Food Guide Pyramid defines a serving of pasta or rice as one half cup, whereas most food labels indicate that a serving is one cup. Pasta, as served in restaurants, is at least 3 cups. Food companies, restaurants, and fast food chains have responded to consumers who think that they are getting better value for their money when the portions are "supersized" [2].

Profits from food items generally rise when manufacturers increase product size. Increasing food contents in a container costs relatively little compared with labor and other costs. Increased quantity and increased container size are used to entice customers.

Food manufacturers, retailers, and food service spent $11 billion in 1997 on mass media advertising. Snacks, prepared convenience foods, and soft drinks were the most heavily advertised. Contrast this with the $1 million spent in 1999 by the National Cancer Institute to promote the "5-a-Day" message that encourages Americans to eat more fruits and vegetables [5].

Energy intake is up

Part of the surge in obesity in the United States reflects an increase in per capita energy intake between 1970 and 1997, from 2220 kilocalories to 2680 kilocalories. These figures are estimated from the total food supply and are adjusted for spoilage and disappearance [6]. The bottom line is that a calorie is a calorie when it comes to fat gain and fat loss. If you consume extra energy in the form of protein (4 kcals/g), fat (9 kcals/g), carbohydrate

(4 kcals/g), or alcohol (7 kcals/g) you will store this extra energy in the form of body fat. Conversely, if you limit energy intake, body fat loss will be in proportion to the energy deficit (approximately 3500 kilocalories are equivalent to a pound of fat). Small changes can make large differences over time. For example, choosing to use one tablespoon of mayonnaise on a sandwich instead of two tablespoons can save 100 kilocalories/day. Over a year the total 36,500 kilocalorie deficit could result in a loss of 10 pounds of body fat. For many people, this change has little or no effect on the enjoyment of a sandwich.

Contributions of dietary fat

The calorie differences among foods are most often related to fat content. Fats, as solid fats and oils, contribute twice as much energy per gram as either carbohydrate or protein. Many studies showed that people consume more total calories with high-fat diets compared with low-fat diets [7]. Furthermore, when excess energy comes from dietary fat, instead of carbohydrate or protein, it is more readily stored in fat cells as adipose tissue [8].

The general public has responded to dietary advice to lower fat intake [9] and results of national dietary surveys indicated that the percentage of total dietary energy from fat has decreased from 42% in 1970 to 38% in 1994. This statistic is misleading because although the percentage of fat has decreased, total energy intake has increased. The result is an increase in absolute fat intake from 154 grams to 159 grams per day. According to the USDA Economic Research Service (USDA-ERS), responsibility for the increased consumption lies in added fats, such as butter, shortening, and oils that are incorporated into commercially-prepared baked goods, snack foods, and fried foods [6]. See Figure 3 for food sources of concentrated fats in the average diet.

The list includes foods that many individuals enjoy and would not want to give up permanently. Actually, for long-term weight management it may be preferable to include a moderate amount of fat with meals. Weight loss

Cooking:	Fried food - chicken, fish, or potatoes
	Baked goods using butter, margarine or shortening- cookies, cakes, pies, biscuits
Snacks:	Chips, crackers and doughnuts
Meats:	High fat cuts such as prime rib or spareribs, sausage and hamburgers
Dairy:	Full fat milk products, cheese, and ice cream
Salad Dressings:	Mayonnaise or made with oil

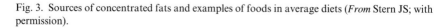

Fig. 3. Sources of concentrated fats and examples of foods in average diets (*From* Stern JS; with permission).

success and overall satisfaction was evaluated in a group of men and women who followed a diet plan that included a moderate fat intake of healthful fats such as olive oil, peanut butter, and nuts. They were compared with a similar group who followed a low-fat plan of less than 30% total kilocalories. At 6 months, both groups had lost about the same amount of weight; after 1 year the group who followed a moderate-fat diet had lost an average of 9 pounds, whereas people who followed the low-fat diet weighed more than at the beginning of the study. It is possible that the moderate-fat plan was more enjoyable, allowed people to include favorite foods, and influenced the participants to stay with the diet. More than half of the participants in the moderate-fat plan remained on the program at the end of 18 months, whereas only 20% of the people on the low-fat plan were still participating [10]. Moderate amounts of fat can be part of a healthful diet as long as consumers have a respect for the power of fat. Dietary fat has the power to add pleasure, taste, and satisfaction, but it also has the power to easily be converted to excess body fat.

As important as fat is, weight loss will not result if total energy intake is not reduced [11,12]. When nutritionists recommended low-fat diets to help combat obesity, the food industry readily produced hundreds of new food products with low fat or no fat. In some of those foods the fat is replaced with energy-dense, refined carbohydrates [13]. Many of the new low-fat cookies, cakes, and frozen desserts are high in sugar so the fat is reduced but the total kilocalories per serving are not.

Table 1 shows that it is possible for low-fat foods to contain as many kilocalories as higher fat items. The problem is aggravated when individuals believe that they can eat much more of a fat-reduced food and not gain

Table 1
Fat-free versus regular calorie comparison

Fat-free or reduced fat	Calories	Regular	Calories
Reduced-fat peanut butter, 2 T	187	Regular peanut butter, 2 T	191
Fat-free fig cookies, 2 cookies (30 g)	102	Regular fig cookies, 2 cookies (30 g)	111
Nonfat vanilla frozen yogurt (<1% fat), 1/2 cup	100	Regular whole milk vanilla frozen yogurt (3–4% fat) 1/2 cup	104
Fat-free caramel topping, 2 T	103	Caramel topping, homemade with butter, 2 T	103
Low-fat blueberry muffin, 1 small (2 1/2 inch)	131	Regular blueberry muffin, 1 small (2 1/2 inch)	138
Low-fat cereal bar, 1 bar (1.3 oz.)	130	Regular cereal bar, 1 bar (1.3 oz.)	140

Data from National Heart, Lung, and Blood Institute. National Institutes of Health. Clinical guidelines on the identification, evaluation, and treatment of overweight and obesity in adults—the evidence report. June 1998.

weight. This misinformed overconsumption could be the reason that the low-fat message is not working. Total fat has increased, energy has increased, and people are getting fatter [14]. Dietary fat may be wrongly accused of singlehandedly promoting obesity. It is possible that food energy density, rather than dietary fat, is responsible for increasing obesity [13].

Energy density defined

Energy density, or the concentration of energy per gram, is increased or decreased by the amount of dietary fat, fiber, water, and air in a given food. For example, orange juice is more energy dense than the whole fruit. Figure 4 shows a range of kilocalories that are contained in 4 ounces of various foods.

The more energy dense the food, the easier it is to consume more of it. In a study of women who were given meals of high- or low-energy density, lean and obese test subjects consumed 20% fewer kilocalories when they ate foods with low energy density, independent of fat content [15]. Subjects tended to eat a constant volume of food for each meal, regardless of the energy density. The amount of food, rather than caloric value, determined how much was eaten [16].

Drinking more calories

Sweetened beverages have a low calorie density per unit, but when the drinks are consumed in large quantities throughout the day, their contribution to total energy intake becomes significant. Sugar-sweetened beverages, including sweetened fruit drinks and carbonated drinks, account for

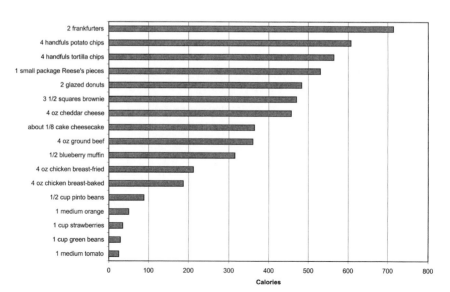

Fig. 4. Energy density calories in 4-ounce servings.

nearly half of the total added sugars in the U.S. diet [17,18] and they are available everywhere. In 1997, 2.8 million vending machines dispensed more than 27 billion drinks. Most of those drinks were 12-ounce cans, but the soft drink trend is toward serving sizes of 20 ounces or more [19]. The larger the container, the more beverage people will drink, especially if they assume that the container is a single serving, whether it is 12 ounces, 20 ounces, or more [20].

Soft drinks contribute extra energy that adds up day-by-day and eventually leads to overweight and obesity. They also displace more nutritious foods that supply essential vitamins, minerals, and other nutrients. High intake of added sugars is correlated with decreased diet quality, an excess in kilocalories, and deficiencies in Vitamin A and C, folic acid, and calcium [9,14]. When the goal is to reduce total calorie intake, a good place to start is with energy-dense, nutrient-poor foods, such as soft drinks. Those beverages can be reasonably consumed less frequently as a smaller part of total energy intake.

Another reason to limit sugar-sweetened drinks is that liquid kilocalories may not be recognized by appetite feedback mechanisms. People normally adjust or moderate energy intake by eating less after a large meals, but that check occurs more readily with meals of solid foods than with beverages. A group of men and women were given 450 extra kilocalories per day, either as a liquid or solid (three 12-ounce cans of soda or 45 large jelly beans) [21]. The people who ate the candy adjusted for the extra energy and later ate less, but those who got the extra liquid kilocalories made no compensation. They simply added those extra kilocalories. The author of the article stated, "Liquid kilocalories don't trip our satiety mechanisms. They just don't register" [18].

Food is conveniently available

Because a large percentage of meals that are eaten away from home allow for easy and inexpensive access to large quantities of energy dense foods, the nutritional quality of those meals must be considered. They can no longer be ignored and thought of as special occasion occurrences because they are now part of our normal patterns of food consumption, whether it is a gourmet dinner, a fast food burger, or a soda from a vending machine. In 1970, away-from-home meals represented 25% of the total food budget; in 1995, it had risen to 40% of total food spending [5]. The National Restaurant Association reported that in 1981 the average American ate 3.7 commercially-prepared meals per week. By 2000, that number had increased to 4.2 per week [22]. All of those meals have contributed to the increase in overweight and obesity, because the frequency of eating in restaurants has been positively associated with body fatness. That result was probably related to evidence that commercially-prepared meals generally have high energy and fat content and low fiber content [23].

Is anyone successful at responding to our food environment?

Even when the food environment presents large portions, energy dense foods, and easy availability of thousands of food choices, some people are successful in losing weight and maintaining weight loss. But for the vast majority, permanent weight loss is an elusive goal. To discover a game plan for long-term weight management that also provides the greatest health benefits, we turn to weight management experts, people who have lost weight and kept it off. The National Weight Control Registry (NWCR) is a database of nearly 3000 people who have been recognized as successful at long-term weight maintenance. To join they must have lost a minimum of 30 pounds and have kept it off for at least a year. Dr. James Hill at the University of Colorado and Dr. Rena Wing, currently at Brown University, founded the registry in 1993 as a way to follow weight loss maintainers and to determine the variables of weight maintenance, or weight regain. A study of the participants in 1997 reported that they had lost an average of 66 pounds and had maintained at least a 30-pound weight loss for an average of 5.5 years [24].

How did they do it?

The key behaviors of these successful weight maintainers were reduced energy intake, reduced dietary fat intake, and increased activity. To reduce energy intake, they became aware of calorie values of food, reduced dietary fat intake, and limited food quantity. The participants ate regular meals, occasionally at restaurants, but most of their meals were self-prepared [24]. In an earlier study [25], another group of women who were successful at weight maintenance devised personalized weight loss and maintenance plans. Some used ideas from their earlier weight loss experience, or ideas from books, but in one way or another increased activity and reduced caloric intake was achieved. They developed new meal patterns with less fat and sugar and more fruits and vegetables. They were conscious of quantity but did not deprive themselves of favorite, high-calorie foods because they were not waiting for the diet to end, but were learning to make choices that could keep them satisfied and healthy for a lifetime. Because successful maintainers differ greatly in the ways that they achieve long-term weight loss, a one-size-fits-all diet plan will not be effective.

What do we tell patients?

We need much more research on how people manage weight and keep it off. We do not have enough evidence from long-term, randomly-controlled, trials to define the best approaches to weight loss and maintenance. In the meantime, we rely on data from studies, such as the NWCR to make educated assumptions about weight management. As professionals we can use the data we have to help people understand their own conditions surrounding overeating, and to help them decide what changes they would be willing to make to lose weight. The list of weight management strategies from the experts can serve as a guide (Box 1) and a summary of these strategies is provided at the end of the following section (Box 2).

Develop an individualized plan

Begin with current diet assessment. The word "diet" brings to mind meals of tuna and carrot sticks or dry toast. A diet is actually defined as all of the food and drink that a person takes in during the course of a day. People often have a difficult time remembering what they ate from one day to the next; a journal of the amounts of all food and beverages consumed can be an effective learning tool. Even though people generally underestimate how much they eat, keeping food records helps to identify the eating patterns that contribute to weight gain.

Food records provide immediate feedback to the individual who can use them to evaluate problem areas and consider changes s/he would be willing to make. In this way, a personalized plan for weight loss begins to emerge. For example, a journal may show that having a doughnut everyday at work may be just a habit and is eaten "because it is there" rather than for hunger or real enjoyment. The individual may want to try having a "doughnut hole," another lower calorie food, or skip it altogether. A journal can be provided by the health care professional or the patient may choose to use another place to record the data, such as a notebook, a Palm Pilot, or even a computerized diet analysis program. The clinician does not have to monitor food records but acts as a coach to provide positive encouragement, knowledge, and referral to other professionals for additional skill building.

Reduce energy intake

Table 2 summarizes ways to reduce energy intake. A 500 to 1000 kilocalorie per day deficit can result in a fat loss of 1 to 2 pounds per week. This type of energy reduction is designed to achieve slow, progressive weight loss.

Box 1. Weight management strategies from the experts

Make individualized plan: include assessment and skill development
Reduce energy intake
Recognize fat as concentrated source of energy
Eat less fat and sugar and more fruits and vegetables
Limit food quantity at home and when eating out

Note: Although increased activity is a major part of weight management, this article focuses on changes in food intake strategies.

Table 2
Ways to reduce energy intake[a]

Description	Advantages	Disadvantages
Fasting: [26] Fewer than 200 kcal/day May be part of religious or spiritual practices	Rapid weight loss	Not nutritionally adequate Loss of fluid, electrolytes, and protein may lead to cardiac complications Cannot be continued for long term weight maintenance Gallstones common during rapid weight loss
Very low calorie diet [11] 200 to 800 kcal/day	Rapid weight loss of 3 to 5 pounds/week	Not nutritionally adequate—must be supplemented with vitamins, minerals, and essential fatty acids Requires medical supervision and frequent monitoring and follow-up Gallstones common during rapid weight loss Rapid initial weight loss usually regained. Long-term weight loss not different from low calorie diets
Low fat diet [11] Fat intake less than 20% of total energy	May be efficient method of reducing total energy intake	Effective only if total energy intake also reduced Decreased long term compliance because of restriction of many foods

Diet	Advantages	Disadvantages
Low calorie diet [11] 800 to 1500 kcal/day or, 500 to 1000 kcal/day deficit	Can produce weight loss of 1 to 2 pounds/week Can be used for long-term weight management Most foods can be included	Lower calorie levels may require vitamin/mineral supplements to assure adequate nutrition
Liquid Meal Replacements [27] 200 to 250 kcal per serving Used for one or more meals	Controlled food servings removes food choice and portion size problems May be useful for people unable to change eating habits Easy to use and inexpensive	Possible decreased long-term compliance because of limited food choice May be hard to follow when eating in social situations
Portion Controlled Meals Pre-measured, individually packaged meals of various calorie and nutrient levels	Controlled food servings removes food choice and portion size problems May be effective way to control calorie intake	Possible decreased long-term compliance because of limited food choices and availability May be low in fiber, fruits, vegetables

a The most healthful weight loss diets are low in energy but not essential nutrients. The diet should lead to modified eating habits that will help maintain weight after the weight loss phase is over.

For most people this means that the reduced energy plan will total about 1000 to 1200 kilocalories for women and 1200 to 1600 kilocalories for men [11]. Very low calorie diets are less than 800 kilocalories per day and usually are not used for long-term weight management. Because they are usually based on liquid supplements, and not familiar food, they are difficult to integrate into a normal lifestyle. Patients on these diets may require frequent monitoring and may not receive adequate amounts of essential nutrients. Most importantly, evidence showed that at the end of 1 year of dieting, moderate kilocalorie deficits are as effective at producing weight loss as severe calorie restriction [28,29].

Evaluating the calorie content of foods takes practice because energy content is not always obvious. Table 3 shows that 4 ounces of pork loin has less potential energy than a medium baked potato. For a woman with a goal of 1200 kilocalories per day, just six chocolate sandwich cookies provide more than one quarter of those kilocalories. Calorie content of foods can be estimated using food labels, restaurant nutrition information sheets, and handbooks of nutrient information. For weight reduction and maintenance, it is worth the initial effort to become acquainted with the energy that is provided by favorite foods. As participants in the NWCR found, weight control becomes easier over time; it becomes second nature to balance higher calorie foods with lower calorie choices to arrive at overall energy goals. Subjects reported that they truly derived pleasure from eating foods that were lower calorie and lower fat [30].

Plan to recognize fat as a concentrated source of energy

Although some fat is necessary for good health, reduction of total fat intake is a strategy that NWCR participants found to be important for their weight management. In the campaign to prevent obesity, the National Heart, Lung, and Blood Institute suggests limiting total fat to 30% or less of total calories [11]. Many studies showed that people consume more total energy with high-fat diets compared with low-fat diets [9]. It is helpful to translate that calculation into equivalent grams of fat as shown in Table 4,

Table 3
Calorie and fat content of selected foods

Food	Calories	Fat grams
Baked pork loin–4 oz	240	11
Baked pork spare ribs–4 oz	450	35
French fries–4 oz.	375	14
Baked potato–8 oz.	250	0
Strawberry ice cream–1 cup	260	10
Fresh strawberries–1 cup	45	0
Chocolate sandwich cookie–6	330	14
Gingersnaps–6	150	5

Data from The NutriBase guide to fat and fiber in your food. New York: Avery Publishing Group; 1995.

Table 4
Fat gram equivalents for 30% of total calories

Total calories	30% of calories	Fat gram equivalent
1000	300	34
1200	360	40
1400	420	47
1600	480	53

because calculating percentages of calorie intake is more complicated than simply looking at the fat gram content listed on food labels and nutrition information sheets.

Eat more fruits and vegetables

Calorie density of menu items can be diluted by the addition of fruits, vegetables, whole grains, and water. For example, extra vegetables and whole grain bread can reduce the calorie density of a meat sandwich. Plant fiber adds volume, provides a feeling of fullness, and fewer overall kilocalories may be consumed. Dietary fibers are plant polysaccharides that are not digested by humans. Eating more plant foods such as fruits, vegetables, grains, and legumes is an effective way to add dietary fiber.

Limit food quantity at home and when eating out

In a survey undertaken by the American Institute of Cancer Research, 78% of adults believed that eating certain kinds of food and avoiding others was more effective for weight loss than eating less food. In other words, they

1 1/2 ounces of cheese is similar to a 9-volt battery

 1 cup of rice or pasta is about the size of a fist

A serving of meat is about 3 ounces or the size of a deck of cards

 A medium sized piece of fruit is about the size of a baseball

A medium sized baked potato is similar to a computer mouse

Fig. 5. Common equivalents of standard food portions ... visualize objects of similar size (*From* Stern JS; with permission).

thought that quantity did not matter if the correct types of food were consumed [31]. The National Weight Control Registry weight-loss experts found that eating less food to reduce energy intake was the strategy that worked best.

By recalibrating portion sizes to fit individual health goals it is possible to enjoy favorite energy dense foods in moderation at home or when eating out. Even without measuring spoons or cups, the amount of a standard food portion may be visualized by comparison with objects of similar size. For example, some common equivalents are shown in Fig. 5.

Long-term success

The available research studies and experiences of people in the National Weight Control Registry showed that success is not based on deprivation. It is not reliance on supreme will power. It is not a focus on just a few foods. Success is awareness of foods that are healthful and good tasting. It is

---

Box 2. Guide to developing your own successful strategies

Make an individualized plan
Keep food records.
Decide what you would be willing to change.

Reduce energy intake
Read food labels and ask for nutrition information when
   eating out
What foods are worth about 500 calories?
Use meal replacements or portion-controlled servings
What calorie changes could you make?

Recognize fat as concentrated source of energy
Set fat gram goal
What favorite foods are high in fat?
What fat changes could you make?

Eat less fat and sugar and more fruits and vegetables
What foods do you eat that are high in concentrated sugar?
How can you eat more fruit each day?
How can you eat more vegetables each day?

Limit food quantity at home and when eating out
Measure some portions of food. Compare with what you
   normally eat
Practice estimating portion sizes using common equivalents
How can you tell when you are satisfied? How much is enough?

enjoyment of a balanced variety of foods that contain fat, protein, and carbohydrates. It is about integration of favorite foods into a dietary scheme, rather than fighting temptation. To maximize the probability of losing weight and keeping it off, clinicians can use these approaches to encourage patients to define weight management objectives and plans of action that allow for enjoyment of favorite meals, and selectivity and discrimination in food and beverage choices. Given the availability of thousands of foods in the marketplace that can combine taste, enjoyment, and nourishment there is no need to consume tasteless food; people can discover the satisfaction and pleasure in maintaining the new, healthier eating habits.

> For bringing people together, for celebrating the most important moments in our lives—nothing pleases us, delights us and unites us like food. Dan Glickman, U.S. Secretary of Agriculture, 2000 [32].

References

[1] Stern J, Dennenberg RV. How to stay slim and healthy on the fast food diet. New Jersey: Prentice Hall; 1980.
[2] Young LR, Nestle M. The contribution of expanding portion sizes to the U.S. obesity epidemic. Am J Public Health 2002;92:246–9.
[3] Carrey B. Pure indulgence. Available at: http://Epinions.com. Accessed July 5, 2002.
[4] Wansink B, Park S. Accounting for taste: prototypes that predict preference. J Database Marketing 2000;7:308–20.
[5] Frazao E. America's eating habits: changes and consequences. AIB-750, USDA, Economic Research Service, 1999.
[6] Putnam J. Major trends in the U.S. food supply. Food Rev 2000;23:8–15.
[7] Hill JO, Peters J. Environmental contribution to the obesity epidemic. Science 1998;280:1371–4.
[8] Horton TJ, Drougas H, Brachey A, et al. Fat and carbohydrate overfeeding in humans: different effects on energy storage. Am J Clin Nutr 1995;62:19–29.
[9] Harnack L, Jeffery RW, Boutelle KN. Temporal trends in energy intake in the U.S.: an ecological perspective. Am J Clin Nutr 2000;71:1478–84.
[10] McManus K, Antinoro L, Sacks F. A randomized controlled trial of a moderate-fat, low-energy diet compared with a low fat, low-energy diet for weight loss in overweight adults. Int J Obes Relat Metab Disord 2001;25:1503–11.
[11] National Heart, Lung, and Blood Institute (NHLBI)—National Institutes of Health. Clinical guidelines on the identification, evaluation, and treatment of overweight and obesity in adults—the evidence report. June 1998.
[12] Pirozzo S, Summerbell C, Cameron C, et al. Advice on low-fat diets for obesity. Cochrane Database Syst Rev 2002;2:CD003640.
[13] Astrup A. The American paradox: the role of energy-dense fat-reduced food in the increasing prevalence of obesity. Curr Opin Clin Nutr Metab Care 1998;6:573–7.
[14] Levine AS. Energy density of foods: building a case for food intake management. Am J Clin Nutr 2001;73:999–1000.
[15] Bell EA, Rolls BJ. Energy density of foods affects energy intake across multiple levels of fat content in lean and obese women. Am J Clin Nutr 2001;73:1010–8.
[16] Bell EA, Rolls BJ. Intake of fat and carbohydrate: role of energy density. Eur J Clin Nutr 1999;53(Suppl 1):S166–173.
[17] Guthrie JF, Morton JF. Food sources of added sweeteners in the diets of Americans. J Am Diet Assoc 2000;100:45–51.

[18] Krebs-Smith SM. Choose beverages and foods to moderate your intake of sugars: measurement requires quantification. J Nutr 2001;131(2S–1):527S–35S.

[19] Center for Science in the Public Interest. In the drink. Nutr Action Healthletter 2000; Nov:7–9.

[20] Johnson R, Frary C. Choose beverages and foods to moderate your intake of sugars: the 2000 dietary guidelines for Americans — What's all the fuss about? J Nutr 2001;131: 2766S–71S.

[21] DiMeglio DP, Mattes RD. Liquid versus solid carbohydrate: effects on food intake and body weight. Int J Obes Relat Metab Disord 2000;24:794–800.

[22] Ebbin R. Americans' dining-out habits. Restaurants USA. Available at: http://www. restaurant.org/rusa. Accessed June 20, 2002.

[23] McCrory MA, Fuss PJ, Hays NP, et al. Overeating in America: association between restaurant food consumption and body fatness in healthy adult men and women ages 19 to 80. Obes Res 1999;7:564–71.

[24] Klem ML, Wing RR, McGuire MT, et al. A descriptive study of individuals successful at long-term maintenance of substantial weight loss. Am J Clin Nutr 1997;66:239–46.

[25] Kayman S, Bruvold W, Stern JS. Maintenance and relapse after weight loss in women: behavioral aspects. Am J Clin Nutr 1990;52:800–7.

[26] Mahan K, Escott-Stump S, editors. Krause's food, nutrition and diet therapy. Philadelphia: WB Saunders; 2000.

[27] Heber D, Ashley JM, Wang HJ, et al. Clinical evaluation of a minimal intervention meal replacement regimen for weight reduction. J Am Coll Nutr 1994;13:608–14.

[28] Wadden TA. Treatment of obesity by moderate and severe caloric restriction. Results of clinical research trials. Ann Intern Med 1993;119:688–93.

[29] Wadden TA, Foster GD, Letizia KA. One-year behavioral treatment of obesity: comparison of moderate and severe caloric restriction and the effects of weight maintenance therapy. J Consult Clin Psychol 1994;62:165–71.

[30] Klem ML, Wing RR, McGuire MT, et al. Does weight loss maintenance become easier over time? Obes Res 2000;8:438–44.

[31] American Institute of Cancer Research. AICR introduces the new american plate. Available at: http://www.aicr.org. Accessed June 20, 2002.

[32] Glickman D. Eating in the 20th century. Food Rev 2000;23:Upfront.

8

Risks of Obesity

George A. Bray

Obesity is a chronic disease in the same sense as hypertension and atherosclerosis. The cause of obesity is an imbalance between the energy ingested in food and the energy expended. The excess energy is stored in fat cells that enlarge or increase in number. This hyperplasia and hypertrophy of fat cells is the pathologic lesion of obesity. Enlarged fat cells produce the clinical problems that are associated with obesity, either because of the weight or mass of the extra fat or because of the increased secretion of free fatty acids and numerous peptides from enlarged fat cells. The consequence of these two mechanisms is other diseases, such as diabetes mellitus, gallbladder disease, osteoarthritis, heart disease, and some forms of cancer. The spectrum of medical, social, and psychological disabilities that are associated with obesity is depicted in Fig. 1.

The effects of excess weight on morbidity and mortality have been known for more than 2000 years. Hippocrates recognized that "sudden death is more common in those who are naturally fat than in the lean," and Malcolm Flemyng in 1760 observed that

corpulency, when in an extraordinary degree, may be reckoned a disease, as it in some measure obstructs the free exercise of the animal functions; and hath a tendency to shorten life, by paving the way to dangerous distempers.

The diseases that are associated with overweight are responsible for significant health care costs [1]. In this cost-conscious era, several analyses of the health costs that are related to obesity have been done around the world. Between 3% and 7% of total health care costs can be attributed to overweight. The direct cost by various disease categories for the United States is shown in Table 1 [2].

Overweight also increases the use of the health care system. In a study of health care expenditures, individuals who were at the extremes of body mass index had the highest expenditures; individuals who were in the middle of

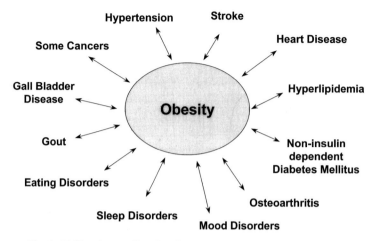

Fig. 1. BMI and mortality. Conditions that are associated with obesity.

the BMI range (26–27 kg/m^2) had the lowest probability of health care expenditures. The probability of health care expenditures increased significantly at both extremes of BMI for subjects with positive baseline expenditures, compared with subjects without baseline expenditures. BMI was associated with the annual number of inpatient days, number and cost of outpatient visits, costs of outpatient pharmacy, and laboratory and total costs in a large health maintenance organization [3]. Mean annual costs were 25% higher in participants with a BMI between 30 kg/m^2 and 35 kg/m^2, and were 44% higher in those with a BMI above 35 kg/m^2, compared with individuals with a BMI of 20 to 25 kg/m^2 [3]. Using data from the National Center for Health Statistics and the Framingham Heart Study, Thompson et al [4] estimated that the costs for lifetime treatment of hypertension, hypercholesterolemia, Type 2 diabetes, heart disease, and stroke in men and women with a BMI of 37.5 kg/m^2 was $10,000 more than for men and women

Table 1
Cost of obesity in the United States (1995)

Disease	Direct cost (in billions of dollars)
Diabetes mellitus	32.4
Coronary heart disease	7.0
Osteoarthritis	4.3
Hypertension	3.2
Gallbladder disease	2.6
Colon cancer	1.0
Breast cancer	0.84
Endometrial cancer	0.29
Total	51.63

Data from Wolf AM, Colditz GA. Current estimates of the economic cost of obesity in the United States. Obes Res 1998;6:97–106.

with a BMI of 22.5 kg/m^2. Sturm [5], in a prospective study, found that health care costs and use for obesity exceeded those of smoking in most of the variables that he examined.

Effects of overweight, body fat distribution, weight gain, and sedentary lifestyle on mortality

Excess body weight

The mortality that is associated with excess weight increases as the degree of obesity and overweight increases. One study estimated that between 280,000 and 325,000 deaths could be attributed to obesity annually in the United States [6]. More than 80% of these deaths occur among people with a BMI that is higher than 30 kg/m^2. The increase in death from obesity has been documented in a number of studies from around the world.

Nurses' Health Study

In the Nurses' Health Study, the risk of death rose progressively in women with a BMI that was higher than 29 kg/m^2 [7]. Mortality was lowest among women who weighed at least 15% less than the U.S. average for women of similar age and among women whose weight had been stable since early adulthood.

American Cancer Society's Cancer Prevention Study I

Among 62,116 white men and 262,019 white women (both groups were healthy, nonsmokers) who were followed for 14 years, a greater body mass index was associated with increased rate of death from all causes and from cardiovascular disease in both groups up to age 75 years. The impact of the excess body weight was higher among younger subjects than older ones [8].

American Cancer Society's Cancer Prevention Study II

In an even larger study (457,785 men and 588,369 women) with a 14-year follow-up, the association of BMI and mortality was affected by smoking status and the history of other disease (Fig. 2). Among the nonsmokers, the lowest mortality for men was in the group that had a BMI that was between 23.5 kg/m^2 and 24.9 kg/m^2 and for women it was in the group that had a BMI from 22.0 kg/m^2 to 23.4 kg/m^2. Among subjects with a BMI that was greater than 40 kg/m^2, the relative risk of death was 2.6 times higher for men and 2.0 times higher for women compared with those having a BMI between 23.5 kg/m^2 and 24.9 kg/m^2. Black men and women had lower risks than corresponding categories of white men and women. Among black persons with a BMI that was higher than 40 kg/m^2, the relative risk of death was 1.4 for men and 1.2 for women. There was no effect of age and the risk of death or cardiovascular disease did not significantly increase over the BMI range

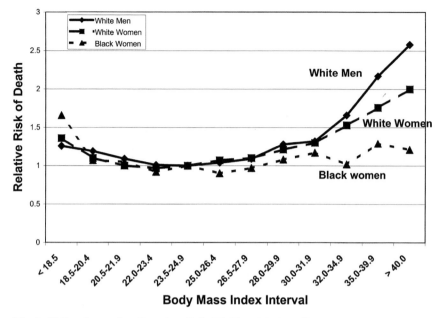

Fig. 2. BMI and mortality. (*Data from* Calle EE, Thun MJ, Petrelli JM, et al. Body-mass index and mortality in a prospective cohort of U.S. adults. N Engl J Med 1999;341:1097–1105).

of 22.0 kg/m^2 to 26.4 kg/m^2 for men and 20.5 kg/m^2 to 24.9 kg/m^2 for women [9].

Aerobics Center Longitudinal Study

In this study, 25,714 men were followed from 1 to 10 years. The all-cause mortality and cardiovascular mortality was highest in men with a BMI that was greater than 30 kg/m^2 and was lowest in those with a BMI between 18.5 kg/m^2 and 24.9 kg/m^2 [10]. In this same population, the deaths from cardiovascular disease increased from just over 5 deaths/10,000 man-years with a body fat of less than 16.7%, to nearly 8 deaths/10,000 man-years in men with a body fat of 16.7% to 25.0%, to nearly 12 deaths/10,000 man-years in men with a body fat above 25.0% [10].

Finnish Heart Study

The association between obesity and the risk of death from CHD was confirmed by a study of 8373 Finnish women (aged 30 to 59 years) who were followed for 15 years [11]. Body weight, cardiovascular risk factors, and coronary mortality were tracked these men and women in eastern Finland. This study found that for each increase in body weight of approximately 1 kg, the risk of coronary mortality increased by 1% to 1.5%. A substantial part of this risk was mediated through the link between body weight and blood pressure.

Regional fat distribution

Regional fat distribution is important in the risk of death [12–14]. The life insurance industry first noted this at the beginning of the twentieth century. This theme was picked up again after World War II, when researchers noted that obese individuals with an android or male distribution of body fat were at higher risk for diabetes and heart disease than those with a gynoid or female type of obesity. Clinical and epidemiologic work in the 1980s convinced the world of the relationship between body fat distribution and risk of excess mortality. The Framingham Study examined the relationship between fat distribution and metabolic risk factors. Three clusters could be detected with some overlap. The metabolic complex of insulin, glucose, triglycerides, and BMI was one constellation. A second cluster included cholesterol, low-density lipoprotein cholesterol, and high-density cholesterol. The final cluster was BMI, systolic blood pressure, and diastolic blood pressure [15].

Weight gain

In addition to overweight and central fatness, the amount of weight gain after age 18 to 20 also predicts mortality. This is clearly illustrated in the Nurses' Health Study and the Health Professionals Follow-up Study, in which a graded increase in mortality from heart disease is associated with increasing degrees of weight gain (Fig. 3) [16]. A weight gain of more than

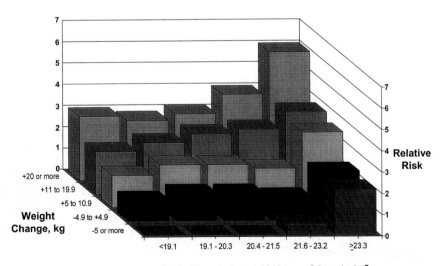

Body Mass Index at 18 Years of Age, kg/m²

Fig. 3. BMI, weight change, and coronary heart disease in women. (*From* Willett WC, Manson JE, Stampfer MJ, et al. Weight, weight change, and coronary heart disease in women. Risk within the "normal" weight range. JAMA 1995;273:461–5; with permission.)

10 kg indicates a higher level of increased risk. Weight gain in men after age 20 in the Health Professionals Follow-up Study showed a similar relationship.

Sedentary lifestyle

A sedentary lifestyle is the final important component in the relationship of excess mortality to obesity. A sedentary lifestyle increases the risk of death at all levels of BMI. Unfit men with a BMI below 25 kg/m^2 had a significantly higher risk than the men with a high level of cardiorespiratory fitness. Obese men with a high level of fitness had risks of death that were not different from the fit men of normal body fat. A similar relationship was found with waist girth. Men who were physically unfit had a significantly higher risk of death at any level of waist circumference than men who were physically fit [17].

Intentional weight loss

If overweight increases risk of mortality, then we would anticipate that intentional weight loss would reduce it. A definitive demonstration of this prediction is not available, but several studies suggested that intentional weight loss does reduce risk [18,19]. Weight loss that is maintained for 2 years following surgical treatment of obesity reduces blood pressure, improves abnormal lipid levels, and reduces the risk of diabetes [18]. Patients who were treated for obesity with gastric operations were reported to have lower rates of death (Fig. 4). A follow-up of women aged 40 to 64 in the American Cancer Society study who intentionally lost weight found a significant reduction of 20% to 25% in all-cause mortality [19].

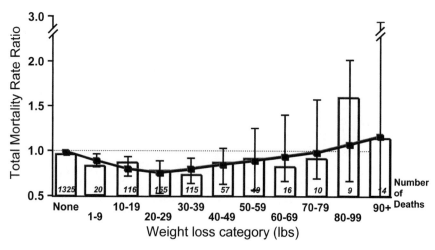

Fig. 4. Assessing intentionality in weight loss and its association with mortality. (*From* Williamson D, Thompson TJ, Thun M, et al. Intentional weight loss and mortality among overweight individuals with diabetes. Diabetes Care 2000;23:1499–1504; with permission.) [38]

Weight loss affects a number of risk factors. The data on participants in the Swedish Obesity Study show the degree of weight loss that is required to affect individual risk factors. Changes in blood pressure and triglycerides are very responsive to weight loss and decrease after a 5% to 10% weight loss. HDL cholesterol increases with a similar weight-related change. Conversely, total cholesterol is not affected until weight loss exceeds 20%. For most comorbidities, however, a 10% weight loss is sufficient to see significant improvement in risk factors [18]. Blood pressure returns to baseline by 4 to 6 years even when weight loss is maintained [20].

Recent studies buttressed the idea that losing about 5% of body weight can significantly reduce the risk of developing Type 2 diabetes in high-risk individuals. In studies from Finland [21] and the United States [22] conversion rates from impaired glucose tolerance to diabetes were reduced by 58%.

Morbidity associated with obesity and increased central fat

Overall morbidity

Fig. 5 shows the relative risks for diastolic blood pressure, BMI along with cutpoints, and hypercholesterolemia among overweight individuals. Overweight obviously affects several diseases, but is only one of several factors. Sjostrom et al [18] evaluated the 2-year incidence rate of new cases of disease in the overweight control group of the Swedish Obese Subjects Intervention Study. In this population, the incidence of new cases of hypertension was 15%, the incidence of new cases of diabetes was 7.8%, the incidence for new cases of hyperinsulinemia was 5.8%, the incidence for new cases of hypertriglyceridemia was 27.8%, and the incidence for new cases of increased HDL cholesterol was 15.9% in this follow-up of untreated patients with a BMI that averaged 38 kg/m^2.

The risk of developing diabetes, hypertension, gallbladder disease, and coronary artery disease differs by ethnic group and by gender within ethnic group. This is particularly evident when the BMI is greater than 40 kg/m^2, but is also present when the BMI is between 30 kg/m^2 and 40 kg/m^2 [23]. In white women, the risk of noninsulin-dependent diabetes mellitus was greater than the risk of hypertension, which, in turn, was greater than the risk of gallbladder disease. Although the risk of diabetes was also high in white men, the risk of gallbladder disease exceeded that of hypertension In black and Mexican-American men, the risk of hypertension was higher than that of diabetes. In black women, the risks of diabetes and gallbladder disease were higher than white women, whereas in Mexican-American women, the risks of coronary heart disease, diabetes, and gallbladder disease were similar; the odds ratio was less than in the corresponding black or white women. These ethnic and gender differences undoubtedly reflect the interaction of genetic and environmental factors.

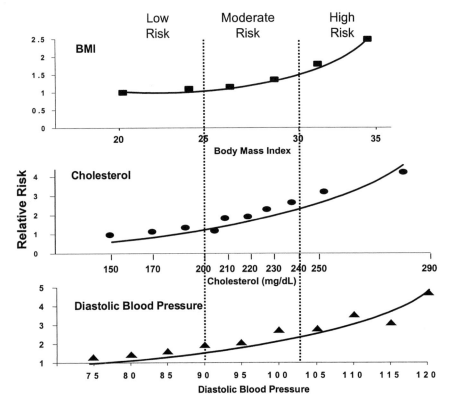

Fig. 5. Relative risk.

Finally, the number of comorbidities tracks the BMI. The prevalence of one comorbidity rises in the group with a BMI higher than 25 kg/m^2, whereas the prevalence of two comorbidities increases with BMI above 35 kg/m^2 [23].

The pathology of excess fat

Each disease whose risk is increased by overweight can be classified into one of two pathophysiologic categories. The first category is risks that result from the metabolic changes that are associated with excess fat. These include diabetes mellitus, gallbladder disease, hypertension, cardiovascular disease, and some forms of cancer. The second group of disabilities arises from the increased mass of fat itself; these include osteoarthritis, sleep apnea, and the stigma of obesity.

The fat cell can be viewed as a type of endocrine cell and adipose tissue can be viewed as an endocrine organ. The hypertrophy or hyperplasia of this organ is the pathologic lesion in obesity. After the identification of adipsin (complement D) in the fat cell, several other secretory peptides were identified. Leptin is clearly the most important, and cements the role of the adipocyte as an endocrine cell and fat as an endocrine organ. From the pathophysiologic perspective, however, the release of free fatty acids may be the most important.

Fat distribution is important in the response to the endocrine products of the fat cell. The accumulation of fat in visceral fat cells is modulated by several factors. Androgens and estrogen that are produced by the gonads and adrenals, as well as peripheral conversion of Δ^4-androstenedione to estrone in fat cells, are pivotal in body fat distribution. Male or android fat distribution, and female or gynoid fat distribution, develop during adolescence. The increasing accumulation of visceral fat in adult life is related to gender, but the effects of cortisol, decreasing growth hormone, and changing testosterone levels are important in age-related fat accumulation. Increased visceral fat enhances the degree of insulin resistance that is associated with obesity and hyperinsulinemia. Together, hyperinsulinemia and insulin resistance enhance the risk of the comorbidities that are described below.

Diseases associated with hypersecretion from enlarged fat cells

Diabetes mellitus, insulin resistance, and the metabolic syndrome

Type 2 diabetes mellitus is strongly associated with overweight in both genders in all ethnic groups [24,25]. The risk of Type 2 diabetes mellitus increases with the degree and duration of overweight, and with a more central distribution of body fat. The relationship between increasing BMI and the risk of diabetes in the Nurses Health Study is shown in Fig. 6 [26]. The risk of diabetes was lowest in individuals with a BMI that was less than 22 kg/m². As BMI increased, the relative risk increased; at a BMI of 35 kg/m², the relative risk of developing Type 2 diabetes mellitus increased 40-fold, or 4000%. A similar, strong curvilinear relationship was observed in men in the Health Professionals Follow-up Study. The lowest risk in men was associated with a BMI that was less than 23 kg/m², and slightly lower for the women in the Nurses Health Study. With a BMI that was greater than 35 kg/m², the age-adjusted relative risk for diabetes in men increased to 60.9, or more than 6000%.

Weight gain also increases the risk of diabetes. Up to 65% of the cases of Type 2 diabetes mellitus can be attributed to overweight. Of the 11.7 million cases of diabetes, overweight may account for two thirds of diabetic deaths. Using the BMI at age 18, a 20-kg weight gain increased the risk for diabetes 15-fold, whereas a weight reduction of 20 kg reduced the risk to almost zero. In the Health Professionals Follow-up Study, weight gain was also associated with an increasing risk of NIDDM, whereas a 3-kg weight loss was associated with a reduction in relative risk.

Weight gain seems to precede the onset of diabetes. Among the Pima Indians, body weight steadily and slowly increased by 30 kg (from 60 kg to

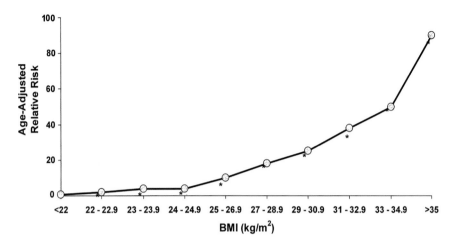

*p < 0.05

Fig. 6. BMI and risk of noninsulin-dependent diabetes mellitus (NIDDM). (*From* Colditz GA, Willett WC, Rotnitzky A, et al. Weight gain as a risk factor for clinical diabetes mellitus in women. Ann Intern Med 1995;122:481–6; with permission.)

90 kg) in the years preceding the diagnosis of diabetes [25]. After the diagnosis of diabetes, body weight decreased slightly. In the Health Professionals Follow-up Study, the relative risk of developing diabetes increased with weight gain, as well as with increased BMI. In long-term follow-up studies, the duration of overweight and the change in plasma glucose during an oral glucose tolerance test were strongly related. When overweight was present for less than 10 years, plasma glucose was not increased. With longer durations, of up to 45 years, a nearly linear increase in plasma glucose occurred after an oral glucose tolerance test. The risk of diabetes is increased in hypertensive individuals who are treated with diuretics or β-blocking drugs; this risk was increased in the overweight.

In the Swedish Obese Subjects Study, Sjostrom et al [18] observed that diabetes was present in 13% to 16% of obese subjects at baseline. Of those who underwent gastric bypass and subsequently lost weight, 69% who initially had diabetes went into remission; only 0.5% of those who did not have diabetes at baseline developed it during the 2 years of follow-up. In contrast, in the obese control group that lost no weight, the remission rate for diabetes was low (16%) and the incidence of new cases of diabetes was 7.8%.

Weight loss or moderating weight gain over years reduces the risk of developing diabetes. This was most clearly shown in the Health Professionals Follow-up Study, in which relative risk declined by nearly 50% with a weight loss of 5 to 11 kg. Type 2 diabetes was almost nonexistent with a weight loss of more than 20 kg or with a BMI that was less than 20 kg/m^2 [23].

Table 2
Clinical features of the metabolic syndrome

Risk factor	Defining level
Abdominal obesity (waist circumference)	
Men	>102 cm (>40 in)
Women	>88 cm (>35 in)
HDL-cholesterol	
Men	<40 mg/dL
Women	<50 mg/dL
Triglycerides	≥150 mg/dL
Fasting glucose	≥110 mg/dL
Blood pressure (SBP/DBP)	≥130/≥85 mmHg

A pathophysiologic model for diabetes is shown in Fig. 7. Increased insulin secretion and insulin resistance result from obesity. The relationship of insulin secretion to BMI has already been noted. A greater BMI correlates with greater insulin secretion. Obesity develops in more than 50% of nonhuman primates as they age. Nearly half of these obese animals subsequently develop diabetes. The time course for the development of obesity in nonhuman primates, as in the Pima Indians, is spread over several years. After the animals gain weight, the next demonstrable effects are impaired glucose removal and increased insulin resistance as measured by impaired glucose clearance with a euglycemic hyperinsulinemic clamp. The hyperinsulinemia, in turn, increases hepatic VLDL triglyceride synthesis and secretion, increases plasminogen activator inhibitor-1 (PAI-1) synthesis, increases sympathetic nervous system activity, and increases renal sodium reabsorption.

Insulin resistance is the hallmark of the metabolic (or dysmetabolic) syndrome. The National Cholesterol Education Program Adult Treatment Panel III recently provided defining values for this syndrome (Table 2). When three of the five criteria that are listed in the table are abnormal, then the patient has the metabolic syndrome. A central feature of this syndrome is increased visceral fat. As noted in Fig. 7 and several later figures, this increased release of free fatty acids impairs insulin clearance by the liver and alters peripheral metabolism. The reduced production of adiponectin by the fat cell is another potential player in the development of insulin resistance.

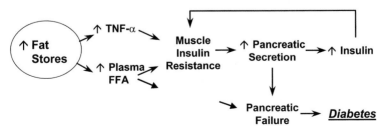

Fig. 7. Obesity and diabetes. Model of type 2 diabetes.

Gallbladder disease

Cholelithiasis is the primary hepatobiliary pathology that is associated with overweight [27]. The old clinical adage "fat, female, fertile, and forty" describes the epidemiologic factors that often are associated with the development of gallbladder disease. This is demonstrated in the Nurses' Health Study [28]. When BMI was less than 24 kg/m², the incidence of clinically symptomatic gallstones was approximately 250 per 100,000 person-years of follow-up. The incidence gradually increased with increased BMI (to 30 kg/m²) and increased very steeply when BMI exceeded 30 kg/m². This confirmed work that was published by many other researchers [27].

Part of the explanation for the increased risk of gallstones is the increased cholesterol turnover that is related to total body fat [27]. Cholesterol production is linearly related to body fat; approximately 20 mg of additional cholesterol is synthesized for each kilogram of extra body fat. Thus, a 10-kg increase in body fat leads to the daily synthesis of the amount of cholesterol that is contained in the yolk of one egg. The increased cholesterol, is, in turn, excreted in the bile. High cholesterol concentrations relative to bile acids and phospholipids in bile increase the likelihood of precipitation of cholesterol gallstones in the gallbladder. Additional factors, such as nidation conditions, are also involved in the formation of gallstones [27].

During weight loss, the likelihood of gallstones increases because the flux of cholesterol is increased through the biliary system. Diets with moderate levels of fat that trigger gallbladder contraction, and thus empty its cholesterol content, may reduce this risk. Similarly, the use of bile acids, such as ursodeoxycholic acid, may be advisable if the risk of gallstone formation is believed to be increased.

The second GI feature that is altered in obesity is the quantity of fat in the liver [27]. Increased steatosis is characteristic of the livers of overweight people and may reflect increased VLDL production that is associated with hyperinsulinemia. The accumulation of lipid in the liver suggests that the secretion of VLDL in response to hyperinsulinemia is inadequate to keep up with the high rate of triglyceride turnover.

Hypertension

Blood pressure is often increased in overweight individuals (Fig. 8) [29]. In the Swedish Obesity Study, hypertension was present at baseline in 44% to 51% of subjects. One estimate suggested that control of overweight would eliminate 48% of the hypertension in whites and 28% of the hypertension in blacks. For each decline of 1 mm Hg in diastolic blood pressure, the risk of myocardial infarction decreases an estimated 2% to 3% [29].

Overweight and hypertension interact with cardiac function. Hypertension in normal-weight people produces concentric hypertrophy of the heart with thickening of the ventricular walls. In overweight individuals, eccentric

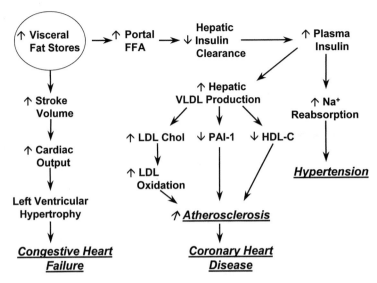

Fig. 8. Obesity and heart disease.

dilatation occurs. Increased preload and stroke work are associated with hypertension. The combination of overweight and hypertension leads to thickening of the ventricular wall and larger heart volume, and thus to a greater likelihood of cardiac failure.

The hypertension of overweight people seems to be strongly related to altered sympathetic activity (Fig. 8). During insulin infusion, overweight subjects have a much greater increase in the muscle sympathetic nerve firing rate than normal-weight subjects, but the altered activity is associated with a lesser change in the vascular resistance of calf muscles.

Hypertension is associated with Type 2 diabetes, impaired glucose tolerance, hypertriglyceridemia, and hypercholesterolemia. Hyperinsulinemia in overweight and hypertensive patients suggests insulin resistance and the metabolic syndrome. An analysis of the factors that predict blood pressure and changes in peripheral vascular resistance in response to body weight gain showed that a key determinant of the weight-induced increases in blood pressure was a disproportionate increase in cardiac output that could not be fully accounted for by the hemodynamic contribution of new tissue. This hemodynamic change may be attributable to a disproportionate increase in cardiac output that is related to an increase in sympathetic activity.

Heart disease

Data from the Nurses' Health Study indicate that the risk for women in the United States to develop coronary artery disease is increased 3.3-fold with a BMI that is greater than 29 kg/m^2, compared with women who have a BMI that is less than 21 kg/m^2 [7]. A BMI of 27 kg/m^2 to less than

$29\,\mathrm{kg/m^2}$ increases the relative risk to 1.8. Weight gain also strongly affects this risk at any initial BMI [15]. That is, at all levels of initial BMI, weight gain was associated with a graded increase in risk of heart disease. This was particularly evident in the highest quintile, in which weight gain was more than 20 kg.

Dyslipidemia may be important in the relationship of BMI to increased risk of heart disease [12]. A positive correlation between BMI and tri-glyceride has been demonstrated repeatedly. The inverse relationship be-tween HDL cholesterol and BMI, however, may be even more important because a low HDL cholesterol carries a greater relative risk than elevated triglycerides. Central fat distribution is also important in lipid abnormal-ities. Waist circumference alone accounted for, as much as, or more of the variance in triglycerides and HDL cholesterol as waist circumference divided by hip circumference (WHR) or sagittal diameter, two other measures of central fat. A positive correlation for central fat and triglyceride and the inverse relationship for HDL cholesterol is evident for all measures.

Increased body weight is associated with several cardiovascular abnor-malities [30]. Cardiac weight increases with increasing body weight which suggests increased cardiac work. Heart weight as a percentage of body weight, however, is lower than in a normal-weight control group. The in-creased cardiac work that is associated with overweight may produce cardiomyopathy and heart failure in the absence of diabetes, hypertension, or atherosclerosis. Weight loss decreases heart weight; this decrease was linearly related to the degree of weight loss in men and women. An echocardiographic study of left ventricular midwall function showed that obese individuals compensated by using cardiac reserve, especially in the presence of hypertension. Heart rate was well within normal limits. A pathophysiologic diagram for the observed changes is shown in Fig. 9.

Portal fatty acids increase insulin, which increases hepatic triglyceride production. This, and the changes in fat cell size, changes cholesterol production, as well as the rate of PAI-1 production. The net effects are re-flected in the increased risk of atherosclerosis. The second effect of en-largement of fat cells is an increased capillary bed and blood flow. This can lead to congestive heart failure. A third component may be inflammation range. C-reactive protein (CRP), an index of inflammation, is increased in patients with obesity and atherosclerosis.

Central fat distribution is associated with small dense low-density lipoproteins as opposed to large fluffy LDL particles [12]. For a similar level of cholesterol, the risk of coronary heart disease is significantly higher in individuals with small dense LDL. Because each LDL particle has a single molecule of apo B protein, the concentration of apo B can be used to estimate the number of LDL particles. Despres et al [12] demonstrated that the level of apo B is a strong predictor of the risk for CHD. Based on a study of French Canadians, these researchers proposed that estimating apo B, the levels of fasting insulin, the concentration of triglyceride, the concentration of HDL cholesterol, and waist circumference could help identify individ-

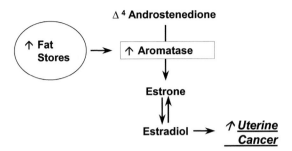

Fig. 9. Obesity and uterine cancer.

uals who are at high risk for the metabolic syndrome and coronary heart disease.

Cancer

Certain forms of cancer are significantly increased in overweight individuals [7,31]. Males face increased risk for neoplasms of the colon, rectum, and prostate. In women, cancers of the reproductive system and gallbladder are more common. One explanation for the increased risk of endometrial cancer in overweight, postmenopausal women is the increased production of estrogens by adipose tissue stromal cells (Fig. 9). This increased production is related to the degree of excess body fat that accounts for a major source of estrogen production in post-menopausal women. Breast cancer is not only related to total body fat, but also may have a more important relationship to central body fat [32]. The increased visceral fat measured by computed tomography shows an important relationship to the risk of breast cancer.

Endocrine changes

A variety of endocrine changes are associated with overweight (Box 1). The changes in the reproductive system are among the most important. Irregular menses and frequent anovular cycles are common, and the rate of fertility may be reduced. Some reports described increased risks of toxemia. Hypertension and cesarean section may also be more frequent in overweight [33].

Diseases associated with increased fat mass

Bones, joints, muscles, connective tissue, and skin

Osteoarthritis is significantly increased in overweight individuals. The osteoarthritis that develops in the knees and ankles may be directly related to the trauma that is associated with the degree of excess body weight [34]. The increased osteoarthritis in other, nonweight-bearing joints suggests that some components of the overweight syndrome alter cartilage and bone

**Box 1. Common hormonal abnormalities
that are associated with obesity**

Increased cortisol production
Insulin resistance
Decreased sex hormone-binding globulin in women
Decreased progesterone levels in women
Decreased testosterone levels in men
Decreased growth hormone production

metabolism, independent of weight bearing. Increased osteoarthritis accounts for a significant component of the cost of overweight.

Several skin changes are associated with excess weight. Stretch marks, or striae, are common and reflect the pressures on the skin from expanding lobular deposits of fat. Acanthosis nigricans, with deepening pigmentation in the folds of the neck, knuckles, and extensor surfaces occurs in many overweight individuals, but is not associated with increased risk of malignancy. Hirsutism in women may reflect the altered reproductive status in these individuals.

Sleep apnea

Alterations in pulmonary function have been described in overweight subjects, but subjects were free of other potential chronic pulmonary diseases in only a few studies. When underlying pulmonary disease was absent, only major degrees of increased body weight significantly affected

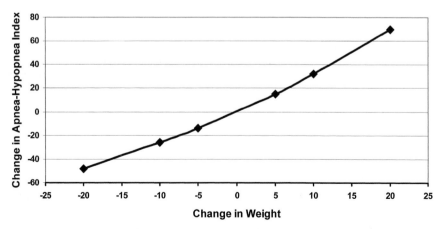

Fig. 10. Model of sleep apnea and body weight change. (*From* Peppard, Young T, Palta M, et al. Longitudinal study of moderate weight change and sleep-disordered breathing. JAMA 2000;284(23):3015–21; with permission.)

pulmonary function. The chief effect is a decrease in residual lung volume that is associated with increased abdominal pressure on the diaphragm [35]. Fat distribution, independent of total fat, also influenced ventilatory capacity in men, possibly through effects of visceral fat level.

In contrast to the relatively benign effects of excess weight on respiratory function, the sleep apnea associated with overweight can be severe [34]. A pathophysiologic sequence is presented in Fig. 10 [36]. Overweight subjects with obstructive sleep apnea showed several significant differences from overweight subjects without sleep apnea. Sleep apnea was considerably more common in men than women and, as a group, subjects were significantly taller than individuals without sleep apnea. People with sleep apnea have an increased snoring index and increased maximal nocturnal sound intensity. Nocturnal oxygen saturation also was significantly reduced. One interesting hypothesis is that the increased neck circumference and fat deposits in the pharyngeal area may lead to the obstructive sleep apnea of obesity.

Psychosocial function

Overweight is stigmatized [37], that is, overweight individuals are exposed to the consequences of public disapproval of their fatness. This stigma occurs in education, employment, health care, and elsewhere. Psychosocial consequences are revealed by examining the education, marital status, and income level in adolescents who were overweight into adult life. These effects were more evident in females than in males.

References

[1] Colditz, GA. Economic costs of obesity and inactivity. Med Sci Sports Exerc 1999; 31(11 Suppl):S663–7.

[2] Wolf AM, Colditz GA. Current estimates of the economic cost of obesity in the United States. Obes Res 1998;6:97–106.

[3] Quesenbery CP Jr. Caan B, Jacobson A. Obesity, health services use, and health care costs among members of a health maintenance organization. Arch Intern Med 1998;158: 466–72.

[4] Thompson D, Edelsberg J, Colditz GA, et al. Lifetime health and economic consequences of obesity. Arch Int Med 1999;159:2177–83.

[5] Sturm R. The effects of obesity, smoking, and drinking on medical problems and costs. Obesity outranks both smoking and drinking in its deleterious effects on health and health costs. Health Aff 2002;21:245–53.

[6] Allison DB, Fontaine KR, Manson JE, et al. Annual deaths attributable to obesity in the United States. JAMA 1999;282:1530–8.

[7] Manson JE, Willett WC, Stampfer MJ, et al. Body weight and mortality among women. N Engl J Med 1995;333:677–85.

[8] Stevens J, Cai J, Pamuk ER, et al. The effect of age on the association between body-mass index and mortality. N Engl J Med 1998;338:1–7.

[9] Calle EE, Thun MJ, Petrelli JM, et al. Body-mass index and mortality in a prospective cohort of US adults. N Engl J Med 1999;341:1097–105.

[10] Wei M, Kampert JB, Barlow CE, et al. Relationship between low cardiorespiratory fitness and mortality in normal-weight, overweight, and obese men. JAMA 1999; 282:1547–53.

[11] Jousilahti P, Tuomilehto J, Vartiainen E, et al. Body weight, cardiovascular risk factors, and coronary mortality. 15 year follow-up of middle-aged men and women in eastern Finland. Circulation 1996;93:1372–9.

[12] Despres JP, Krauss RM. Obesity and lipoprotein metabolism. In: Bray GA, Bouchard C, James WP, editors. Handbook of obesity. New York: Marcel Dekker; 2003.

[13] Kissebah AH, Krakower GR. Regional adiposity and morbidity. Physiol Rev 1994; 74:761–811.

[14] Lapidus L, Bengtsson C, Larsson B, et al. Distribution of adipose tissue and risk of cardiovascular disease and death: a 12 year follow up of participants in the population study of women in Gothenburg, Sweden. Br Med J (Clin Res Ed) 1984;289:1257–61.

[15] Meigs JB, D'Agostino RB Sr, Wilson PW, et al. Risk variable clustering in the insulin resistance syndrome. The Framingham Offspring Study. Diabetes 1997;46:1594–600.

[16] Willett WC, Manson JE, Stampfer MJ, et al. Weight, weight change, and coronary heart disease in women. Risk within the 'normal' weight range. JAMA 1995;273:461–5.

[17] Lee CD, Blair SN, Jackson AS. Cardiorespiratory fitness, body composition, and all-cause and cardiovascular disease mortality in men. Am J Clin Nutr 1999;69:373–80.

[18] Sjostrom CD, Lissner L, Sjostrom L. Relationships between changes in body composition and changes in cardiovascular risk factors: the SOS Intervention Study. Obes Res 1997;5:519–30.

[19] Williamson DF, Pamuk E, Thun M, et al. Prospective study of intentional weight loss and mortality in never-smoking overweight US white women aged 40–64 years. Am J Epidemiol 1995;141:1128–41.

[20] Sjostrom CD, Peltonen M, Wedel H, et al. Differentiated long-term effects of intentional weight loss on diabetes and hypertension. Hypertension 2000;36:20–5.

[21] Tuomilehto J, Lindstrom J, Eriksson JG, et al. Prevention of type 2 diabetes mellitus by changes in lifestyle among subjects with impaired glucose tolerance. N Engl J Med 2001;344:1343–50.

[22] Diabetes Prevention Program Research Group. Reduction in the incidence of type 2 diabetes with lifestyle intervention or metformin. N Engl J Med 2002;346:393–403.

[23] Must A, Spadano J, Coakley EH, et al. The disease burden associated with overweight and obesity. JAMA 1999;282:1523–9.

[24] Albu J, Pi-Sunyer FX. Obesity and diabetes. In: Bray GA, Bouchard C, James WP, editors. Handbook of obesity. New York: Marcel Dekker; 2003.

[25] Ravussin E. Energy metabolism in obesity. Studies in the Pima Indians. Diabetes Care 1993;16:232–8.

[26] Colditz GA, Willett WC, Rotnitzky A, et al. Weight gain as a risk factor for clinical diabetes mellitus in women. Ann Intern Med 1995;122:481–6.

[27] Ko CW, Lee SP. Obesity and gallbladder disease. In: Bray GA, Bouchard C, James WP, editors. Handbook of obesity. New York: Marcel Dekker; 2003.

[28] Stampfer MJ, Maclure KM, Colditz GA, et al. Risk of symptomatic gallstones in women with severe obesity. Am J Clin Nutr 1992;55:652–8.

[29] Rocchini AP. Obesity and blood pressure regulation. In: Bray GA, Bouchard C, James WP, editors. Handbook of obesity. New York: Marcel Dekker; 2003.

[30] Alpert MA, Hashimi MW. Obesity and the heart. Am J Med Sci 1993;306:117–23.

[31] Lew EA. Mortality and weight: insured lives and the American Cancer Society studies. Ann Intern Med 1985;103:1024–9.

[32] Schapira DV, Clark RA, Wolff PA, et al. Visceral obesity and breast cancer risk. Cancer 1994;74:632–9.

[33] Baeten JM, Bukusi EA, Lambe M. Pregnancy complications and outcomes among overweight and obese nulliparous women. Am J Public Health 2001;91(3):436–40.

[34] Felson DT, Anderson JJ, Naimark A, et al. Obesity and knee osteoarthritis. The Framingham Study. Ann Intern Med 1988;109:18–24.

[35] Strohl KP, Strobel RJ, Parisi RA. Obesity and pulmonary function. In: Bray GA, Bouchard C, James WP, editors. Handbook of obesity. New York: Marcel Dekker; 1997. p. 725–39.

[36] Gortmaker SL, Must A, Perrin JM, et al. Social and economic consequences of overweight in adolescence and young adulthood. N Engl J Med 1993;329:1008–12.

[37] Peppard PE, Young T, Palta M, et al. Longitudinal study of moderate weight change and sleep-disordered breathing. JAMA 2000;284(23):3015–21.

[38] Williamson DF, Thompson TJ, Thun M, et al. Intentional weight loss and mortality among overweight individuals with diabetes. Diabetes Care 2000;23:1499–504.

9

The Office Approach to the Obese Patient

Robert F. Kushner

With nearly 60% of US adults and 13% of children and adolescents currently categorized as overweight or obese, this condition represents one of the most common chronic medical problems seen by the primary care physician [1]. And because obesity is associated with an increased risk of multiple health problems, these patients are also more likely to present with silent diseases, such as hypertension, type 2 diabetes, or dyslipidemia, or with a variety of complaints requiring further medical attention. It is important for physicians to routinely identify, evaluate, and treat patients for obesity in the course of daily practice. In actuality, however, less than half of obese adults report being advised to lose weight by health care professionals [2–6]. Failure of health care providers to initiate or to intensify therapy when indicated has recently been called *clinical inertia* by Phillips et al [7]. The low rate of identification and treatment of obesity is believed to be due to several factors, including inadequate reimbursement, limited time during office visits, competing demands, lack of training in counseling, and low confidence in the ability to treat and change behaviors. These barriers are similar to the provision of several other preventive care services, such as smoking cessation and counseling on domestic violence. Physicians cannot rely on intuition, convenience, and habit to address obesity. Successful treatment requires systematic organization of office-based processes and functions along with training in patient counseling. Put Prevention into Practice (PPIP), a national campaign by the Agency for Health Care Policy and Research to improve the delivery of clinical preventive services such as counseling for health behavior change, provides a useful framework for analyzing the office systems designed to deliver patient care [8]. The office audit (Table 1), adapted from PPIP, can be used for assessing current obesity care. It is recommended that the audit be completed before reading this chapter because it will serve to highlight

Table 1
Office audit for delivery of office-based obesity care

Do you routinely assess and evaluate patients for overweight and obesity?
What kinds of services or programs do you routinely provide to your overweight patients,
  for example, dietary and exercise counseling, group support, referral to a registered
  dietitian, use of anti-obesity medications?
Are the services or programs recorded in the patient's chart?
What policies and procedures do you have in place for providing obesity care, for example,
  all patients have a height, weight, and BMI measured and recorded in the chart,
  the patient's readiness is assessed before initiating treatment, weight-loss goals are
  established and tracked in the progress notes?
What forms, patient handouts, and educational materials are you using?
How does your office environment support or inhibit delivery of obesity care, for example,
  sturdy armless chairs, large and thigh blood pressure cuffs, large gowns, measuring
  of body weight in a private setting, a sensitive and informed office staff?
What functions do staff currently serve in the provision of obesity care, for example,
  office nurse obtains weight, height, and BMI; physician's assistant reviews food and
  activity diaries and medication side effects; receptionist schedules referral appointments
  with dietitian and clinical psychologist?
What can you do differently?

Adapted from "10 Steps: Implementation Guide. Put Prevention into Practice" In: The
clinicians' handbook of preventive services. 2nd edition. Publication no. 98-0025. Rockville
(MD): Agency for Healthcare Research and Quality; 1998. Available at: http://www.ahrq.
gov/ppip/impsteps.htm.

current strengths and deficiencies in the office and help focus on targeted information needed to improve obesity care.

Put Prevention into Practice identifies key components that can either expedite or hinder the care of patients in the office. They include organizational commitment, clinicians' attitudes, staff support, establishing policies and protocols, using simple office tools, and delegating tasks among others. Although currently there are only limited evidence-based interventions shown to specifically improve health professionals' management of obesity [9,10], this chapter reviews the office-based systems that should be considered when caring for the obese patient (Table 2). Jaen et al [11] conceptualize the office-based delivery of care as an interaction among the patient, the clinician, and the practice environment (Fig. 1). This integrative model provides a useful framework to address the issues and concerns involved in obesity care.

The practice environment

Accessibility to the office is critical for the obese patient. Facility limitations include difficult access from the parking lot or stairs, narrow doors and hallways, and cramped restrooms. These problems are the same ones that face other patients with disabilities and are covered under the regulations of the Americans with Disabilities Act of 1990. The National Association to Advance Fat Acceptance, an advocate group for overweight

Table 2
Office-based obesity care

The physical environment
 Accessibility and comfort: Stairs, doorways, hallways, restrooms, waiting room chairs
 and space; magazines and pictures
Equipment
 Large adult and thigh blood pressure cuffs, large gowns, step stools, weight and
 height scales, tape measure
Materials
 Educational and behavior-promoting brochures; pamphlets and handouts on BMI,
 obesity-associated diseases, diet, exercise, medications, and surgery
Tools
 Pre-visit questionnaires, BMI chart stamps, body weight flow sheets, food and
 activity diaries, pedometers
Protocols
 Patient care treatment protocols for return-visit schedule and medications; referrals to
 dietitians, exercise specialists, psychologists, and commercial programs
Staffing
 Team approach to include office nurse, physician assistant, nurse practitioner,
 health advocate or educator

persons, provides useful guidelines for health care providers in dealing with obese patients [12]. Recommendations for the waiting room include having several sturdy armless chairs with at least 6 to 8 inches of space between them, and firm high sofas if possible. Although often thought insignificant, hanging artwork and having magazines in the waiting and examination rooms can convey misinterpreted messages to patients. Magazines, newspapers, television, movies, and billboards constantly remind overweight

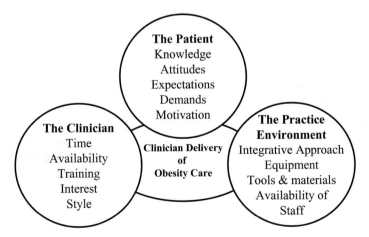

Fig. 1. Conceptualization of office-based delivery of obesity care. Interrelated factors involving the patient, the physician, and the practice environment determine overall effectiveness. (Reprinted with permission from Jaen CR, Stange KC, Nutting PA. Competing demands of primary care: a model for the delivery of clinical preventive services. J Fam Pract 1994;38:166–71; Dowden Health Media.)

individuals of society's beauty ideals. Magazines, newsletters, and artwork can be chosen that do not contribute to these unattainable images.

Equipment

Measurement of an accurate height and weight is paramount to treating patients with obesity. All too often, the physician's office has a scale that does not measure more than 350 pounds, or the foot platform is too narrow to securely balance the overweight individual. Although a wall-mounted sliding statiometer is the most accurate instrument, a firm height meter attached to the scale will suffice. The weight scale preferably should have a wide base with a nearby handle bar for support if necessary. Depending on the patient population, it is reasonable to select a scale that measures in excess of 350 pounds. To protect privacy, consider placing the scale in a private area of the office to avoid unnecessary embarrassment.

Examination rooms should have large gowns available to wear and a sturdy step stool to mount the examination tables. In addition to the standard adult size, each room should be equipped with large adult and thigh blood pressure cuffs for measurement of blood pressure. A bladder cuff that is not the appropriate width for the patient's arm circumference will cause a systematic error in blood pressure measurement; if the bladder is too narrow, the pressure will be overestimated and lead to a false diagnosis of hypertension. To avoid errors, the bladder width should be 40% of the circumference of the upper arm at the midpoint, and the length of the bladder should be 80% of the circumference of the arm [13]. A large adult cuff (16 cm wide) should be chosen for patients with mild to moderate obesity (or arm circumference 14–17 inches), whereas a thigh cuff (20 cm wide) will need to be used for patients whose arm circumferences are greater than 17 inches. Lastly, a cloth or metal tape should be available for measurement of waist circumference, as per the National Heart, Lung, and Blood Institute Practical Guide for obesity classification [14].

Tools, protocols, and procedures

A significant portion of the time spent in the evaluation and treatment of the obese patient can be expedited by the use of tools, protocols, and procedures. Tools assist in patient risk assessment, prompting and tracking of counseling and referral, and education [15]. Perhaps the most commonly used tool is a questionnaire. A self-administered medical history questionnaire can be either mailed to the patient before the initial visit or completed in the waiting room. At the Wellness Institute at Northwestern Memorial Hospital, the initial six-page questionnaire is posted on the center's Internet Web site for easy accessibility [16]. In addition to standard questions, sections of the form could inquire about past obesity treatment programs, a body weight history, current diet and physical activity levels, social support, and goals and expectations. The review-of-systems section can include medical prompts that are more commonly seen among the obese, such as snoring, morning headaches, daytime sleepiness (for obstructive sleep apnea); urinary incontinence; skin fold infections; sexual dysfunction; and symptoms of binge-eating disorder, among others.

Periodic measurement of height and weight along with recording of the body mass index (BMI) is recommended by the US Preventive Services Task Force [17], the National Institutes of Health [14], the American Heart Association [18], the American Academy of Family Physicians [19], the American College of Preventive Medicine [20], the American Medical Association [21], and the American Dietetic Association [22]. Despite the uniformity of these recommendations, the single best strategy to ensure ongoing performance of the measurements is not certain. One approach is to have a laminated BMI table immediately adjacent to the height and weight scale for easy determination and documentation of BMI in the patient's chart. Tables are available free from several Internet sites and pharmaceutical companies. Identifying BMI as a fifth vital sign also may increase physician awareness and prompt counseling. This method was used successfully in a recent study in which a smoking-status stamp was placed on the patient chart, alongside blood pressure, pulse, temperature, and respiratory rate [23]. A 1998 public education campaign by the American College of Physicians called "High BMI Spells Risk" fostered a similar heightened awareness. Use of prompts, alerts, or other reminders has been shown to significantly increase physician performance of other health maintenance activities as well [24,25]. Once the patient is identified as overweight or obese, printed education tools, such as brochures and pamphlets, can be provided. Food and activity diaries and patient information sheets on a variety of topics, such as the food guide pyramid, deciphering food labels, healthy snacking, dietary fiber, aerobic exercise and resistance training, and dealing with stress can be used to support behavior change and facilitate patient education. Ready-to-copy materials can be obtained from a variety of sources free of charge, such as those found in the Practical Guide [14], or for a minimal fee from other public sites and commercial companies. Additional Internet resources for the patient are listed in the Appendix at the end of this chapter.

Based on the health promotion literature, use of written materials and counseling protocols should lead to more effective and efficient obesity care. In a study of community-based family medicine physicians, Kreuter et al [26] showed that patients are more likely to reduce smoking, increase physical activity, and limit dairy fat consumption when physician advice is supported by health education materials. In another randomized intervention study by Swinburn et al [27], a written goal-oriented exercise prescription, in addition to verbal advice, was more effective than verbal advice alone in increasing the physical activity level of sedentary individuals over a 6-week period. Several exercise assessment and counseling protocols have been developed that can be incorporated easily into obesity care. These protocols include Project PACE (Provider-based Assessment and Counseling for Exercise) [28], ACT (The Activity Counseling Trial) [29], and STEP (The Step Test Exercise Prescription) [30]. Protocols and procedures for various treatment pathways can be established for obtaining periodic laboratory monitoring and referral to allied health professionals, such as registered dietitians, exercise specialists, and clinical psychologists. The Practical Guide provides a treatment algorithm called "A Quick Reference Tool to ACT," an acronym standing for *a*ssessment, *c*lassification, and *t*reatment. Other treatment algorithms have been developed by the American Medical Association [21] and the American Pharmaceutical Association [31]. The treatment algorithm from the National, Heart, Lung, and Blood Institute's "Clinical guidelines on the identification, evaluation, and treatment of overweight and obesity in adults"[32] is shown in Fig. 2.

Using an integrated team approach

How practices operate on a day-to-day basis is extremely important for the provision of effective obesity care. Establishing an integrative team approach is one such strategy [24,33,34]. Teamwork entails coordination and delegation of tasks among providers and staff [15]. Starfield [35] defines a *patient care team* as "a group of diverse clinicians who communicate with each other regularly about the care of a defined group of patients and participate in that care." Such teams ensure that key elements of care that doctors may not have the training or time to do well are performed competently [36]. Other personnel are often better qualified to deliver the dietary, physical activity, and behavioral counseling. Accordingly, there is an opportunity for other office staff to play a greater role in the care of obese patients. A sense of "groupness," defined as the degree to which the group practice identifies itself and functions as a team, will enhance the quality and efficiency of care [37].

The optimal team composition and management structure varies among practices; however, as an example of an integrative model, receptionists can provide useful information about the program, including general philosophy, staffing, fee schedules, and other written materials; registered nurses can obtain vital measurements, including height and weight (for BMI), waist circumference, instruction on and review of food and activity journals, and other educational materials; and physician assistants can monitor the progress of treatment and assume many of the other responsibilities of care. A new position of health advocate, whose role is to serve as a resource to the physician and to patients by providing additional information and assisting in arranging recommended follow-up, may be particularly useful [38]. Regardless of how the work load is delegated, the power of the physician's voice should not be underestimated. The physician should be perceived as the team leader and the source of common philosophy of care [39]. According to Crabtree et al [37], the keys to success include physician commitment and a supportive organizational structure.

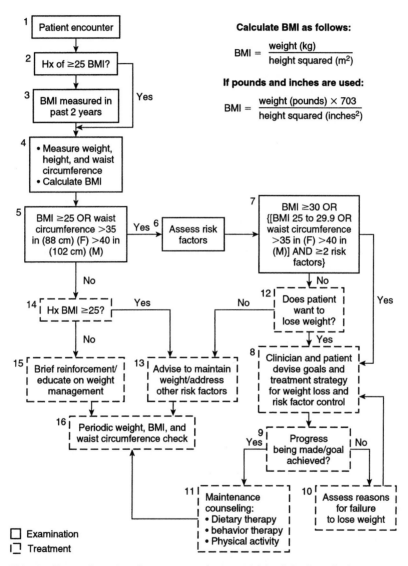

Calculate BMI as follows:

$$BMI = \frac{weight\ (kg)}{height\ squared\ (m^2)}$$

If pounds and inches are used:

$$BMI = \frac{weight\ (pounds) \times 703}{height\ squared\ (inches^2)}$$

This algorithm applies only to the assessment for overweight and obesity and subsequent decisions based on that assessment. It does not reflect any initial overall assessment for other cardiovascular risk factors that are indicated.

Fig. 2. Treatment algorithm for obesity. Ht = height; Hx = history; Wt = weight. (*From* the Expert Panel. Clinical guidelines on the identification, evaluation, and treatment of overweight and obesity in adults: the evidence report. National, Heart, Lung, and Blood Institute, Public Health Service, US Department of Health and Human Services; 1998.)

The patient-physician encounter

Although all of the office-based systems reviewed in the preceding paragraphs are important, the cornerstone of effective treatment for obesity is grounded in skillful and empathetic physician-patient communication. This vital interaction is affirmed by Balint's assertion that "the most frequently used drug in medical practice is the doctor himself" [40]. From the patient's perspective, a caring physician is compassionate, supportive, trustworthy, open-minded, and nonjudgmental. He or she takes into account the patient's needs, values, beliefs, goals, personality traits, and fears [41]. In a review of the literature, Stewart [42] found that the quality of communication between the physician and patient directly influenced patient health outcomes. A large body of literature has described key elements of communication that foster behavior change. Because the primary aim of obesity counseling is to influence what the patient does *outside* of the office, the time spent in the office needs to be structured and effective.

Effective counseling begins with establishing rapport and soliciting the patient's agenda. Attentively listening to the patient to understand his or her goals and expectations is the first essential step. Asking the patient, "How do you hope that I can help you?" is an information-gathering, open-ended question that directly addresses his or her concerns [43]. Among 28 identified elements of care that were inquired about with patients before the office visit, Kravitz [44] found that "discussion of own ideas about how to manage condition" was ranked as the highest pre-visit physician expectation. Interestingly, this step is not always done in the primary care office. In a survey of 264 patient-physician interviews, patients completed their statement of concern only 28% of the time, being interrupted by the physician after an average duration of 23 seconds [45]. Physicians were found to redirect the patient and focus the clinical interviews before giving patients the opportunity to complete their statement of concern. Obesity interviewing and counseling should be patient-centered, allowing the patient to be an active participant in setting the agenda and having his or her concerns heard. This process requires skillful management by the physician to structure the interview within the time allocated.

The style of communication used by the physician refers to the approach taken when interacting with and counseling patients. Roter [46] defines four prototypes of doctor-patient relationships using a "power" balance sheet. In this model, power relates to who sets the agenda, whether the patient's values are expressed and considered, and what role the physician assumes. As shown in Fig. 3, high physician and high patient power (*upper left*) depicts a relationship of mutuality and balance: a "working together in partnership." High physician and low patient power (*lower left*) is when the doctor sets the agenda and prescribes the treatment: "Do as I say." In the low physician and high patient power relationship (*upper right*), the patient sets the agenda and takes sole responsibility for decision making: "Whatever

Provider Power/Interest

		High	Low
	High	Mutuality "We'll work as partners"	Consumerism "What ever you want"
Patient Power/ Interest			
	Low	Paternalism "Do what I say"	Dysfunctional "Don't ask:Don't tell"

Fig. 3. Four prototypes of physician-patient relationships are depicted using a "power/interest" balance sheet. In this model, power/interest relates to who sets the agenda, whether the patient's values are expressed and considered, and what role the physician assumes. (*From* Roter D. The enduring and evolving nature of the patient-physician relationship. Patient Educ Couns 2000;39:5–15; with permission.)

you want." Roter calls this interaction *consumerism*. In a low physician and low patient power relationship (*lower right*), the role of the doctor and the patient is unclear and undefined, which is a dysfunctional relationship: "Don't ask—don't tell." According to Roter, the optimal relationship is that of mutuality or what is called *relationship-centered medicine*. Another term for this mutual relationship is *shared decision making* [47]. The physician

Table 3
Therapeutic aspects of the clinical encounter

Cognitive strategies
  Negotiation of priorities
  Giving an explanation
  Suggestion
  Patient education
  Giving a prognosis
Affective strategies
  Empathy
  Encouragement of emotional expression
  Encouragement
  Offering hope
  Touch
  Reassurance
Behavioral strategies
  Emphasis of patient's active role
  Praising desired behaviors
  Suggesting alternative behaviors
  Attending to compliance
Social strategies
  Use of family and social supports
  Use of community agencies and other health care providers

Adapted from Novack DH. Therapeutic aspects of the clinical encounter. J Gen Intern Med 1987;2:346–55.

Table 4
Chart audit for obesity care

	Yes	No	D/N/A*
Weight noted in medical record.			
Height noted in medical record.			
BMI documented in medical record.			
Patient weighed at follow-up office visits.			
Obesity included on the patient problem list.			
Weight loss addressed with overweight/obese patient without existing comorbid medical conditions.			
Dietary counseling provided to overweight/obese patient.			
Exercise counseling provided to overweight/obese patient.			
Weight management provided to patient with a diagnosis of diabetes, hypertension, or hyperlipidemia.			
Weight-loss goal set for overweight/obese patient.			
Weight-loss counseling provided to overweight/obese patient.			
Referral to ancillary staff (dietitians, psychologists, exercise specialists) for obese patient.			

Adapted from the Centers for Obesity and Research and Education (CORE).
* D/N/A = does not apply.

and patient should work as partners, developing strategies that give the patient the best chance to control his or her own weight-management problem [48]. In the course of providing obesity care, it is likely that more than one relationship is used among patients because the tasks of management are largely unique to each person. The important point is that the encounter should be functional, informative, respectful, and supportive.

The desire for a "patient-centered" or "relationship-centered" interaction is supported by a large quantitative study of 824 patients who completed a pre-visit and post-visit questionnaire pertaining to their physician's consultation style [49]. Patients valued three elements of the office encounter: communication, which included listening, exploration of concerns, and requirements for information; partnership, which included finding a common ground for discussion and mutual agreement about patients' ideas, the problem, and treatment; and health promotion, which included how to stay healthy and reduce risks of future illnesses.

Depending on the patient's course of treatment and response, various strategies and techniques are used during the visit. The traditional therapeutic role of the physician is to address concerns, build trust, give advice, and be supportive [50]. Novack [51] describes four therapeutic interventions that support patient behavior change. Each of the therapeutic strategies listed in Table 3 is directed toward keeping the patient motivated and providing a sense of control. Among the components of effective counseling, empathy is perhaps the most important. In clinical practice, empathy is the ability to understand the patient's situation, perspective, and feelings and to communicate that understanding to the patient [52]. The feeling of being understood is intrinsically therapeutic. Patients with obesity typically provide emotionally laden testimony about the frustration, anger, and shame of losing (and gaining) weight, the discrimination they feel in the workplace and society for being overweight, and the ridicule they may have experienced with other health care providers. Recognizing and acknowledging the patient's concerns and experiences is an extremely important element in communication [53]. It is important for the patient to have the opportunity to tell the story of his or her weight journey in his or her own words and for the physician to validate the patient's experience.

Summary

Effective obesity care will not be accomplished without the implementation of a well-planned, office-based organizational system designed to address the assessment, evaluation, and treatment of the overweight and obese patient. Completing an office audit, as shown in Table 1, should be useful for triggering quality improvement opportunities regarding obesity care. Similarly, the chart audit in Table 4 can be used to assess current and future practice behavior. This chapter has reviewed the key office-based components for the delivery of obesity care. The strategies and techniques used for treatment are addressed in the remaining chapters in this book.

References

[1] US Department of Health and Human Services. The Surgeon General's call to action to prevent and decrease overweight and obesity. Rockville (MD): US Department of Health and Human Services, Public Health Service, Office of the Surgeon General; 2001.

[2] Kristeller JL, Hoerr RA. Physician attitudes toward managing obesity: differences among six specialty groups. Prev Med 1997;26:542–9.

[3] Galuska DA, Will JC, Serdula MK, Ford ES. Are health care professionals advising obese patients to lose weight? JAMA 1999;282:1576–8.

[4] Nawaz H, Adams ML, Katz DL. Weight loss counseling by health care providers. Am J Public Health 1999;89:764–7.

[5] Sciamanna CN, Tate DF, Lang W, Wing RR. Who reports receiving advice to lose weight? Results from a multistate survey. Arch Intern Med 2000;160:2334–9.

[6] Stafford RS, Farhat JH, Misra B, Schoenfeld DA. National patterns of physician activities to obesity management. Arch Fam Med 2000;9:631–8.

[7] Phillips LS, Branch WT, Cook CB, Doyle JP, El-Kebbi IM, Gallina DL, et al. Clinical inertia. Ann Intern Med 2001;135:825–34.

[8] 10 Steps: implementation guide. Put prevention into practice. In: The clinicians' handbook of preventive services. 2nd edition. Publication no. 98–0025. Rockville (MD): Agency for Healthcare Research and Quality; 1998. Available at: http://www.ahrq.gov/ppip/impsteps.htm. Accessed March 16, 2003.

[9] Harvey EL, Glenny AM, Kirk SFL, Summerbelt CD. A systematic review of interventions to improve health professionals' management of obesity. Int J Obes 1999;23:1213–22.

[10] Harvey EL, Glenny AM, Kirk SFL, Summerbelt CD. Improving health professionals' management and the organization of care for overweight and obese people. The Cochrane database of systematic reviews. The Cochrane Library; 2002.

[11] Jaen CR, Stange KC, Nutting PA. Competing demands of primary care: a model for the delivery of clinical preventive services. J Fam Pract 1994;38:166–71.

[12] NAAFA. National association to advance fat acceptance. Available at: http://www. naafa.org. Accessed March 16, 2003.

[13] Perloff D, Grimm C, Flack J, Frohich ED, Hill M, McDonald M, et al. Human blood pressure determination by sphygmomanometry. Circulation 1993;88(Part 1):2460–70.

[14] The practical guide to identification, evaluation, and treatment of overweight and obesity in adults. NIH publication no. 00–4084. US Department of Health and Human Services, Public Health Service, National Institutes of Health, Bethesda (MD): National Heart, Lung, and Blood Institute, October, 2000.

[15] Dickey LL, Gemson DH, Carney P. Office system interventions supporting primary care–based health behavior change counseling. Am J Prev Med 1999;17:299–308.

[16] Northwestern Memorial Wellness Institute. Available at: http://www.nmh.org/wellness.

[17] Guide to clinical preventive services. Report of the US Preventive Services Task Force. 2nd edition. Baltimore: Williams & Wilkins; 1996. Accessed March 16, 2003.

[18] Pearson TA, Blair SN, Daniels SR, Eckel RH, Fair JM, Fortmann SP, et al. AHA guidelines for primary prevention of cardiovascular disease and stroke: 2002 update. Consensus panel guide to comprehensive risk reduction for adult patients without coronary or other atherosclerotic vascular diseases. Circulation 2002;106:388–91.

[19] American Academy of Family Physicians. Recommendations for periodic health examination (RPHE) of the American Academy of Family Physicians. Leawood (KS): American Academy of Family Physicians; 1997.

[20] Nawaz H, Katz DL. American College of Preventive Medicine practice policy statement: weight management counseling of overweight adults. Am J Prev Med 2001;21:73–8.

[21] Lyznicki JM, Young DC, Riggs JA, Davis RM. Obesity: assessment and management in primary care. Am Fam Physician 2001;63:2185–96.

[22] Cummings GP, Coulston AM, Dalton S, Hayes D, Ikeda JP, Manore M. Position of the American Dietetic Association: weight management. J Am Diet Assoc 2002;102:1145–55.

[23] Ahluwalia JS, Gibson CA, Kenney E, Wallace DD, Resnicow K. Smoking status as a vital sign. J Gen Intern Med 1999;14:402–8.

[24] Yano EM, Fink A, Hirsch SH, Robbins AS, Rubenstein LV. Helping practices reach primary care goals: lessons from the literature. Arch Intern Med 1995;155:1146–56.

[25] Balas EA, Weingarten S, Garb CT, Blumenthal D, Boren SA, Brown GD. Improving preventive care by prompting physicians. Arch Intern Med 2000;160:301–8.

[26] Kreuter MW, Chheda SG, Bull FC. How does physician advice influence patient behavior? Evidence for a priming effect. Arch Fam Med 2000;9:426–33.

[27] Swinburn BA, Walter LG, Arroll B, Tilyard MW, Russell DG. The green prescription study: a randomized controlled trial of written advice provided by general practitioners. Am J Public Health 1998;88:288–91.

[28] Calfas KJ, Long BJ, Sallis JF, Wooten WJ, Fratt M, Patrick K. A controlled trial of physician counseling to promote the adoption of physical activity. Prev Med 1996;25:225–33.

[29] Albright CL, Cohen S, Gibbons L, Miller S, Marcus B, Sallis J, et al. Incorporating physical activity advice into primary care: physician-delivered advice within the Activity Counseling Trial. Am J Prev Med 2000;18:225–34.

[30] Petrella RJ, Wight D. An office-based instrument for exercise counseling and prescription in primary care: the Step Test Exercise Prescription (STEP). Arch Fam Prac 2000;9: 339–44.

[31] Albrant DH, Fernstrom MH, Foster GD, Jorgensen A, Kushner RF. AphA Drug treatment protocols: comprehensive weight management in adults. J Am Pharm Assoc 2001; 41:25–31.

[32] Expert Panel. Clinical guidelines on the identification, evaluation, and treatment of overweight and obesity in adults: the evidence report. National, Heart, Lung, and Blood Institute, Public Health Service, Bethesda (MD): US Department of Health and Human Services; 1998.

[33] Kushner R, Pendarvis L. An integrated approach to obesity care. Nutr Clin Care 1999; 2:285–91.

[34] Frank A. A multidisciplinary approach to obesity management: the physician's role and team care alternatives. J Am Diet Assoc 1998;98(Suppl 2):S44–8.

[35] Starfield B. Primary care concepts, evaluation, and policy. New York: Oxford University Press; 1992.

[36] Wagner EH. The role of patient care teams in chronic disease management. BMJ 2000; 320:569–72.

[37] Crabtree BF, Miller WL, Aita VA, Flocke SA, Stange KC. Primary care practice organization and preventive services delivery: a qualitative analysis. J Fam Pract 1998;46: 404–9.

[38] Scholle SH, Agatisa PK, Krohn MA, Johnson J, McLaughlin MK. Locating a health advocate in a private obstetrics/gynecology office increases patient's receipt of preventive recommendations. J Womens Health & Gender-Based Medicine 2000;9:161–5.

[39] Dickey L, Frame P, Rafferty M, Wender RC. Providing more—and better—preventive care. Patient Care 1999;November 15:198–210.

[40] Balint M. The doctor, his patient, and the illness. New York: International University Press; 1972.

[41] Groopman JE, Kunkel EJ, Platt FW, White MK. Sharing decision making with patients. Patient Care 2001;April 15:21–35.

[42] Stewart MA. Effective physician-patient communication and health outcomes: a review. Can Med Assoc J 1995;15:1423–33.

[43] Platt FW, Gaspar DL, Coulehan JL, Fox L, Adler AJ, Weston WW, et al. "Tell me about yourself": the patient-centered interview. Ann Intern Med 2001;134:1079–85.

[44] Kravitz RL. Measuring patients' expectations and requests. Ann Intern Med 2001;134 (9 Part 2):881–8.

[45] Marvel MK, Epstein RM, Flowers K, Beckman HB. Soliciting the patient's agenda: have we improved? JAMA 1999;281:283–7.

[46] Roter D. The enduring and evolving nature of the patient-physician relationship. Patient Educ Couns 2000;39:5–15.

[47] Frosch DL, Kaplan RM. Shared decision making in clinical medicine: past research and future directions. Am J Prev Med 1999;17:285–94.

[48] Clark NM, Gong M. Management of chronic disease by practitioners and patients: are we teaching the wrong things? BMJ 2000;320:572–5.

[49] Little P, Everitt H, Williamson I, Warner G, Moore M, Gould C, et al. Preferences of patients for patient centred approach to consultation in primary care: observational study. BMJ 2001;322:1–7.

[50] Branch WT, Malik TK. Using "windows of opportunities" in brief interviews to understand patients' concerns. JAMA 1993;269:1667–8.

[51] Novack DH. Therapeutic aspects of the clinical encounter. J Gen Intern Med 1987;2: 346–55.

[52] Coulehan JL, Platt FW, Egener B, Frankel R, Lin CT, Lown B, et al. "Let me see if I have this right..." Words that help build empathy. Ann Intern Med 2001;135:221–7.

[53] Suchman AL, Markakis K, Beckman HB, Frankel R. A model of empathic communication in the medical interview. JAMA 1997;277:678–82.

Appendix

Selected Internet resources for patients

1. www.collagevideo.com. Collage Video sells exercise videotapes and includes detailed information and reviews to assist in selecting videotapes based on preferences and physical limitations.

2. www.eatright.org. The American Dietetic Association offers information on nutrition, healthy lifestyle, and how to find a registered dietitian.
3. www.fitday.com. FitDay.com gives nutrition analysis of calories, fat, protein, carbohydrates, and fiber in table and graph form and offers journals, goal setting, and activity-tracking tools.
4. www.healthetech.com. Healthetech offers information on its Palm or Windows software program for personalized weight management.
5. www.nal.usda.gov/about/oei/index.htm. The National Heart, Lung, and Blood Institute Obesity Education Initiative offers information on selecting a weight-loss program, menu planning, food-label reading, and BMI calculation and interpretation.
6. www.niddk.nih.gov/health/nutrit/win.htm. The Weight Control Information Network has weight-loss articles from the National Institutes of Health.
7. www.eDiets.com. Subscription-based online diet, fitness, and counseling network providing a personal profile. Management team consists of licensed dietitians and psychologists.
8. www.Cyberdiet.com. This site provides free planning for meals and exercise profile designed by a registered dietitian.
9. www.efit.com. A free E-newsletter on nutrition tips; it also offers weight-loss counseling services by a registered dietitian.
10. www.obesityhelp.com. This site provides information for and by patients who have undergone gastric bypass surgery and individuals considering weight-loss surgery. All aspects of the surgical process are discussed, including insurance issues, through chat rooms and message boards.

10

Clinical Evaluation of the Obese Patient

Frank Greenway

Obesity is a disease, but it was not recognized as one until the National Institutes of Health (NIH) consensus conference of 1985 [1]. This 1985 paradigm shift had important implications for evaluation and treatment. Before 1985, obesity was believed to be the result of bad habits. Psychologists advised that habits are formed or broken within a 12-week period. Thus, the medications approved for obesity before 1985 were tested and recommended for use over a 12-week period of time. Now that obesity is known to be a chronic disease, one needs to view it as one does hypertension or diabetes. The goal is long-term control, rather than cure. Drugs that have been approved since 1985 reflect this change in thinking and are approved for long-term use.

In treating any disease, but particularly a chronic disease, one needs to think in terms of a risk-to-benefit ratio. One needs to assess the risks of the disease and weigh those risks against the risks and benefits of treatment. The chapter on evaluation of the obese patient (elsewhere in this book) will be directed toward the assessment of those risks. Because diabetes, hypercholesterolemia, and hypertension have been recognized as chronic diseases longer than obesity has, one can learn from the approaches that have been taken with them.

Diastolic blood pressure and serum cholesterol can be plotted against relative mortality risk. If a diastolic blood pressure of 75 mm Hg is assigned a risk of 1, then a diastolic blood pressure of 90 mm Hg carries approximately a 1.5 to 2 times greater risk of death (Fig. 1) [2]. Below a diastolic blood pressure of 90 mm Hg, people are encouraged to reduce salt intake, maintain their best weight, and exercise regularly. When the diastolic blood pressure exceeds 90 mm Hg, the risks become high enough to justify intervention with medication. A similar analogy applies in the case of total cholesterol. A total cholesterol that exceeds 240 mg/dL carries a 1.5–2 times

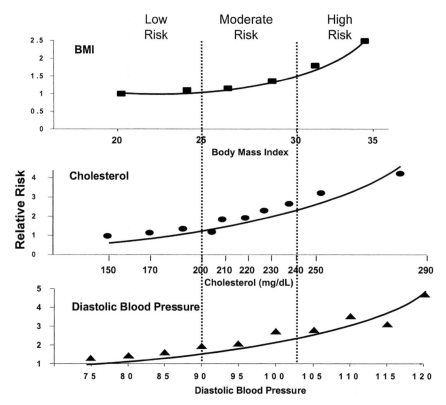

Fig. 1. The curvilinear increase in relative risk associated with body weight, cholesterol, and blood pressure (*From* Bray GA. Contemporary diagnosis and management of obesity. Handbooks in Healthcare. Newtown (PA). 1998. p. 74; with permission).

greater mortality risk and justifies intervention with medication, whereas lower levels are treated with diet and lifestyle changes (see Fig. 1).

Body mass index

Obesity is an excess of body fat, something that is difficult and expensive to measure directly. Dual energy x-ray absorbtiometry is an accurate way to measure total body fat, and CT scanning can quantify the amount of visceral fat in the abdomen. Both are expensive, and the machinery is not available in most office settings [3].

Body mass index is the weight in kilograms divided by the height in meters squared. The BMI correlates with body fat in people with a muscle mass within the normal range. Muscular people, like some professional football players, will have BMI values that overestimate their body fat. Conversely, people with muscle-wasting disease will have BMI values that underestimate their body fat content. Within these limitations, however, the BMI is a good tool for estimating body fat [4]. This is important, because although we often think of weight in estimating obesity, body fat carries the medical risk.

Unfortunately, calculating BMI can be inconvenient, especially for those in a country that does not use the metric system in daily life. This problem can be approached in different ways. One can divide the weight in pounds by 2.2 to derive the weight in kilograms and multiply inches by 0.0254 to derive the height in meters. Dividing the kilograms by the square of the height (in meters) will give the BMI. A second method uses the weight in pounds multiplied by 703, which is then divided by the square of the height in inches [5]. Fortunately, there are tables that one can use to read off a BMI knowing the height and weight. One advantage of using the BMI rather than the old height and weight chart is that BMI is gender nonspecific. Because BMI is an assessment of body fat, it gives a first approximation of mortality risk for obesity just as diastolic blood pressure does for hypertension. A BMI of 30 kg/m^2 carries a 1.5 to 2 times greater mortality risk, is comparable to a diastolic blood pressure of 90 mm Hg, and is the level at which medication treatment is usually considered (see Fig. 1) [2].

A BMI between 18.5 kg/m^2 and 25 kg/m^2 is considered normal. A BMI below 18.5 kg/m^2 is considered underweight, a BMI between 25 kg/m^2 and 30 kg/m^2 is considered overweight, and a BMI above 30 kg/m^2 is considered obese. A classification of risk has been developed based upon BMI (Table 1). The categories of obesity risk are important in selecting appropriate obesity treatments. High-risk obesity corresponds to a BMI between 30 kg/m^2 and 35 kg/m^2, very high-risk obesity is a BMI between 35 kg/m^2 and 40 kg/m^2, and a BMI greater than 40 kg/m^2 is considered extremely high-risk obesity [5]. These classes can be modified by waist circumference, as will become apparent.

Table 1
Classification of overweight and obesity by BMI, waist circumference, and associated disease risk

	BMI kg/m^2	Obesity class	Disease risk[a] relative to normal weight and waist circumference	
			Men ≤102 cm (≤40 in) Women ≤88 cm (≤35 in)	>102 cm (>40 in) >88 cm (>35 in)
Underweight	18.5		—	—
Normal[b]	18.5–24.9		—	—
Overweight	25.0–29.9		Increased	High
Obesity	30.0–34.9	I	High	Very high
	35.0–39.9	II	Very high	Very high
Extreme obesity	≥40	III	Extremely high	Extremely high

[a] Disease risk for type 2 diabetes, hypertension, and cardiovascular disease (CVD).

[b] Increased waist circumference can also be a marker for increased risk even in persons of normal weight.

Data from Clinical guidelines on the identification, evaluation, and treatment of overweight and obesity in adults—The Evidence Report. National Institutes of Health. Obes Res 1998; 6(Suppl 2):51S–209S.

Fat distribution

The distribution of body fat determines the severity of the health risk posed by obesity. Fat inside the abdomen that has venous drainage through the liver is associated with insulin resistance. This visceral fat can be estimated by measuring the waist circumference [6]. The waist circumference defines risk above that which is measured by the BMI. To measure the waist circumference, one should measure at the level of the iliac crest in a plane parallel with the floor while the patient is standing (Fig. 2) [5].

After the BMI exceeds 35 kg/m^2 visceral fat will be increased; measuring the waist circumference is an important part of the clinical evaluation only when the BMI is less than 35 kg/m^2. A waist circumference that is greater than 40 inches (102 cm) in men and greater than 35 inches (88 cm) in women indicates an excess of visceral fat. A large waist circumference increases the mortality risk in those with a BMI that is less than 35 kg/m^2 and elevates them to the next higher class of obesity (see Table 1). In fact, waist circumference may be a better way to assess risk in Asians and in older populations [7].

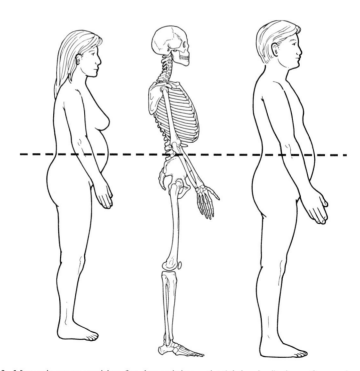

Fig. 2. Measuring tape position for determining waist (abdominal) circumference in adults.

The metabolic syndrome

The metabolic syndrome is a constellation of findings that is related to insulin resistance. The metabolic syndrome has also been called syndrome X. This insulin-resistance syndrome has several components and is now recognized with a separate billing code, ICD 277.7. As one can see from Table 2, the waist circumference is one criterion for the presence of the metabolic syndrome and the risk that is associated with the metabolic syndrome increases as obesity increases. The metabolic syndrome relates obesity to diabetes, hypertension, low HDL cholesterol, and high triglycerides. The high triglycerides are associated with a lipoprotein phenotype that is atherogenic and is a cardiovascular risk factor. Compared with a body mass index that is less than 25 kg/m^2, the prevalence of hypertension doubles, and

Table 2
Definitions of the metabolic syndrome

Organization	AACE[a]	WHO[b]	ATPIII[c]
1. High insulin: glucose ratio	x		
2. Acanthosis Nigricans	x		
3. Waist men	>102 cm		>102 cm
4. Waist women	>88 cm		>88 cm
5. Waist/hip men		>0.9	
6. Waist/hip women		>0.85	
7. HDL men	<35 mg/dL	<35 mg/dL	<40 mg/dL
8. HDL women	<45 mg/dL	<39 mg/dL	<50 mg/dL
9. Triglycerides	>150 mg/dL	>15 mg/dL	>150 mg/dL
10. Hypertension	x	>169/90	>130/85
11. Insulin resistance (clamp)		low 25%	
12. Impaired glucose tolerance 2 hr)		>140 mg/dL	
13. Impaired fasting glucose	x	>110 mg/dL	>110 mg/dL
14. Type 2 diabetes (FBS/2 hr)	x	>126/200 mg/dL	
15. Hyperuricemia	x		
16. Hypercoagulability	x		
17. Polycystic ovary disease	x		
18. Vascular endothelial dysfunction	x		
19. Microalbuminuria	x	>20 mcg/min	
20. Coronary heart disease	x		
21. BMI		>30 kg/m^2	

Abbreviations: CDC, Centers for Disease Control; FBS, fasting blood sugar.

[a] The American Association of Clinical Endocrinologists (AACE) divides the syndrome into major criteria (items 1–15 denoted by x in second column) and minor criteria (items 16–20 denoted by x in second column). No given number of components are required to make the diagnosis, because the CDC has suggested diagnosis based on physician judgement.

[b] The World Health Organization (WHO) requires glucose intolerance, impaired glucose tolerance or diabetes and or insulin resistance together with two or more of the other items checked. The definition of insulin resistance is glucose disappearance with a hyperinsulinemic, euglycemic clamp in the lowest quartile of the population being studied.

[c] The Adult Treatment Panel III (ATPIII) requires three of the items checked to make the diagnosis.

the prevalence of low HDL cholesterol triples over a BMI of 30 kg/m^2 [8]. Thus, the association between obesity and the metabolic syndrome becomes stronger as obesity becomes more severe.

Disease-associated obesity (Box 1)

The relationship between obesity and atherosclerotic vascular disease, including coronary artery disease, seems to be mediated by dyslipidemia [9]. As obesity increases, so do triglycerides. This is a manifestation of insulin resistance and correlates with waist circumference and visceral fat. Because triglycerides and HDL cholesterol compete for the same carrier lipoproteins, as triglycerides go up, HDL cholesterol comes down. This interferes with reverse cholesterol transport, which increases the risk of atherosclerotic disease. Increases in obesity are associated with increases in the size of the vascular bed in fat tissue which puts a strain on the heart and increases the risk of congestive heart failure. As fat cells increase in size, the production of cholesterol and plasminogen activator inhibitor-1 (PAI-1) increase. Cholesterol further stimulates atherosclerosis and the increase in PAI-1 acts as a procoagulant.

Diabetes is the disease that is most closely related to obesity. In the Nurses Health Study, a BMI of 35 kg/m^2 increased the risk of diabetes more than 60 fold compared with a BMI of 22 [10]. Diabetes follows obesity by 10 to 20 years based on data from the Pima Indians [11]. Evidence from the Diabetes Prevention Program confirmed that weight loss and increased physical activity can prevent diabetes [12]. The relation between diabetes and obesity seems to be linked through insulin resistance and fat cell size. If fat cells reach their maximal size and cannot divide, fat becomes stored in muscle cells which creates insulin resistance [13]. Evidence for this relationship is seen in the rare cases of complete lipodystropy where essentially no fat storage sites exist and insulin resistance is extreme [14]. The reversal of insulin resistance with thiazoladienedione medications is further evidence, because these drugs reverse insulin resistance by causing fat cells to divide. Small fat cells are associated with less insulin resistance, presumably because fat can be redirected from muscle sites to the fat cell again.

Box 1. Obesity-associated diseases that require more aggressive treatment

Established coronary artery disease
Other atherosclerotic disease
Type 2 diabetes mellitus
Sleep apnea

Loud snoring and the cessation of breathing during sleep characterize sleep apnea. Frequent brief awakenings during sleep that are associated with these apnea periods often result in daytime drowsiness. Sleep apnea is believed to result from an obstruction of the upper airway because of the deposition of fat. The risk is higher in those with greater neck circumference [15]. Because patients may not know what they sound like during sleep, the physician must have a high index of suspicion and consider a consult with the patient's sleep partner, if one exists. In addition to a large neck, ankle edema, especially in the face of pulmonary hypertension, is associated with sleep apnea [16].

Other factors that increase obesity risk

In addition to the four problems listed above, less serious, obesity-associated diseases are listed in Box 2. The presence of three or more of these less serious problems is equivalent to having a high-risk obesity condition, and necessitates more aggressive intervention. On average, smokers are 4 kg lighter than nonsmokers [17]. Stopping cigarette smoking is more important medically than gaining back the 4 kg that is the likely result of doing so. Although some individuals gain much more weight after stopping smoking, the use of smoking to help maintain a lower weight cannot be justified medically [17].

Having high-risk obesity carries recommendations from expert panels to increase the intensity of treatment for hypertension, hyperlipidemia, and other cardiovascular risk factors [18,19]. Conversely, these panels also recommended the maintenance of a healthy weight.

Although physical inactivity is not one of the risk factors that calls for an increase in the intensity of treatment nor a disease in itself, it does increase the risk for cardiovascular disease and type 2 diabetes [20]. Physical activity is an important component of the treatment recommendations by the expert

---

Box 2. Factors that increase obesity risk

Cigarette smoking
Hypertension (blood pressure higher than 140/90 or the use of antihypertensive agents)
High LDL cholesterol (higher than 160 mg/dL)
Low HDL cholesterol (lower than 35 mg/dL)
Impaired fasting glucose (110–125 mg/dL)
Family history of premature coronary heart disease
Age older than 45 years in men and 55 years in women

panels that recommend treatment for hypertension and hyperlipidemia, as well as for obesity [18,19].

Physical inactivity and obesity-related diseases can be divided into three broad categories. The first of these is related to the metabolic syndrome, the second is related to increased intra-abdominal pressure, and the third is related to mechanical stress. Gallstones have some unique aspects. The increase in fat that accompanies obesity increases cholesterol production and increases bile saturation [21]. Although gallstones are highly associated with obesity and the risk of their occurrence is decreased when obesity is reduced, the process of weight loss increases the risk of gallstone formation [21]. The increased risk of gallstone formation with weight loss is proportional to the rapidity of the weight reduction. During weight reduction, the bile saturation increases in proportion to the caloric deficit; if the fat in the diet is less than 10 grams in a single meal, gallbladder stasis will also play a role in gallstone formation [21]. The relationship of gallstones to the rapidity of weight loss is one of the reasons that weight losses in excess of 1% of body weight per week is not recommended.

In addition to the increased risk of diabetes, dyslipidemia, and hypertension, insulin resistance creates a prothrombotic state, increases uric acid, and predisposes to the development of gout. Insulin resistance or the metabolic syndrome also affects reproductive function and increases the risk of certain cancers. Insulin resistance is associated with high insulin levels. These high insulin levels stimulate growth in the skin that result in acanthosis nigricans [22]. Insulin also stimulates androgen production and fat tissue increases the conversion of androgen to estrogen. The increased androgen levels are responsible for the hirsutism that is associated with insulin resistance in women, and the decrease in sex hormone binding globulin increases the amount of free sex hormones. The increased estrogen suppresses FSH, suppresses ovulation, impairs fertility, and is associated with the polycystic ovary syndrome [23].

Obesity is associated most strongly with cancers of the breast, endometrium, and colon. Insulin stimulates the receptor for insulin-like growth factor and reduces the binding protein for insulin-like growth factor-1. The higher levels of insulin-like growth factor increase the growth of cancer cells and inhibit their death or apoptosis [24]. In addition to this role played by insulin and insulin-like growth factor in obesity-related cancer, estrogen also plays a role in breast cancer and cancer of the uterine endometrium [25].

Breast cancer is common in women and rare in men, a fact that is attributed to the different circulating levels of estrogen. Diet also influences estrogen levels and this difference was suggested to explain why women in Los Angeles have a 20% greater incidence of breast cancer than women in Shanghai [26]. Endometrial cancer is associated with estrogen stimulation unopposed by progesterone, a situation that results from anovulation and estrogen replacement without progesterone [27].

Increased intra-abdominal pressure was shown to be present in obesity by measuring the pressure inside the urinary bladder. The pressure is often higher than that seen with the acute abdominal compartment syndrome that is associated with trauma, for which surgical decompression is indicated. The reason why the obese can tolerate higher intra-abdominal pressure, presumably, is because of its development over a longer period, which gives the body a chance to compensate. Increased intra-abdominal pressure is associated with stress incontinence, gastroesophageal reflux, lower extremity edema, and a propensity to stasis changes in the lower extremities [16]. More serious disabilities associated with increased intra-abdominal pressure include hypertension and pseudotumor cerebri. Pseudotumor cerebri has been treated with shunting of the cerebrospinal fluid, but a recent study suggested that weight reduction by obesity surgery is much more effective [28].

Obesity, especially when severe, puts mechanical stresses on the body. Breathing becomes more difficult and obstructive sleep apnea can result, as well. Although sleep apnea can be treated with continuous positive airway pressure (CPAP), many patients cannot tolerate a mask on their face during sleep; the weight loss that is associated with obesity surgery has cured 40% to 76% of those who have sleep apnea. Obesity also increases the incidence and severity of osteoarthritis and low back pain. Table 3 lists the diseases that are associated with obesity and categorizes them by mechanism and the strength of the association.

Secondary causes of obesity

Although we know relatively little about the cause of most obesity, there are exceptions to this general rule. It is, of course, important clinically to identify the secondary causes because some have specific treatments.

Hypothalamic obesity

Hypothalamic obesity is rare and is caused by bilateral injury to the ventromedial hypothalamus, the paraventricular hypothalamus, or the amygdala.

Table 3
Diseases associated with obesity

Relative risk	Metabolic syndrome	Increased intra-abdominal pressure	Mechanical
>3	Diabetes	Hypertension	
	Gallstones	Sleep apnea	
	Dyslipidemia	Pseudotumor cerebri	
2–3	Coronary disease		Osteoarthritis
1–2	Impaired fertility		Low back pain
	Cancer		

Symptoms consist of signs of increased intracranial pressure (headache, vomiting, blurred vision), hypopituitarism, and neurologic problems (seizures, coma, somnolence, temperature disregulation). Hypothalamic obesity is caused by an increase in the early phase of insulin secretion in the face of insulin sensitivity [29]. Because sites in the brain, upon which appetite suppressant drugs act are destroyed in hypothalamic obesity, other avenues of treatment are required. Treatment with somatostatin reduces the first phase of insulin secretion and has successfully reversed the steady weight gain that is typical of this condition [30].

Endocrine obesity

Endocrine causes of obesity are often in the forefront of obese subject's thoughts. Although known endocrine diseases account for only a small proportion of obesity, identifying patients who have them is important, because they have specific treatments. Although hypothyroidism is associated with a small weight gain, much of the weight gain is not fat. Hypothyroidism is common, especially in older women and measuring TSH can make the diagnosis. Instituting treatment with thyroid hormone replacement will treat the hypothyroidism, but one may need to treat the obesity with other interventions.

Cushing's syndrome is characterized in adults by central obesity, hypertension, and plethoric facies. The central obesity and thin extremities with atrophic skin is sometimes striking in adults. Children, however, present differently. Obese children grow in height and weight and are taller than their peers. Children with Cushing's syndrome become obese without an advance in height. When Cushing's syndrome is suspected, a 24-hour urine free cortisol or an overnight dexamethasone suppression test should be considered. The overnight dexamethasone suppression test is performed by giving the patient 1 mg of dexamethasone to take orally at 11 PM with serum cortisol measured the following morning (normal is suppression to less than 5 mcg/dL) [31]. A positive screening test should trigger a definitive evaluation for Cushing's disease.

Polycystic ovarian disease is a manifestation of insulin resistance. It improves with weight loss and interventions that decrease insulin resistance, like metformin and thiazolidenediones [23].

Genetic syndromes with hypogonadism

Five genetic syndromes are associated with obesity, all of which are associated with hypogonadism. Like the endocrine causes of obesity in children, these genetic syndromes are associated with short stature whereas obesity in normal children is associated with an advance in height-age. Prader-Willi syndrome is the most common of these and is associated with mental retardation, temper tantrums, hyperphagia, nasal speech, and tooth enamel hypoplasia. Prader-Willi syndrome is caused by an abnormality on chromosome 15 and is associated with hypotonia at birth that requires gavage feeding followed later by hyperphagia and obesity. Bardet-Biedl syndrome, Ahlstrom syndrome, Cohen syndrome, and Carpenter syndrome are other obesity syndromes, but they are seen much less commonly [32].

Weight gain

Weight gain after the age of 20 is an important health risk [33]. Most adults will remember what they weighed on completion of high school. Gaining less than 5 kg puts one at low risk and gaining more than 10 kg puts one at high risk. The most concerning pattern of weight gain has been termed progressive obesity. In this condition, children start to gain weight between the ages of 3 and 10 years. They gain a steady amount each year and usually reach 300 pounds before the age of 30 years [34].

Other aspects of weight history are clinically important. Children of diabetic mothers are at higher risk of being overweight as children and adults [35]. Children that were small for gestational age are at greater risk of developing abdominal obesity and insulin resistance in later life [36]. Children of two overweight parents are at an 80% risk of becoming obese as adults, but have only a 40% risk with one obese parent [35]. Children who are overweight between 3 and 10 years of age have a 75% risk of becoming obese as adults, if they have one or more overweight parents [34]. Overweight in adolescence continues into adulthood 80% of the time [34,35]. Other times of higher risk for weight gain in adulthood are during the time when athletic activities decline in the third decade of life for men. Some women can gain significant weight through pregnancy and at menopause, but these have small effects over a population. Women have a redistribution of body fat at menopause to a more central pattern that is partially inhibited by estrogen [37]. Oral contraceptives were associated with weight gain in the past, but this effect seems to be minimal with the lower doses that are now used.

Drug-induced weight gain

Certain drugs that are used to treat other conditions can have the side effect of weight gain (Box 3). These weight gains are small for most medications, but one occasionally sees a patient who is sensitive to the weight gain effects of medications. Glucocorticoids have the greatest propensity for weight gain and result in an iatrogenic Cushing's syndrome. Megace, a progestational agent that is used to induce weight gain in cancer patients works through the glucocorticoid receptor [38]. Cyproheptadine, an antihistamine with antiserotonin properties, increases food intake and has been used to treat weight loss that is associated with tuberculosis and anorexia nervosa [39].

Box 3. Drugs that are associated with weight gain

Glucocorticoids
Megace
Cyproheptadine
Phenothizianes and other antipsychotics
Sedating tricyclic antidepressants
Antiepileptic medications (topiramate is an exception)
Beta-adrenergic blocking drugs
Insulin and drugs that stimulate insulin release

Antipsychotic medications are also associated with weight gain. Phenothiazines gave a 3.2 kg weight gain during three years of observation in a mental institution [40]. Tricyclic antidepressants cause weight gain that is proportional to their sedating effect. Protryptyline, a tricyclic with stimulant properties, was reported to cause weight loss [41]. Antiepileptic medications, especially valproic acid and carbamazepine, have been associated with weight gain. Topiramate, however, another antiepileptic medication, was reported to be associated with weight loss [42].

Caffeine and ephedrine are sold to induce weight loss and stimulate the alpha and beta adrenergic receptors. Phenylpropanolamine, an appetite suppressant that was recently removed from the market, stimulates the alpha-1 adrenergic receptor. It is no surprise, therefore, that blockers of the beta and alpha-1 adrenergic receptors are associated with weight gain. Hypothalamic obesity is associated with increased insulin secretion. Antidiabetic drugs, insulin, sulfonylureas, and thiazolidinediones, induce weight gain. In fact, insulin, gibenclamide, and chlorpropamide were associated with a 3.5 to 4.8 kg weight gain in 6 years whereas there was no weight change with metformin [43].

Food intake considerations

High-fat diets have been associated epidemiologically with obesity; this is one of the reasons why most recommendations for obesity treatment suggest a reduction in dietary fat [44]. Binge eating disorder can be accompanied by obesity. This is a psychiatric illness that is characterized by eating large amounts of food at a single meal. This condition is best treated with drugs that inhibit serotonin reuptake.

Readiness for weight loss

Because obesity is stigmatized in our society and is harder to hide than a disease like hypertension, one might think that all people with obesity would be ready to attempt weight loss. Practicing physicians, however, diagnose obesity in many individuals who do not place a high priority on losing weight. Because the successful treatment of obesity requires a high level of patient cooperation, the patient must be ready to attempt weight loss before treatment is instituted.

Table 4
Evaluating the obese patient

	Comments
History	
Age	>55 yr. (men) or >65 yr. (women) is a cardiac risk factor
Weight at age 18 to 20 years	Gain >10 kg increases health risk
Bulimia or history of anorexia nervosa	Referral to specialized care indicated
Nursing or pregnant	Defer weight loss
Sleep apnea	High risk (high risk indicates more intensive treatment of associated diseases)
Coronary artery disease (CAD)	High risk
Arteriosclerotic vascular disease	High risk
Diabetes	High risk
Physical activity	Low activity increases risk
Diet	High fat correlated with obesity
Smoke	Risk factor (three risk factors = high risk*)
Family history of premature CAD	Risk factor
Taking drugs in Box 3	Consider alternative drug
Readiness for weight loss	Important for timing therapy
Physical examination	
Height, weight, and BMI	Major determinants of therapy
Waist circumference	Increases treatment category less than a BMI of 35 kg/m^2
Blood pressure	Elevation with plethora – consider Cushing's
Funduscopic exam	Is intracranial pressure increased?
Hirsutism	Metabolic syndrome – consider polycystic ovary syndrome
Acanthosis nigricans	High insulin levels
Plethora and thin skin	Consider Cushing's syndrome
Abdominal examination	Aneurysm/atherosclerosis – high risk
Hypogonadism	Consider genetic syndrome
Peripheral edema	Consider sleep apnea, increased intra-abdominal pressure, or heart failure
Pedal pulses	Atherosclerotic vascular disease is a risk factor
Arrest of linear growth	Consider childhood Cushing's or other endocrine cause for obesity
Laboratory	
Fasting blood glucose	Diabetes high-risk, impaired glucose tolerance a risk factor
Triglycerides, HDL cholesterol	Risk factor
LDL cholesterol	Risk factor
Electrocardiogram	Myocardial infarction is high risk

* 3 risk factors equate to high-risk obesity (see Box 1) justifying more aggressive treatment.

Therefore, the physician must determine the receptivity of the patient to weight loss, and encourage those who are not ready to lose weight to contemplate losing weight in the future. Sometimes convincing patients not to gain more weight is all the cooperation for which one can hope. The physician, however, does have a great deal of influence over the attitudes of the patients. Avoiding the subject of obesity in a patient who is at risk for obesity-related disease, but not ready to lose weight, means missing an opportunity to shape that patient's future receptiveness to obesity treatment. Weight, like blood pressure, is routinely measured during visits to physicians. Addressing obesity with the same degree of concern with which blood pressure is addressed should be a goal for physicians who treat patients.

Contraindications to weight loss

Pregnant or lactating women are not candidates for obesity treatment. Weight loss can put the fetus at risk and reduce milk production. Because pregnancy and lactation are temporary conditions, weight loss can await their termination. People with an uncontrolled psychiatric condition, such as major depression or other serious illnesses for which calorie restriction might be detrimental, should have weight loss attempts deferred until the more pressing problems are under control. Obese subjects with a history of anorexia nervosa, bulimia, or who have active substance abuse represent difficult problems and should be referred to specialized care.

Evaluation of the obese patient, like the evaluation of any medical patient, involves a medical history, physical examination, and laboratory evaluation. As with any chronic illness, certain aspects of the history, physical, and laboratory evaluation deserve special emphasis. Those that deserve special emphasis in the case of obesity are described in this and are summarized in Table 4.

References

[1] NIH Consensus Development Conference Statement. Health implications of obesity. Ann Intern Med 1985;103:1973–7.
[2] Bray GA. Coherent preventive and management strategies for obesity. In: Chadwick DJ, Cardew G, editors. The origins and consequences of obesity. Ciba Foundation Symposium 201. London: John Wiley; 1996. p. 228–46.
[3] Heymsfield SB, Allison DB, Wang ZM. Evaluation of total and regional body composition. In: Bray GA, Bouchard C, James WP, editors. Handbook of obesity. New York: Marcel Dekker; 1998. p. 41–77.
[4] Bray GA. In defense of a body mass index of 25 as the cut-off point for defining overweight. Obes Res 1998;6(6):461–2.
[5] National Institutes of Health. National Heart, Lung, and Blood Institute and the North American Association of the Study of Obesity. The practical guide: identification,

evaluation and treatment of overweight and obesity in adults. NIH publication number 00–4084, 2000.

[6] Rankinen T, Kim SY, Perusse L, et al. The prediction of abdominal visceral fat level from body composition and anthropometry: ROC analysis. Int J Obes Relat Metab Disord 1999;23(8):801–9.

[7] Fujimoto WY, Newell-Morris LL, Grote M, et al. Visceral fat obesity and morbidity: NIDDM and atherogenic risk in Japanese-American men and women. Int J Obes 1991; 15(Suppl 2):41–4.

[8] Brown CD, Higgins M, Donato KA, et al. Body mass index and the prevalence of hypertension and dyslipidemia. Obes Res 2000;8(9):605–19.

[9] Despres JP, Krauss RM. Obesity and lipoprotein metabolism. In: Bray GA, Bouchard C, James WP, editors. Handbook of obesity. New York: Marcel Dekker; 1998. p. 651–75.

[10] Colditz GA, Willett WC, Rotnitzky A, et al. Weight gain as a risk factor for clinical diabetes mellitus in women. Ann Intern Med 1995;122(7):481–6.

[11] Ravussin E. Energy metabolism in obesity. Studies in the Pima Indians. Diabetes Care 1993;16(1):232–8.

[12] Knowler WC, Barrett-Connor E, Fowler SE, et al. Reduction in the incidence of type 2 diabetes with lifestyle intervention or metformin. N Engl J Med 2002;346(6):393–403.

[13] Danforth E Jr. Failure of adipocyte differentiation causes type II diabetes mellitus? Nat Genet 2000;26(1):13.

[14] Oseid S, Beck-Nielsen H, Pedersen O, et al. Decreased binding of insulin to its receptor in patients with congenital generalized lipodystrophy. N Engl J Med 1977;296(5):245–8.

[15] Sharma SK, Reddy TS, Mohan A, et al. Sleep disordered breathing in chronic obstructive pulmonary disease. Indian J Chest Dis Allied Sci 2002;44(2):99–105.

[16] Sugerman H, Windsor A, Bessos M, et al. Intra-abdominal pressure, sagittal abdominal diameter and obesity comorbidity. J Intern Med 1997;241(1):71–9.

[17] Flegal KM, Troiano RP, Pamuk ER, et al. The influence of smoking cessation on the prevalence of overweight in the United States. N Engl J Med 1995;333(18):1165–70.

[18] National Cholesterol Education Program. Second report of the Expert Panel on Detection, Evaluation, and Treatment of High Blood Cholesterol in Adults (Adult Treatment Panel II). Circulation 1994;89:1333–445.

[19] The sixth report of the Joint National Committee on Prevention. Detection, evaluation, and treatment of high blood pressure. Arch Intern Med 1997;157:2413–46.

[20] Blair SN, Kohl HW III, Barlow CE, et al. Changes in physical fitness and all-cause mortality. A prospective study of healthy and unhealthy men. JAMA 1995;273(14): 1093–8.

[21] Ko CW, Lee SP. Obesity and gallbladder disease. In: Bray GA, Bouchard C, James WP, editors. Handbook of obesity. New York: Marcel Dekker; 1998. p. 709–24.

[22] Stoddart ML, Blevins KS, Lee ET, et al. Association of acanthosis nigricans with hyperinsulinemia compared with other selected risk factors for type 2 diabetes in Cherokee Indians: the Cherokee diabetes study. Diabetes Care 2002;25(6):1009–14.

[23] Veldhuis JD, Zhang G, Garmey JC. Troglitazone, an insulin-sensitizing thiazolidinedione, represses combined stimulation by LH and insulin of de novo androgen biosynthesis by thecal cells in vitro. J Clin Endocrinol Metab 2002;87(3):1129–33.

[24] Giovannucci E. Insulin, insulin-like growth factors and colon cancer: a review of the evidence. J Nutr 2001;131(Suppl 11):3109S–20S.

[25] Gupta K, Krishnaswamy G, Karnad A, et al. Insulin: a novel factor in carcinogenesis. Am J Med Sci 2002;323(3):140–5.

[26] Berstein L, Yuan JM, Ross RK, et al. Serum hormone levels in pre-menopausal Chinese women in Shanghai and white women in Los Angels: results from two breast cancer case-control studies. Cancer Causes Control 1990;1(1):51–8.

[27] Purdie DM, Green AC. Epidemiology of endometrial cancer. Best Pract Res Clin Obstet Gynaecol 2001;15(3):341–54.

[28] Sugerman HJ, Felton III WL, Sismanis A, et al. Gastric surgery for pseudotumor cerebri associated with severe obesity. Ann Surg 1999;229(5):634–40discussion 640–2.

[29] Bray GA, Gallagher III TF. Manifestations of hypothalamic obesity in man: a comprehensive investigation of eight patients and a review of the literature. Medicine (Baltimore) 1975;54:301–30.

[30] Lustig RH, Rose SR, Burghen GA, et al. Hypothalamic obesity caused by cranial insult in children: altered glucose and insulin dynamics and reversal by a somatostatin agonist. J Pediatr 1999;135(2 Pt 1):162–8.

[31] Carlson HE. Functioning pituitary tumors. In: Hershman JM, Mellinkoff S, Solomon DH, editors. Practical endocrinology. New York: John Wiley; 1981. p. 52–76.

[32] Bray GA. Contemporary diagnosis and management of obesity. Newtown: Handbooks in Health Care; 1998.

[33] Willett WC, Manson JE, Stampfer MJ, et al. Weight, weight change, and coronary heart disease in women. Risk within the 'normal' weight range. JAMA 1995;273:461–5.

[34] Bray GA. The obese patient: major problems in internal medicine. 9th edition. Philadelphia: WB Saunders; 1976.

[35] Bray GA. The syndromes of obesity: an endocrine approach. In: DeGroot LJ, Besser M, Burger HB, et al, editors. Endocrinology. Philadelphia: WB Saunders; 1995. p. 2624–62.

[36] Yanovski SZ, Gormally JF, Leser MS, et al. Binge eating disorder affects outcome of comprehensive very-low-calorie diet treatment. Obs Res 1994;2:205–12.

[37] Aloia JF, Vaswani A, Russo L, et al. The influence of menopause and hormonal replacement therapy on body cell mass and body fat mass. Am J Obstet Gynecol 1995;172:896–900.

[38] Jatoi A, Windschitl HE, Loprinzi CL, et al. Dronabinol versus megestrol acetate versus combination therapy for cancer-associated anorexia: a North Central Cancer Treatment Group study. J Clin Oncol 2002;20(2):567–73.

[39] Saleh JW, Yang MU, van Itallie TB, et al. Ingestive behavior and composition of weight change during cyporheptadine administration. Int J Obes 1979;3(3):213–21.

[40] Waitzkin L. Weight gain among hospitalized, mentally ill men. Behav Neuropsychiatry 1969;1(7):15–8.

[41] Cohen GL. Protriptyline, chronic tension-type headaches, and weight loss in women. Headache 1997;37(7):433–6.

[42] Ketter TA, Post RM, Theodore WH. Positive and negative psychiatric effects of antiepileptic drugs in patients with seizure disorders. Neurology 1999;53(5)(Suppl 2): S53–67.

[43] United Kingdom Prospective Diabetes Study Group. United Kingdom Prospective Diabetes Study 24: a 6-year, randomized, controlled trial comparing sulfonylurea, insulin, and metformin therapy in patients with newly diagnosed type 2 diabetes that could not be controlled with diet therapy. Ann Intern Med 1998;128:165–75.

[44] Bray GA, Popkin BM. Dietary fat intake does affect obesity. Am J Clin Nutr 1998;68(6):1157–73.

11

Behavioral Techniques for Treating the Obese Patient

Rena R. Wing

Amy A. Gorin

Evidence of the effectiveness of behavioral approaches to weight loss

Obesity is important to address in primary care because of the negative health consequences of excessive weight and the increasing evidence that even modest weight losses result in significant health benefits. For example, modest weight losses were shown to lower cardiovascular disease (CVD) risk factors and reduce the risk of developing hypertension and the need for hypertension medicine [1–3]. The most impressive evidence of the positive health impact of weight loss comes from the Diabetes Prevention Program (DPP). DPP [4] examined the effect of a lifestyle intervention for prevention or delay of type 2 diabetes in individuals with impaired glucose tolerance (IGT). The 3234 participants in DPP were recruited from 27 centers across the country. Forty-five percent of study participants were from minority groups who are disproportionately affected by type 2 diabetes (20% were black, 16% were Hispanic American, 5% were American Indian, and 4% were Asian). Moreover, 20% were over the age of 60. All participants had a BMI that was greater than 25 kg/m^2 (mean was 34.0 ± 6.7) and had IGT that defined by a glucose of 95 to 125 mg/dL fasting and 140 to 199 mg/dL 2 hours after a 75 g glucose load.

Participants in the DPP were randomly assigned to one of three interventions: intensive weight loss program (lifestyle intervention), standard lifestyle instruction plus metformin (850 mg, twice daily), or standard lifestyle instruction plus placebo, given in a double-blinded fashion. The participants in the intensive weight loss program met regularly with an individual case manager. They were taught strategies to help them lose at least 7% of their initial body weight and maintain the loss and to achieve at least 150 minutes of physical activity each week, using activities similar in intensity to brisk walking.

Participants in the lifestyle intervention reported an average of 225 minutes of activity per week; 74% met or exceeded the 150-minute exercise goal at 6 months and 58% exceeded the goal at study end (an average of approximately 3 years of follow-up). On average, self-reported caloric intake decreased by 450 kcal/day in the participants in the intensive weight loss program (compared with 296 kcal/day in the patients who took metformin and 249 kcal/day in those who took placebo). The percent of calories from fat decreased from 34% to 28% in the participants in the intensive weight loss program (a 6.6% decrease compared with a 0.8% decrease in the patients who took metformin and placebo). Weight losses for participants in the lifestyle intervention group averaged 7 kg at 6 months; 50% lost 7% or more of their body weight. At the end of the study, the average weight loss was 4 kg and 38% of patients met or exceeded the 7% weight loss goal [4].

These relatively modest changes in diet, weight, and physical activity led to a dramatic 58% decrease in the risk of developing diabetes in participants in the lifestyle intervention group. Lifestyle intervention was more effective than placebo and was twice as effective as metformin, which produced a 31% decrease in risk of diabetes. Lifestyle intervention worked in all ethnic groups, in both genders, in all BMI groups, and in all age groups. Of particular interest was the fact that lifestyle intervention was effective in those over age 60.

Because of the success of the DPP lifestyle intervention, it is important to identify some key components that were used that can be translated into the primary care setting. These components (Box 1) will be described in more detail later because they form the basis of all behavioral interventions.

Evidence of long-term, weight loss success

Despite the positive impact that weight loss can have on health, many physicians are pessimistic about the chances of producing long-term changes in the diet and exercise behaviors of their patients. They point to the statistic that 95% of individuals will regain their weight; however, this statistic is based on a small study that was conducted many years ago [5]. More recent studies suggested that approximately 20% of overweight individuals are successful at long-term maintenance of weight loss [6,7].

Epidemiological studies of weight loss

McGuire et al [6] conducted a random-digit dialing survey of 500 adults in the United States. Among overweight individuals, 62% had lost at least

---

Box 1. Key aspects of DPP lifestyle intervention

• **Goal-based intervention:** each participant was given a goal of losing 7% of their weight and achieving 150 minutes/week of physical activity
• **Focus on diet and physical activity:** recommended diet was low in calories and low in fat; brisk walking and other activities of similar intensity were recommended
• **Behavioral strategies:** therapists introduced strategies to change diet and exercise behavior, including self-monitoring, goal-setting, problem solving, stimulus control, contingency contracting, and self-reinforcement
• **Intensive, on-going contact:** participants were seen individually for 16 sessions over the first 24 weeks and then contacted at least once a month (with an in-person contact at least every 2 months)
• **Individualization of treatment:** through identification of personal motivation for weight loss, specific barriers to success, and problem solving of solutions to these barriers

---

10% of their maximum weight at some time in their life and 38% reported that they were currently at least 10% below their maximum weight. More than 20% reported meeting a strict criterion of success: that they had intentionally lost weight and had maintained a weight loss of at least 10% for at least 1 year. McGuire et al [7] compared the behaviors of these successful weight loss maintainers with regainers (who lost more than 10% of their body weight but regained it) and weight stable, nonobese controls (never weighed more than 10% above their current weight). Successful weight loss maintainers reported eating less fat, with more avoidance of fried foods and more substitution of low-fat for high-fat foods than regainers or weight stable controls. Similarly, weight loss maintainers reported higher levels of physical activity (especially strenuous activity) and greater frequency of self-weighing. Thus, long-term weight losses are possible and seem to result from long-term changes in behavior.

There is also evidence that people who lose weight, even if they regain it, may be healthier than those who do not lose weight. In the Nurses Health Study, for example, 8% of women with a BMI of 25 to 29.9 lost 5% of their weight over a 2-year period and 1% of women with a BMI of 30 or higher lost 5% of their weight over a 2-year period [8]. Women who lost weight during this 2-year period regained more weight over the next 4 years, but their overall weight gain from years 1 through 6 was less than other women (Fig. 1). Thus, one would expect that their cardiovascular risk factors would be improved relative to those who had not lost weight.

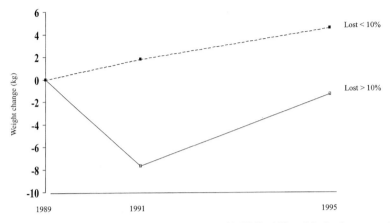

Fig. 1. Long-term weight pattern in 13,349 women with BMI of 22 to 25 who lost more than 10% of their original weight between 1989 and 1991 compared with those who did not. The same pattern was observed in thinner and heavier women.

The National Weight Control Registry

Perhaps the most impressive evidence that long-term weight maintenance is possible comes from the National Weight Control Registry (NWCR). The NWCR includes more than 3000 individuals who meet the eligibility criteria of having lost at least 10% of their initial body weight and kept it off for at least 1 year [9]. Registry members have been more successful than these minimum eligibility criteria; they have lost an average of 30 kg, reduced from a BMI of 35 to 25, and have kept the weight off for 5.5 years [10]. Thus, by any criteria one might use, registry participants have been clearly successful at long-term weight control. Although registry members are a self-selected sample, the similarities in the behaviors that they reported and the behaviors that were noted in a population-based sample of successful weight losers [7] increases our confidence in the representative nature of these individuals.

Findings from this registry provide encouragement to physicians and patients. Almost all (90%) of NWCR members had previously tried to lose weight without success. Thus, past failure does not mean that the individual cannot lose weight and maintain it successfully in their next attempt. NWCR members indicated that their current successful effort was distinguished from previous, unsuccessful attempts because it involved a greater commitment, stricter dieting, and a greater emphasis on exercise.

Also encouraging is the fact that almost half of NWCR subjects reported having been overweight as a child. Forty-six percent reported that one parent was overweight or obese and 27% report that both parents were overweight or obese [10]. Thus, neither childhood-onset obesity nor strong genetic predisposition to obesity precludes success.

NWCR members were asked about how they lost the weight and what they do now to maintain it. The approach to weight loss varied; 60% of

---

Box 2. Key strategies of successful weight-loss maintainers

Consume low-fat, low-calorie diet
Achieve high levels of physical activity
Weigh self frequently
Eat regular meals, including breakfast

---

women and 37% of men used some type of formal program for weight loss, but the remainder reported losing weight on their own. A triggering event often initiated the weight loss effort [10]. For approximately one third of the sample, the triggering event related to their own health (eg, being diagnosed with hypertension); therefore, physicians may be in an unique position to motivate patients to initiate weight loss efforts.

Changes in diet and exercise were reported almost universally by NWCR members (Box 2). When asked about their current diet, NWCR members report consuming 1381 kcal/day with 24% of calories from fat, 19% of calories from protein, and 56% of calories from carbohydrate (CHO). Although these figures may underestimate actual intake (as is often observed), it is clear that these individuals are following a low-calorie, low-fat eating style. Less than 1% of registry members reported eating a diet with less than 24% of carbohydrates, which is similar to the type of regimen recommended by Atkins (less than 90 g of CHO on a 1500 kcal diet would represent a 24% CHO diet) [9]. On average, registry members reported eating 4.7 meals or snacks per day. Almost 80% reported eating breakfast every day of the week [11]. Moreover, they continued to eat at restaurants 2.5 times per week and ate fast food 0.7 times per week.

Ninety-one percent of registry members reported engaging in regular physical activity as part of their weight loss maintenance routine; the level of activity reported was higher than expected. On average, registry members reported expending about 2700 kcal/week in physical activity [9]. Seventy-two percent of registry members expended more than 1000 kcal/week in physical activity; 52% expended more than 2000 kcal/week in activity. These activity levels represent about 60 to 90 minutes of moderate activity per day. Walking was an important part of the activity regimen that was described by the participants (76% report walking) but 20% reported cycling, 20% reported weight lifting, 18% reported aerobics, 10% reported running, and 9% reported stair climbing.

The long-term weight loss maintenance of NWCR members seems to require ongoing vigilance. Most (75%) NWCR members weigh themselves at least once per week. Moreover, they reported high levels of dietary re-straint, similar to levels reported by patients who have recently completed a weight loss program.

This ongoing vigilance and continued adherence to a low-fat, low-calorie diet and high exercise level should not be interpreted to mean that these individuals are obsessive, depressed, or experiencing symptoms of eating disorders. Rather, NWCR members reported marked improvements in the quality of their life since losing weight. More than 90% reported increased energy, mobility, general mood and self-confidence; overall quality of life wass considered to have improved by 95% of the sample.

Translating the research to clinical practice

These exciting new findings from the DPP and NWCR underscore the health benefits of weight loss and the possibility of long-term weight loss success. A common theme in both of these studies is a behavioral approach to weight loss. Elements from a behavioral approach can be easily adapted for use in primary care settings. Before discussing specific behavioral strategies that can be used in patient care, it is important to understand the theoretical underpinnings of the approach.

Overview

Behavioral treatment for obesity is based on a functional analysis, or A-B-C model, of behavior change. The goal of treatment is to produce weight loss by changing the behaviors (B) related to body weight, namely energy intake and physical activity, and by modifying environmental antecedents (A) and consequences (C) that influence these behaviors. Introduced in the late 1960s, early behavioral weight control programs were short (typically 10 weeks in length) and focused on moderately overweight patients. Patients were taught to monitor their eating and activity, but attention was directed at cues surrounding these behaviors (when and where they occurred) rather than on changing caloric balance. These early programs produced average weight losses of 3.8 kg [12,13]. Over time, the length of treatment has been extended, heavier patients with medical comorbidities have been treated, and more attention has been directed at decreasing caloric intake and increasing expenditure, with specific, more aggressive goals given for both behaviors. With these changes, average weight losses have increased substantially. State-of-the-art behavioral weight loss programs now produce average weight losses of 9.7 kg [14]. When restudied 1 year later, patients have retained approximately two-thirds of their initial weight loss.

Treatment format

Behavioral treatment for obesity is typically delivered to groups of 10 to 15 overweight individuals using a closed-group format (all patients begin the group at the same time and progress throughout treatment together). Patients often express a preference for individual counseling; however, a group format produces greater weight losses, regardless of stated preference [15], and is more cost effective. For the first 6 months of treatment, groups are typically held once a week for approximately 60 to 90 minutes. This initial phase is often followed by an additional 6 to 12 months' of bi-monthly or monthly maintenance meetings. Lengthening the treatment from 20 to 40 weeks and continuing to see participants monthly during follow-up have been shown to improve treatment outcome [16,17]. Treatment is typically conducted by multidisciplinary teams of health care professionals with training in nutrition, exercise physiology, or behavioral psychology.

Before the start of each session, a brief weight check-in is conducted with each patient individually. Group time is devoted to reviewing homework assignments from the previous week, discussing problems and barriers encountered by patients, and generating solutions to these problems. New material is presented in a lecture-discussion format, with a presentation by group leaders and opportunity for discussion of the topic by group members.

Treatment goals

Patients who enter weight loss treatment often want to lose 30% or more of their initial body weight [18]. Current programs are not able to achieve such large weight losses, and if achieved, maintenance is often poor. Moreover, as found in DPP and other randomized controlled trials, more modest weight losses can produce significant health benefits, including improvements in blood sugar control, blood pressure, and cholesterol levels [2–4]. Therefore, patients should be encouraged to aim for a 10% weight loss at a rate of approximately 1 kg per week. To achieve these goals, behavioral weight control treatment focuses on decreasing caloric intake by 500 to 1000 kcal/day and increasing physical activity (Table 1).

Dietary recommendations

Patients in behavioral weight control programs are prescribed a daily caloric intake goal, typically 1200 to 1500 kcal/day for individuals who weigh less than 200 pounds and 1500 to 1800 kcal/day for individuals who weigh more than 200 pounds. These caloric guidelines should produce daily deficits of 500 to 1000 calories and corresponding weight losses of .5–1 kg (1–2 pounds) per week. Caloric goals can subsequently be adjusted up or down if weight losses do not approximate these rates.

Most behavioral programs also recommend a dietary fat goal that is designed to produce a 20% or 25% fat diet (eg, if the patient is consuming

Table 1
Standard dietary and physical activity recommendations

	Daily caloric intake	Daily fat intake	Weekly physical activity
If patient weighs:			
Less than 200 pounds	1200–1500 kcals	27–33 grams	150 minutes
More than 200 pounds	1500–1800 kcals	33–40 grams	150 minutes

1500 kcal/day, they would be given a fat goal of 33 to 42 g/day). Restricting fat is considered important because fat has 9 calories/gram whereas protein and carbohydrates have 4 calories/gram. Thus, it is easy to overeat when consuming a high-fat diet. Previous studies that compared low-fat ad libitum diets, low-calorie diets, or the combination suggested that the combination produced the best long-term weight losses [19,20]. Such diets should also help to lower cholesterol levels and are consistent with the American Heart Association recommendations. Further, National Weight Control Registry members reported consuming 24% of their calories from fat, compared with 36% that was reported by average American adults.

During the 1980s, there was a great deal of interest in very low calorie diets (VLCDs). VLCDs are diets of approximately 400 kcal/day, consumed as liquid formula or lean meat, fish, and fowl ("protein-sparing modified fasts") [21,22]. These diets were found to be well-tolerated by patients and produced 20 kg weight losses over 12 weeks. Despite combining these diets with behavior modification approaches and providing extensive, ongoing contact, maintenance of these weight losses was poor [21,23–26]. At 1-year follow-up, patients typically had regained significant amounts of weight and returned to levels comparable to those achieved with low calorie diets of 1200 to 1800 kcal/day. Because of this finding and the medical monitoring that is required with 400 kcal/day diets, they are no longer commonly used.

Strategies to improve adherence to dietary recommendations

Providing structure to patients on the types and amounts of food that they should eat seems to promote adherence to dietary recommendations (Table 2). One approach to creating such structure is to provide patients with the foods that they should be eating. The other approach is to use portion-controlled foods (eg, Slimfast, Lean Cuisine) for 1 or 2 meals per day. In two studies, patients were given a 1200 to 1500 kcal/day goal as part of a behavioral treatment program and were asked to self-select the food items they desired within this goal or to consume the foods that met this dietary goal that were specifically provided to them by the study [27,28]. Providing patients with the foods that they should eat increased weight losses at 12 months (9.1 kg versus 4.5 kg) and 18 months (6.4 versus 4.1 kg). Similar positive effects were achieved in other studies with food provision [29] and through the use of specific meal plans and grocery lists [28]. Similarly, the use of Slimfast for 2 meals/day was shown to promote initial weight loss; using 1 Slimfast/day may improve the maintenance of weight loss [30]. Wadden, et al [31] used a 900 kcal/day diet, in which patients were instructed to consume four daily servings of liquid meal replacement with a shelf-stable dinner entrée and salad. This diet, used as one component of a behavioral weight loss program, was associated with weight losses of 16.5 kg at 6 months. Thus, these approaches that provide structure to patients on the types of foods that they should be eating and the appropriate portion

Table 2
Specific strategies to improve dietary adherence

If patient reports:	Some suggestions to improve adherence
Boredom with diet	Emphasize portion control, rather than limiting types of food Try new recipes Encourage increased variety in fruit and vegetable consumption
Lack of structure in food choices	Provide meal plans or grocery lists as guidance Promote use of portion-controlled food choices
Excessive restaurant eating	Counsel patients on high calorie content of large portion sizes Provide patients list of better restaurant choices and menu selections within restaurants Teach patient assertiveness skills to ask for menu modifications
Tempted by high-fat and high-calorie foods at home	Have patient change their environments to support better food selections, for example, keep high calorie snacks in paper bag, out of sight and display fruits and vegetables in prominent location
Not achieving weight loss	Review accuracy of self-monitoring (consider portion sizes; items omitted) Promote use of portion-controlled food choices Decrease the prescribed calorie and fat goals

sizes to consume, may be helpful in increasing the magnitude of weight loss that is achieved.

A common barrier to dietary adherence is boredom [32]. This is an interesting concern, because, in truth, weight loss can be produced by continuing to eat the same foods one did before, but limiting the portion sizes. To address boredom, patients can be encouraged to experiment with new and varied ways of preparing low-fat, healthy foods, such as chicken. In an early study, Nowalk and colleagues [33] showed that having patients taste sample foods that are prepared in new ways and giving them copies of the recipe maximized the chance that they would try the new foods. Encouraging patients to increase the variety of fruits and vegetables, but decrease the variety in high-fat items (eg, desserts) should be most effective in promoting long-term weight loss [34].

Restaurants and dining out frequently are often cited as other barriers to weight loss. Portion sizes have become increasingly large; patients should be encouraged to share their entrées with others in their group or to save part for a subsequent meal. It is also important for patients to recognize that "super-sizing" may be a good deal financially, but is a bad caloric decision [35]. Assertiveness techniques, which help patients learn to be able to request specific food items and methods of preparation, can also be important.

Exercise recommendations

The other side of the energy balance equation is physical activity. The standard exercise prescription in behavioral weight loss treatment, which is consistent with public health guidelines, is for overweight patients to engage in 150 minutes of moderate intensity exercise per week. Moderate intensity exercise is akin to brisk walking; 150 minutes per week equates to approximately 1000 kcals of energy expenditure (walking 1 mile equals 100 calories and takes approximately 15 minutes).

Although this level of physical activity is sufficient to produce health benefits, such as improvements in cardiorespiratory fitness, a convergence of empirical evidence suggests that a higher level of exercise is more conducive to weight loss and maintenance. In a recent, randomized, controlled trial [36], the greatest weight losses (mean 13 kg) at 18 months were observed in patients who exercised 200 minutes per week, compared with weight losses of 6.5 kg in patients who exercised 150 to 200 minutes per week, and 3.5 kg in patients who exercised less than 150 minutes per week. A similar post-hoc analysis of another weight loss intervention found the greatest weight loss (7.6 kg) in individuals in the top quartile of physical activity (average 2550 kcals/wk) with no differences in weight loss (3.0 to 4.8 kg) between individuals in the bottom three quartiles (250 to 1300 kcals/wk) [37]. A high level of physical activity also seems important to long-term weight maintenance. Participants in the NWCR reported an average of 2800 kcals of physical activity per week [9].

Based on these observations, Jeffery et al [38] conducted a randomized, controlled trial that examined whether a high level of physical activity (2500 kcals/wk) produced better weight losses than the standard recommendations (1000 kcals/wk). Although initial weight losses were similar across groups, individuals with high physical activity achieved greater weight losses at 18 months (6.7 kg) than individuals in standard treatment (4.1 kg). Together with the post-hoc data from previous trials and reports from the NWCR, the results of this study strongly suggest that exercise prescriptions in behavioral weight loss treatments should be higher (ie, 2000–2500 kcal/wk or approximately 60 min/day).

Strategies to improve adherence to physical activity recommendations

Regardless of the specific energy expenditure goal, a major challenge to health professionals is helping patients adopt and maintain an exercise program (Table 3). Several barriers to becoming physically active are reported by patients; the most common is lack of time. With competing demands of work and family life, patients often state that it is not feasible to devote 30 minutes or more per day to exercise. A positive message to share with patients who face this issue is that exercise can be accumulated in 10 minute bouts throughout the day (eg, four 10-minute bouts for a total of 40 minutes) with the same weight loss benefits as one continuous bout of equal duration. The

Table 3
Specific strategies to improve exercise adherence

If patient reports:	Suggestions to improve adherence:
Lack of time to exercise	Break exercise into short bouts of 10 minutes throughout the day Incorporate more lifestyle activity into daily routine, for example, park further away from work to increase walking
No access to exercise equipment	Emphasize brisk walking as the primary mode of exercise
Weather prohibits outdoor activity	Advise patients to keep aerobic exercise tapes at home Walk at malls
Too tired at the end of the day to exercise	Exercise in the morning Lay out exercise clothes and shoes as visual cues in evening to exercise Find an exercise partner to help with motivation
Doesn't like to exercise	Identify new types of activity that the patient might try Increase social aspects of exercise by joining a gym

strategy of using short bouts, also referred to as intermittent exercise, was shown to improve initial adherence to exercise in behavioral weight loss treatment, with no negative impact on long-term weight loss or fitness results [36,39].

Another barrier that is commonly reported by patients is lack of access to a supervised exercise setting (eg, aerobics classes, personal trainer). For these individuals, it is important to acknowledge that although a supervised setting does have some benefits, research indicates that home-based exercise is at least as effective in promoting long-term weight loss [40–42]. Patients should be counseled that the setting of the exercise is not crucial, rather the key is initiating and maintaining an exercise program long-term. To facilitate adoption of such a program, patients should be advised that the amount of exercise equipment in the home is positively correlated with activity level. Moreover, in a randomized controlled trial, better exercise adherence and weight losses were observed at 18 months in women who were provided a treadmill for use at home compared with women who were given the same exercise prescription but who were not provided a treadmill [36]. Lack of access to a supervised setting should not be a barrier to adoption of physical activity; patients should be informed that keeping more exercise equipment in their homes may facilitate weight loss.

Behavioral strategies

Several behavioral modification strategies are taught to patients to increase their adherence to the dietary and exercise recommendations. These strategies are described below:

DATE: Tuesday, 3/21/00

TIME	FOOD OR BEVERAGE	CAL.	FAT
8a	4 oz. orange jc.	60	0
"	3/4 c special'K cereal	80	0
"	4 oz skim milk	45	.5
"	8 oz coffee	0	0
	TOTAL	185	.5
12p	Lean Cuisine	270	7
	vegetable lasagna		
	frozen entrée		
"	10 grapes	50	0
"	12J oz diet coke	0	0
	TOTAL	505	7.5
4p	6 animal crackers	50	1.5
	TOTAL	555	9
6³⁰p	4 oz. skinless chick brst	190	4
"	1/2 c cooked rice	90	0
"	1/2 c mixed vegetables	60	0
"	1/2 tsp margarine	20	2.0
"	salad	0	0
"	vinegar - balsamic	0	0
	TOTAL	915	15
8p	1/2 c jello instant red.cal	80	0
	choc fudge pudding prep.		
	w/ skim milk — TOTAL CALORIES AND FAT	995	15

Fig. 2. Sample food diary.

Keeping track of progress

The cornerstone of the behavioral approach to weight loss is self-monitoring, or teaching individuals to observe and record their eating and exercise behaviors. A sample entry from a self-monitoring diary is shown in Fig. 2.

Self-monitoring involves recording the type and amount of food eaten, the number of calories and fat grams consumed, and the type and amount of physical activity that is engaged in each day. For the initial 6 months of treatment, patients are instructed to self-monitor their behaviors every day. During maintenance, the frequency of self-monitoring is usually decreased (eg, 3 days of every week, or 1 week during the month). Throughout the course of treatment, therapists provide written feedback on completed diaries, focusing on what the patient is doing well and what the patient can improve upon. There is significant empirical support for the use of self-monitoring in behavioral treatment for obesity; the greatest weight loss is observed in individuals who are the most consistent in their recording [43].

Modifying the environment

In the A-B-C model, emphasis is placed on modifying environmental antecedents or cues to eating and exercise [44]. If a patient is surrounded by cues for overeating or inactivity (eg, cookie jar on the countertop), then long-term success is unlikely. In contrast, if the patient is surrounded by cues that promote healthy eating and activity (eg, fruit bowl on the countertop, sneakers displayed in prominent location), then positive behavior change is more likely to occur. Patients in behavioral weight control treatment are taught how to modify their environment to improve their weight loss outcomes. These stimulus control techniques can be applied to any environment, including the home and workplace.

Navigating social settings

Because eating and exercise does not occur in a vacuum but within a larger social context, it is important for patients to enlist the support of family and friends in the weight loss process. Specifically, patients are taught how to communicate their needs about eating and exercise in a clear and effective manner. These assertiveness skills can be used in many situations, from asking a family member to help with household chores so that a 30-minute walk is possible to asking for a lower-fat substitution at a restaurant. Recruiting patients with their friends and family and working to increase intragroup support and healthy intergroup competition has been shown to promote maintenance of weight loss [45].

Overcoming barriers

Throughout treatment, patients face barriers that limit their potential for long-term weight loss success. To overcome these barriers, patients are taught a core set of problem-solving skills that can be applied to a variety of situations. The 5-step problem-solving process includes: (1) clearly defining the problem; (2) generating several possible solutions; (3) evaluating the solutions and selecting one to implement; (4) implementing the selected solution; and (5) evaluating the outcome and implementing a new solution if necessary [46]. There is time during the individual check-ins and during the group for problem-solving skills to be reviewed.

Managing negative thinking

A common type of barrier that is faced during weight loss is negative thinking. Maladaptive thoughts about eating and exercise, such as "I blew my diet at lunch, I might as well forget the rest of the day and start again tomorrow," and "If I can't get a full 30-minute walk in today, it is not worth it," make positive behavior change difficult. Patients in behavioral weight control treatment are taught cognitive restructuring skills to change negative

Table 4
Managing negative thinking

Common negative thoughts	More positive alternatives
"I overdid it at lunch, I might as well forget the rest of the day and start again tomorrow."	"Every meal counts. I will make better choices the rest of the day."
"I can't do my standard 2-mile walk today so I am not going to go at all."	"Although I'd like to exercise more, I will start with a 10 minute-bout right now and see if I can get more exercise in later."
"I've had a stressful day. I deserve a piece of cake."	"The cake might taste good but it will not make me feel better about the day. I am going to take a hot bath instead to relax."
"I didn't lose any weight this week. Why do I even bother trying?"	"Although I'm not at my goal weight yet, I feel much better about myself for taking these positive steps. I am confident the scale will move if I stick with my diet and exercise plan."

thoughts to more realistic ones. After learning about the common types of negative thinking that occur during weight loss (Table 4), patients identify the specific negative thoughts that they are having that might interfere with their progress. Patients are taught how to challenge these thoughts and substitute them with more realistic or neutral ones.

Planning for slips and lapses

A final step in behavioral weight control treatment is preparing patients to deal with the inevitable slips and lapses that will occur over time. Drawing on Marlatt and Gordon's [47] addiction work, patients are taught to anticipate future high-risk situations and have a plan in place for dealing with these challenges. Emphasis is not placed on avoiding slips entirely, which is unrealistic, but on getting back on track quickly to avoid a major lapse.

Summary

With more than 50% of American adults overweight or obese, primary care physicians should play an active role in helping overweight patients lose weight. Modest weight losses of as little as 7% to 10% can produce significant health benefits, such as preventing the development of diabetes. To help individuals achieve this weight loss, behavior change strategies should be emphasized with all overweight patients. Changes in diet and exercise can produce long-term weight loss with tremendous positive impact. Primary care physicians are well positioned to support these behavior changes in their overweight patients.

References

[1] NHLBI. Clinical guidelines on the identification, evaluation, and treatment of overweight and obesity in adults-The evidence report. Obes Res 1998;6(S2):51S–210.

[2] Whelton PK, Appel LJ, Espeland MA, et al. Sodium reduction and weight loss in the treatment of hypertension in older persons: a randomized controlled trial of non-pharmacologic interventions in the elderly (TONE). JAMA 1998;279(11):839–46.

[3] Wing RR, Koeske R, Epstein LH, et al. Long-term effects of modest weight loss in type II diabetic patients. Arch Intern Med 1987;147:1749–53.

[4] Diabetes Prevention Program Research Group. Reduction in the incidence of type 2 diabetes with lifestyle intervention or Metformin. N Engl J Med 2002;346:393–403.

[5] Stunkard AJ, McLaren-Hume M. The results of treatment for obesity. Arch Intern Med 1959;103:79–85.

[6] McGuire M, Wing R, Hill J. The prevalence of weight loss maintenance among American adults. Int J Obes 1999;23:1314–9.

[7] McGuire MT, Wing RR, Klem ML, et al. Behavioral strategies of individuals who have maintained long-term weight losses. Obes Res 1999;7(4):334–41.

[8] Field AE, Wing RR, Manson JE, et al. Relationship of a large weight loss to long-term weight change among young and middle-aged US women. Int J Obes Relat Metab Disord 2001;25(8):1113–21.

[9] Wing RR, Hill JO. Successful weight loss maintenance. Annu Rev Nutr 2001;21: 323–41.

[10] Klem ML, Wing RR, McGuire MT, et al. A descriptive study of individuals successful at long-term maintenance of substantial weight loss. Am J Clin Nutr 1997;66:239–46.

[11] Wyatt HR, Grunwald GK, Mosca CL, et al. Long-term weight loss and breakfast in subjects in the National Weight Control Registry. Obes Res 2002;10(2):78–82.

[12] Brownell KD, Jeffery RW. Improving long-term weight loss: pushing the limits of treatment. Behavior Therapy 1987;18:353–74.

[13] Wadden TA. The treatment of obesity: an overview. In: Stunkard AJ, Wadden TA, editors. Obesity: theory and therapy, vol 2. New York: Raven Press Ltd.; 1993. p. 197–218.

[14] Wing RR. Behavioral approaches to the treatment of obesity. In: Bray G, Bouchard C, James P, editors. Handbook of obesity. New York: Marcel Dekker Inc.; 1998. p. 855–73.

[15] Renjilian DA, Perri MG, Nezu AM, et al. Individual versus group therapy for obesity: effects of matching participants to their treatment preferences. J Consult Clin Psychol 2001;69(4):717–21.

[16] Perri MG, Nezu AM, Patti ET, et al. Effect of length of treatment on weight loss. J Consult Clin Psychol 1989;57(3):450–2.

[17] Perri MG, Sears SF, Clark JE. Strategies for improving maintenance of weight loss: toward a continuous care model of obesity management. Diabetes Care 1994;16(1):200–10.

[18] Foster GD, Wadden TA, Vogt RA, et al. What is a reasonable weight loss? Patients' expectations and evaluations of obesity treatment outcomes. J Consult Clin Psychol 1997; 65(1):79–85.

[19] Jeffery RW, Hellerstedt WL, French SA, et al. A randomized trial of counseling for fat restriction versus calorie restriction in the treatment of obesity. Int J Obes 1995;19: 132–7.

[20] Pascale RW, Wing RR, Butler BA, et al. Effects of a behavioral weight loss program stressing calorie restriction versus calorie plus fat restriction in obese individuals with NIDDM or a family history of diabetes. Diabetes Care 1995;18(9):1241–8.

[21] Wadden TA, Stunkard AJ. Controlled trial of very low calorie diet, behavior therapy, and their combination in the treatment of obesity. J Consult Clin Psychol 1986;54:482–8.

[22] National Task Force on the Prevention and Treatment of Obesity. Very low-calorie diets. JAMA 1993;270(8):967–74.

[23] Wadden TA, Sternberg JA, Letizia KA, et al. Treatment of obesity by very low calorie diet, behaviour therapy, and their combination: a five-year perspective. Int J Obes 1989;13: 39–46.

[24] Wadden TA, Foster GD, Letizia KA. One-year behavioral treatment of obesity: comparison of moderate and severe caloric restriction and the effects of weight maintenance therapy. J Consult Clin Psychol 1994;62:165–71.

[25] Wing RR, Marcus MD, Salata R, et al. Effects of a very-low-calorie diet on long-term glycemic control in obese type 2 diabetic subjects. Arch Intern Med 1991;151:1334–40.

[26] Wing RR, Blair E, Marcus M, et al. Year-long weight loss treatment for obese patients with Type II diabetes: does inclusion of an intermittent very low calorie diet improve outcome? Am J Med 1994;97:354–62.

[27] Jeffery RW, Wing RR, Thorson C, et al. Strengthening behavioral interventions for weight loss: a randomized trial of food provision and monetary incentives. J Consult Clin Psychol 1993;61:1038–45.

[28] Wing RR, Jeffery RW, Burton LR, et al. Food provision vs. structured meal plans in the behavioral treatment of obesity. Int J Obes 1996;20:56–62.

[29] Metz JA, Kris-Etherton PM, Morris CD, et al. Dietary compliance and cardiovascular risk reduction with a prepared meal plan compared to a self-selected diet. Am J Clin Nutr 1997; 66:373–85.

[30] Ditschuneit HH, Flechtner-Mors M, Johnson TD, et al. Metabolic and weight-loss effects of a long-term dietary intervention in obese patients. Am J Clin Nutr 1999;69:198–204.

[31] Wadden TA, Vogt RA, Andersen RE, et al. Exercise in the treatment of obesity: effects of four interventions on body composition, resting energy expenditure, appetite, and mood. J Consult Clin Psychol 1997;65:269–77.

[32] Smith C, Wing R, Burke L. Vegetarian and weight loss diets among young adults. Obes Res 2000;8(2):123–9.

[33] Nowalk MP, Wing RR, Koeske R. The effect of tasting food samples on the use of recipes distributed in nutrition counseling. Am Dietetic Assoc 1986;86:1715–6.

[34] McCrory M, Fuss P, McCallum J, et al. Dietary variety within food groups: association with energy intake and body fatness in men and women. Am J Clin Nutr 1999;69:440–7.

[35] Young LR, Nestle M. The contribution of expanding portion sizes to the US obesity epidemic. Am J Public Health 2002;92(2):246–9.

[36] Jakicic J, Wing R, Winters C. Effects of intermittent exercise and use of home exercise equipment on adherence, weight loss, and fitness in overweight women. JAMA 1999; 282(16):1554–60.

[37] Jeffery RW, Wing RR, Thorson C, et al. Use of personal trainers and financial incentives to increase exercise in a behavioral weight-loss program. J Consult Clin Psychol 1998; 66:777–83.

[38] Jeffery RW, Wing RR. The effects of an enhanced exercise program on long-term weight loss. Obes Res 2001;9(Suppl 3):100S.

[39] Jakicic JM, Wing RR, Butler BA, et al. Prescribing exercise in multiple short bouts versus one continuous bout: effects on adherence, cardiorespiratory fitness, and weight loss in overweight women. Int J Obes 1995;19:893–901.

[40] Dunn AL, Marcus BH, Kampert JB, et al. Comparison of lifestyle and structured interventions to increase physical activity and cardiorespiratory fitness: a randomized trial. JAMA 1999;281:327–34.

[41] Andersen R, Frankowiak S, Snyder J, et al. Effects of lifestyle activity vs. structured aerobic exercise in obese women: a randomized trial. JAMA 1998;281(4):335–40.

[42] Perri MG, Martin AD, Leermakers EA, et al. Effects of group- versus home-based exercise in the treatment of obesity. J Consult Clin Psychol 1997;65:278–85.

[43] Baker RC, Kirschenbaum DS. Self-monitoring may be necessary for successful weight control. Behav Ther 1993;24:377–94.

[44] Stuart RB. Behavioral control of overeating. Behav Res Ther 1967;5:357–65.

[45] Wing RR, Jeffery RW. Benefits of recruiting participants with friends and increasing social support for weight loss maintenance. J Consult Clin Psychol 1999;67(1):132–8.

[46] D'Zurilla TJ, Goldfried MR. Problem solving and behavior modification. J Abnorm Psychol 1971;78:107–26.

[47] Marlatt GA, Gordon JR. Relapse prevention: maintenance strategies in addictive behavior change. New York: Guilford; 1985.

12

Exercise Strategies for the Obese Patient

John M. Jakicic

It has been suggested that exercise is a behavior that is critically important for the management of body weight. The role of exercise may be important for initial weight loss [1], prevention of weight regain [2–4], and prevention of initial weight gain [5,6]. Although each of these areas is uniquely important, the impact of exercise during each of these phases of weight management may vary. The dose and mode of exercise also may have differential effects on weight loss and factors that contribute to weight control. Although exercise is important for weight control, the benefits of exercise can be realized only if patients adopt and maintain adequate levels of exercise. Effective strategies for adoption and maintenance of exercise ultimately must be developed and implemented.

The role of exercise in weight loss and the prevention of weight regain

It has been suggested that the combination of changes in both diet and exercise behaviors is most effective for initial weight loss [1]. In short-term studies that are typically less than 6 months in duration, the effect of exercise on weight loss is somewhat controversial. Data from intervention trials have shown that exercise alone has minimal impact on weight loss, with most weight loss resulting from changes in energy intake. For example, Hagan et al [7] have shown that weight loss in men after 12 weeks of treatment was 0.3%, 8.4%, and 11.4% resulting from exercise alone, diet alone, and diet plus exercise, respectively. For women, these interventions resulted in reductions in body weight of 0.6%, 5.5%, and 7.5%, respectively. This pattern of results has been reported by other investigators [8] and suggests that the combination of both diet and exercise is most effective for initial weight loss.

Despite these findings, it has been suggested that exercise can be as effective as diet provided that the dose of exercise is sufficient to provide an adequate energy deficit. For example, Ross et al [9] have reported that across a period of 3 months, a 700-kcal/d (2930 kJ/d) deficit from diet or exercise resulted in weight loss of 7.4 kg or 7.6 kg, respectively. Although these results are promising and support the use of exercise without modifications to diet for weight loss, the amount of exercise necessary to elicit an energy deficit of 700 kcal/d is substantial (approximately 7 miles of brisk walking per day). Because this level of exercise may be unrealistic for most overweight individuals, the combination of changes in both energy intake (diet) and energy expenditure (exercise) seems to be the most appropriate approach for initial weight loss.

Exercise may play a much more important role in long-term weight loss and the prevention of weight regain after initial weight loss. The literature review conducted by Pronk and Wing [10] concluded that exercise is one of the best predictors of long-term weight loss. Evidence to support this conclusion can be drawn from the National Weight Control Registry. In this registry of individuals who have lost a minimum of 30 pounds and have maintained this weight loss for at least 1 year, 89% of individuals reported participating in both exercise and dietary modification to maintain their weight loss [3]. In a 1-year follow-up study, McGuire et al [4] reported that individuals in the National Weight Control Registry who maintained their exercise maintained their weight loss, whereas those individuals who decreased their exercise showed increases in body weight.

The role of exercise in the primary prevention of weight gain

Although exercise may be an important component of interventions for weight loss, there is also a growing body of literature to support the role of exercise in the prevention of weight gain. Initial data to support this concept come from observational data across subjects in various age groups. Data from the National Health Interview Survey and the Behavioral Risk Factor Surveillance System demonstrate that the percent of adults meeting the minimal public health recommendation for physical activity (30 minutes of moderate-intensity activity on most days of the week) decreases from young adulthood (18–29 years of age) to middle age (45–64 years of age) [11]. In comparison, there is an increase in the prevalence of obesity in adults across these same age groups [12,13]. As obesity increases with age, there seems to be a corresponding decrease in physical activity, and this decrease in activity may contribute partially to the increase in body weight.

There is additional evidence to support the relationship between physical activity and weight gain in adults. For men in the National Health and Nutrition Examination Survey I follow-up study (1971–1975 to 1982–1984), the relative odds of gaining 8.1 to 13.0 kg increased to 2.0 and 3.9 for those reporting moderate or low levels of physical activity at both assessments compared with those reporting high levels of physical activity [6]. For women, the relative odds of gaining more than 13.0 kg were 3.4 if moderate activity was reported at both assessments and 7.1 if low levels of activity were reported at both assessment periods [6]. Data from the Pound of Prevention Study showed that body weight for women was lower by 0.10 kg for each additional moderate-intensity exercise session per week and by 0.15 kg for each high-intensity exercise session per week [5]. This effect also was demonstrated in men, with body weight being 0.54 kg lower for each additional high-intensity exercise session per week [5]. Encouraging adults to engage in adequate levels of exercise may be important for prevention of weight gain.

It may be important to engage in exercise that sufficiently increases cardiorespiratory fitness to elicit the desired outcomes relative to prevention of weight gain. Data from the Aerobics Center Longitudinal Study have demonstrated that a 1-minute increase during a graded exercise test for assessing cardiorespiratory fitness reduces weight gain by approximately 0.6 kg in both men and women [14]. With this level of improvement in fitness, the odds of gaining greater than or equal to 5 kg or greater than or equal to 10 kg were reduced by 9% to 14% and 21%, respectively, in both men and women.

The health impact of exercise independent of body weight

Exercise participation may have important impacts on health-related outcomes independent of the effect of exercise on body weight. Interesting and compelling findings to support this concept have been published by Barlow et al [15], Lee et al [16], and Wei et al [17] from data collected at the Cooper Center for Aerobics Research. Wei et al [17] reported that the relative risk of cardiovascular disease was 3.1 for unfit compared with fit individuals who were of normal body weight. The relative risk of cardiovascular disease in unfit individuals increased to 4.5 and 5.0 for overweight and obese individuals, respectively. These findings suggest that clinicians should promote participation in exercise that results in an improvement in cardiorespiratory fitness regardless of the impact of this level of exercise on changes in body weight and regardless of initial body weight of patients.

Clinical exercise-prescription considerations

As demonstrated, exercise should be included within clinical programs for the prevention and treatment of overweight and obesity. To prescribe an appropriate exercise program for individuals in a clinical setting, physicians and health practitioners need to consider a number of factors in a systematic manner. These factors include assessment (what is the current level of exercise), prescription (what level and what type of exercise are recommended), and compliance (how to address factors that may influence adoption and maintenance of exercise).

Assessment of patient before making exercise recommendations

When making exercise recommendations to patients, it is important to consider their current activity level, the level of medical clearance that may be necessary before engaging in an exercise program, and factors that may impact adoption and maintenance of an exercise program. Each of these issues is addressed briefly below.

Assessing current activity level

Information related to a patient's current activity level may prove to be extremely valuable to the clinician who is making exercise recommendations. A clinician can adequately assess this information by asking simple yet important questions that include the following:

1. *"Do you participate in physical activity similar to brisk walking for at least 10 continuous minutes on a regular basis?"* It has been shown that physical activity that is of the same intensity as brisk walking can have significant health benefits if done regularly and in adequate duration. It is important for the clinician to anchor this intensity of activity so that the patient clearly understands the type of information that the clinician is seeking. It may be important for clinicians to describe brisk walking as walking that is done at the same speed that a person would walk at when he or she is late for an important meeting or engagement. The concept of 10 continuous minutes helps the patient identify periods of purposeful and meaningful activity that can have a health benefit.

2. *"When you participate in activities similar to brisk walking, on how many days per week do you accumulate at least 30 minutes of this type of activity?"* It is important that patients eventually participate in at least 30 minutes of moderate-intensity activity on 5 or more days per week. Knowledge about these parameters allows the clinician to set clear, achievable, and progressive goals with the patient. For example, for an individual who is somewhat active, it will be important to discuss issues related to increasing further his or her level of activity. For individuals who are extremely inactive, however, the first step is to engage the patient in some level of activity while working to overcome the barriers that have prevented prior participation in physical activity.

3. *"What type of physical activity do you currently participate in or enjoy doing?"* Acquiring this information is important for numerous reasons. First, it provides information related to the patient's perception of the types of activity that he or she believes is similar to brisk walking. This information may indicate that the patient needs further counseling related to activities that are most appropriate and provide adequate

health and weight-loss benefits. Knowing the types of activity that the patient finds enjoyable is invaluable. It is important to include these forms of activity in the physical activity recommendations that are made to the patient. It is likely that compliance may be enhanced when the patient is permitted to participate in an activity that he or she reports enjoying.

4. *"What are the most common barriers that you face that affect your ability to be physically active or to participate in regular exercise?"* When discussing exercise with a patient, this component is one of the most important yet overlooked areas that can be addressed. Simply prescribing exercise may not be adequate if there are barriers that prohibit participation in this level or type of activity. For example, simply telling a patient to take a brisk walk around his or her neighborhood may be ineffective if he or she lives in a neighborhood that is unsafe because of traffic patterns, lack of sidewalks, or crime. Knowing this information would most likely allow the clinician to work with the patient to develop an activity program that presents the fewest barriers, which may maximize compliance.

Medical clearance before exercise

Moderate-intensity physical activity is relatively safe for most individuals if appropriately screened and provided that the exercise is progressed in a reasonable manner. The American College of Sports Medicine [18] has established guidelines for when more extensive medical screening, including exercise testing, is necessary before beginning an exercise program. This additional screening is typically necessary when the individual has multiple risk factors or medical conditions (eg, diabetes, previous heart disease, and so forth) that increase the risk associated with exercise participation. It is recommended that clinicians become familiar with these guidelines to reduce unnecessary screening procedures of relatively healthy patients while ensuring the safety of higher-risk patients.

Barriers to exercise participation

As indicated previously, it is important for the clinician to understand that the barriers of individual patients affect their ability to adequately participate in physical activity and regular exercise. These barriers can vary from work-related barriers, to personal barriers, to environmental barriers. Consideration of these factors can make a significant difference between having a patient who is successful or not successful when adopting and maintaining the exercise program. A standard exercise prescription can have differential effects on patients depending on these barriers. Ultimately, exercise adoption and maintenance is based on the ability to overcome current barriers and plan for future barriers, regardless of the nature of the specific barrier. The role of the clinician is to assist patients in addressing these issues.

Exercise-prescription considerations

Exercise volume

There is overwhelming evidence that exercise is beneficial for improving health and that it can impact body weight significantly. These benefits may be realized only if adequate levels of exercise are adopted and maintained, however. Current public health recommendations are for individuals to participate in a minimum of 30 minutes of moderate-intensity activity on most, preferably all, days of the week [19]. This recommendation typically is interpreted as participation in a minimum of 150 minutes of moderate-intensity physical activity per week. Although there is evidence to support this recommendation when considering changes in risk factors for many chronic diseases, the scientific evidence seems to indicate that a higher level of exercise is necessary to enhance and maintain long-term weight loss. The scientific evidence available to date suggests that approximately 300 minutes per week or 2000 to 2500 kcal/d (8372–10465 kJ/d) of exercise may be necessary to improve long-term weight loss in previously overweight adults [2,3,20].

Although it is important to strive for this higher level of exercise, initial exercise goals may need to be somewhat less aggressive. For example, because it seems that significant improvements in health can be achieved with an amount of exercise equivalent to 150 minutes per week, it may be important to initially progress individuals to this exercise goal. Once this goal is achieved and maintained, it then may be beneficial to work with overweight patients to achieve a goal closer to 300 minutes per week of exercise. Individuals should be encouraged to engage in moderate-intensity exercise at least 5 days per week while gradually increasing the duration of exercise performed each day.

Exercise intensity

Current public health recommendations are for individuals to engage in adequate levels of moderate-intensity physical activity to elicit health benefits. Moderate-intensity physical activity typically is described as activity that is similar to brisk walking. Although more vigorous-intensity physical activity may result in greater improvements in physical fitness, vigorous-intensity physical activity may not be more effective than moderate-intensity physical activity when energy expenditure is equated. For example, Duncan et al [21] examined overweight adult women and randomly assigned them to different intensities of exercise based on walking speed (strollers, brisk walkers, or aerobic walkers) but varied the duration of the exercise sessions to equate energy expenditure across the groups. Results after 24 weeks of treatment showed no significant difference in change in percent body fat among the exercise groups, with changes varying from 4% to 6%. Energy expenditure rather than exercise intensity seems to be important for weight control. Because of the association between physical fitness and health, however, patients should be encouraged to exercise at a level to elicit optimal changes in physical fitness along with optimal levels of energy expenditure.

Exercise mode

It is also important to consider different modes of activity that can be beneficial for the treatment of obesity. Aerobic forms of exercise have been the most commonly studied modes of exercise for the management of body weight. Aerobic exercise can significantly increase total energy expenditure while also affecting risk factors for chronic diseases such as heart disease and diabetes. Walking seems to be one of the most popular forms of aerobic exercise [11]. A recent behavioral weight-loss study conducted by Jakicic et al [2] showed that walking was selected for approximately 75% of the exercise sessions during the initial 6 months of treatment. Because walking is a weight-bearing activity, it may be difficult for some obese individuals because of the added stress placed on the lower extremities. In these situations, non–weight-bearing forms of exercise, such as stationary cycling, may be recommended, and this form of exercise has been shown to be effective for reducing body weight. Selection of an appropriate form of aerobic exercise should be based on factors related to the individual client that may include physical limitations, patient enjoyment, and access to the selected exercise.

During periods of energy intake restriction and weight loss, lean body mass and resting energy expenditure typically are reduced. Because lean body mass is associated with resting energy expenditure, it could be hypothesized that maintaining or increasing lean body mass during weight loss could result in the maintenance or increase of resting energy expenditure. Because resistance exercise has been shown to increase lean body mass, resistance exercise commonly is recommended as a method of offsetting the changes in lean body mass and resting energy expenditure; however, randomized studies have not supported this recommendation [22,23]. Resistance exercise may improve strength and may lead to improvements in physical function in overweight adults. During periods of energy restriction, however, resistance exercise may not be capable of totally preventing the reductions in lean body mass and resting energy expenditure that are commonly observed.

Strategies that affect exercise adoption and maintenance

Intermittent versus continuous exercise

Perceived lack of time is a commonly reported barrier that affects exercise adoption and maintenance [24]. The physical activity recommendations proposed by the Centers for Disease Control and Prevention and the American College of Sports Medicine [19] indicate that a minimum of 30 minutes of exercise can be accumulated throughout the day rather than occur in one continuous bout. Data from DeBusk et al [25] and Ebisu [26] initially demonstrated that exercise performed in multiple bouts per day that were 10 to 15 minutes in duration elicited significant improvements in cardiorespiratory fitness in men. Jakicic et al [2,27] have confirmed these findings in overweight women. Jakicic et al [27] also have shown that prescribing intermittent exercise may be effective for enhancing initial exercise adoption in sedentary overweight women. For individuals who have difficulty adopting continuous bouts of exercise, an effective alternative may be to encourage multiple 10- to 15-minute bouts of exercise.

Lifestyle approaches to exercise

An alternative to supervised, structured exercise may be a lifestyle approach to physical activity. Studies by Dunn et al [28] and Andersen et al [29] support the effectiveness of lifestyle approaches to modifying physical activity behaviors. In both studies, supervised exercise sessions were compared with a lifestyle approach for modifying exercise behaviors. The lifestyle approach incorporated the use of behavioral strategies into the intervention to address barriers to exercise participation. It has been inferred that these studies show that lifestyle forms of moderate-intensity physical activity (eg, house chores, gardening, and so forth) are as effective as more traditional forms of exercise (eg, cycling, aerobics, and so forth) for modifying health and fitness outcomes. Neither Dunn et al [28] nor Andersen et al [29] reported the type, duration, or intensity of the activity that actually was performed by individuals receiving the lifestyle approach, however. Therefore, although these studies show that teaching behavioral strategies can be effective for modifying exercise behaviors, conclusions regarding the specific activities that can be effective are not supported by these studies. Clinicians are encouraged to engage in discussions with patients regarding barriers to participation in exercise and to provide guidance for overcoming these barriers. As illustrated in Fig. 1, the role of

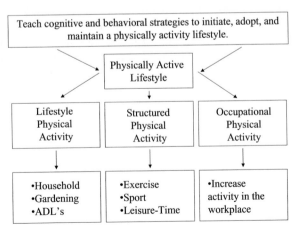

Fig. 1. Framework for effectively increasing physical activity adoption and maintenance in patients.
Abbreviation: ADLs, activities of daily living.

the clinician is to facilitate compliance to exercise and physical activity recommendations by integrating intervention strategies based on effective behavioral modification theories (eg, social cognitive theory, transtheoretical model, and so forth). These strategies may improve participation in all forms of activity that can affect body weight, including structured exercise, activities of daily living, and occupational activities.

Intervention delivery channels

Continued contact with patients is important for changing and maintaining health-related behaviors for weight loss, including exercise; however, achieving this level of contact can be extremely challenging in clinical settings where patients are seen infrequently, and when seen, the visit lasts only 10 to 15 minutes. Incorporating innovative methods of increasing patient-clinician contact, without overburdening the clinician, may play an important role in modifying exercise and other weight-loss behaviors. For example, Marcus et al [30] have shown that providing written materials matched to stage of readiness for change can effectively increase exercise participation. Telephone contact from a paraprofessional has been shown by Lombard et al [31] to be an effective technique of increased physical activity participation in adults. More recently, Tate et al [32] have reported that computer-based Internet interventions can be an effective channel for effectively modifying weight-loss and related behaviors. Using innovative intervention channels seems to be promising for modifying weight loss–related behaviors (eating and exercise) and should be considered by clinicians.

Summary

Exercise is an important component of weight-control programs, yet the impact of exercise for weight control is based on the ability of patients to engage in adequate levels of activity. The minimal level that should be recommended is at least 30 minutes of moderate-intensity physical activity on most days of the week. Although this level of physical activity may improve health-related factors, there is some evidence to support the recommendation of higher levels of exercise for weight-control purposes. The role of the clinician is to provide adequate guidance to patients regarding issues related to the intensity, duration, and mode of exercise that may be most appropriate. When addressing these issues, it is also important to consider the barriers that individual patients may encounter that will have an effect on adoption and maintenance of exercise behaviors.

References

[1] National Institutes of Health, National, Heart, Lung, and, Blood, and Institute. Clinical guidelines on the identification, evaluation, and treatment of overweight and obesity in adults: the evidence report. Obes Res 1998;6(Suppl 2):83S–1015.

[2] Jakicic JM, Winters C, Lang W, Wing RR. Effects of intermittent exercise and use of home exercise equipment on adherence, weight loss, and fitness in overweight women: a randomized trial. JAMA 1999;282:1554–60.

[3] Klem ML, Wing RR, McGuire MT, Seagle HM, Hill JO. A descriptive study of individuals successful at long-term maintenance of substantial weight loss. Am J Clin Nutr 1997; 66:239–46.

[4] McGuire MT, Wing RR, Klem ML, Lang W, Hill JO. What predicts weight regain in a group of successful weight losers? J Consult Clin Psychol 1999;67:177–85.

[5] Sherwood NE, Jeffery RW, French SA, Hannan PJ, Murray DM. Predictors of weight gain in the Pound of Prevention study. Int J Obes 2000;24:395–403.

[6] Willamson DF, Madans J, Anda RF, Kleinman JC, Kahn HS, Byers T. Recreational physical activity and ten-year weight change in a US national cohort. Int J Obes 1993;17: 279–86.

[7] Hagan RD, Upton SJ, Wong L, Whittam J. The effects of aerobic conditioning and/or calorie restriction in overweight men and women. Med Sci Sports Exerc 1986;18:87–94.

[8] Wing RR, Venditti EM, Jakicic JM, Polley BA, Lang W. Lifestyle intervention in overweight individuals with a family history of diabetes. Diabetes Care 1998;21:350–9.

[9] Ross R, Dagnone D, Jones PJH, Smith H, Paddags A, Hudson R, et al. Reduction in obesity and related comorbid conditions after diet-induced weight loss or exercise-induced weight loss in men. Ann Intern Med 2000;133:92–103.

[10] Pronk NP, Wing RR. Physical activity and long-term maintenance of weight loss. Obes Res 1994;2:587–99.

[11] US Department of Health and Human and Services. Physical activity and health: a report of the Surgeon General. Atlanta (GA): US Department of Health and Human Services, Centers for Disease Control and Prevention, National Center for Chronic Disease Prevention and Health Promotion; 1996.

[12] Flegal KM, Carroll MD, Kuczmarski RJ, Johnson CL. Overweight and obesity in the United States: prevalence and trends. Int J Obes 1998;22:39–47.

[13] Kuczmarski RJ, Carroll MD, Flegal KM, Troiano RP. Varying body mass cutoff points to describe overweight prevalence among US adults: NHANES III (1988–1994). Obes Res 1997;5:542–8.

[14] DiPietro L, Kohl HW, Barlow CE, Blair SN. Improvements in cardiorespiratory fitness attenuate age-related weight gain in healthy men and women: the Aerobics Center Longitudinal Study. Int J Obes 1998;22:55–62.

[15] Barlow CE, Kohl HW, Gibbons LW, Blair SN. Physical activity, mortality, and obesity. Int J Obes 1995;19:S41–4.

[16] Lee CD, Blair SN, Jackson AS. Cardiorespiratory fitness, body composition, and all-cause and cardiovascular disease mortality in men. Am J Clin Nutr 1998;69:373–80.

[17] Wei M, Kampert J, Barlow CE, Nichaman MZ, Gibbons LW, Paffenbarger RS, et al. Relationship between low cardiorespiratory fitness and mortality in normal-weight, overweight, and obese men. JAMA 1999;282:1547–53.

[18] American College of Sports Medicine. Guidelines for exercise testing and prescription. Phildelphia (PA): Lippincott, Williams and Wilkins; 2000.

[19] Pate RR, Pratt M, Blair SN, Haskell WL, Macera CA, Bouchard C, et al. Physical activity and public health: a recommendation from the Centers for Disease and Prevention and the American College of Sports Medicine. JAMA 1995;273:402–7.

[20] Schoeller DA, Shay K, Kushner RF. How much physical activity is needed to minimize weight gain in previously obese women. Am J Clin Nutr 1997;66:551–6.

[21] Duncan JJ, Gordon NF, Scott CB. Women walking for health and fitness: how much is enough? JAMA 1991;266:3295–9.

[22] Geliebter A, Maher MM, Gerace L, Gutin B, Heymsfield SB, Hashim SA. Effects of strength or aerobic training on body composition, resting metabolic rate, and peak oxygen consumption in obese dieting subjects. Am J Clin Nutr 1997;66:557–63.

[23] Kraemer WJ, Volek JS, Clark KL, Gordon SE, Puhl SM, Koziris LP, et al. Influence of exercise training on hysiological and performance changes with weight loss in men. Med Sci Sports Exerc 1999;31:1320–9.

[24] Dishman RK. Determinants of participation in physical activity. In: Bouchard C, Shephard RJ, Stephens T, Sutton JR, McPherson BD, editors. Exercise, fitness, and health: a consensus of current knowledge. Champaign (IL): Human Kinetics; 1990.

[25] DeBusk R, Stenestrand U, Sheehan M, Haskell W. Training effects of long versus short bouts of exercise in healthy subjects. Am J Cardiol 1990;65:1010–3.

[26] Ebisu T. Splitting the distances of endurance training: on cardiovascular endurance and blood lipids. Jap J Phys Educ 1985;30:37–43.

[27] Jakicic JM, Wing RR, Butler BA, Robertson RJ. Prescribing exercise in multiple short bouts versus one continuous bout: effects on adherence, cardiorespiratory fitness, and weight loss in overweight women. Int J Obes 1995;19:893–901.

[28] Dunn A, Marcus B, Kampert J, Garcia M, Kohl H III, Blair S. Comparison of lifestyle and structured interventions to increase physical activity and cardiorespiratory fitness. JAMA 1999;281:327–34.

[29] Andersen R, Wadden T, Bartlett S, Zemel B, Verde T, Franckowiak S. Effects of lifestyle activity vs structured aerobic exercise in obese women: a randomized trial. JAMA 1999;281:335–40.

[30] Marcus BH, Bock BC, Pinto BM, Forsyth LH, Roberts MB, Traficante RM. Efficacy of an individualized, motivationally-tailored physical activity intervention. Ann Behav Med 1998;20:174–80.

[31] Lombard DN, Lombard T, Winett RA. Walking to meet health guidelines: the effect of prompting frequency and prompt structure. Health Psychol 1995;14:164–70.

[32] Tate DF, Wing RR, Winett RA. Using internet technology to deliver a behavioral weight loss program. JAMA 2001;285:1172–7.

13

Orlistat in the Treatment
of Obesity

Priscilla Hollander

Pharmacotherapy is currently regarded as the second line of treatment for obesity [1]. If an individual has not met his or her goal for weight loss with lifestyle intervention, most algorithms for the treatment of obesity suggest that the next step is the addition of a weight loss drug. Until recently there has been a lack of effective and safe antiobesity drugs. Historically, the search for such drugs has been rife with problems. Drugs, such as amphetamines, or combinations of drugs, such as phentermine and fenfluramine, have shown short-term efficacy, but their side effect profiles have been unacceptable, if not dangerous [2]. Moreover, the desire for major cosmetic weight loss and the lack of understanding of the benefits of modest weight loss led to unrealistic expectations for weight-loss drugs [3,4]. This perception is unfortunate, because antiobesity drugs can and should be an important option in the treatment of obesity. Obesity has been identified as a major health problem in the United States and a variety of approaches are needed for successful treatment [5,6].

Recently, a new approach to establishing the efficacy and safety of weight-loss drugs was established by the Federal Food and Drug Administration (FDA). This process specifies that long-term, randomized, placebo-controlled trials must demonstrate short-term weight loss as well as long-term maintenance and safety. Two drugs have been developed that meet these specifications and are currently available for treatment of obesity. One is orlistat, a gastric lipase inhibitor, and the other is sibutramine, a serotonin-norepinephrine uptake-blocking agent [7,8].

This chapter focuses on the role of orlistat in the treatment of obesity. Orlistat was approved by the FDA in 1999 for the treatment of obesity (body mass index >30 kg/m^2) and for overweight individuals (body mass index >27 kg/m^2) with obesity-related comorbidity such as hypertension, dyslipidemia, diabetes, and sleep apnea [9]. The efficacy and safety of orlistat has been studied extensively in clinical trials in obese patients who do and do not have type 2 diabetes [8–13]. It has been available by prescription in United States and Europe for approximately 4 years; there have been no reports of a serious adverse event profile.

Mechanisms of action

The causes of obesity are multifactorial and its pathophysiology is complex. Absolute or excessive intake of calories is a major factor in weight gain. More specifically, calorie-dense foods, especially foods that are high in fat, play a disproportionate role in the development of obesity. Orlistat decreases the absorption of dietary fat in the gut through its interaction with the gastric and pancreatic lipases. The hydrolysis of triglycerides is decreased when orlistat forms a covalent bond with the active serine residue site of the lipases. By limiting the production of absorbable free fatty acids and monoglycerols, orlistat indirectly inhibits the absorption of dietary fat [14]. When compared with placebo, administration of 120 mg orlistat, given with a high fat meal, can reduce pancreatic lipase activity in the small intestine by approximately 75% [15]. Uptake of absorbable fat from the gut may be decreased by a maximum of 30% in patients who ingest between 50 grams and 80 grams of fat per day. [16]

Orlistat is usually administered orally with a 120 mg dosage at each meal. The systemic absorption of the drug is low; in general, approximately 95% to 97% of the administered dose is found in the feces. The elimination half-life is approximately 1 to 2 hours [17]. Metabolites of orlistat have been detected in the plasma, but in small amounts, and seem to be eliminated in the urine [18]. Although not systemically absorbed, orlistat therapy has a favorable effect on the postprandial triglyceride curve in healthy adults when given in combination with a low- or high-fat meal [19]. There is also intriguing evidence that orlistat may have an independent effect on insulin resistance aside from its effect on weight loss. In a 3-month treatment study of six obese men where weight was held constant, insulin sensitivity as assessed by a euglycemic hyperinsulinemic glucose clamp significantly improved from baseline [20].

Therapeutic potential in general obesity

A successful antiobesity drug should be effective and not be associated with adverse effects. Evidence indicates that a weight loss that is equal to 5% to 10% of basal body weight is the goal to maximize health benefits [5,21]. Obesity has been related to cardiovascular disease in men and women [22,23]. Much of this effect is mediated though the effect of weight on cardiovascular risk factors, such as lipid abnormalities, hypertension, glucose intolerance, and abnormalities of the hemostatic/fibrinolytic systems. These risk factors are often clustered in the same individual; this grouping has been called the insulin resistance syndrome, metabolic syndrome, or syndrome X. Weight loss was shown to have a beneficial effect on most of these cardiovascular parameters [24].

Two-year studies with orlistat

The efficacy and safety of orlistat have been evaluated extensively in numerous clinical trials in the United States and Europe. Of key interest are three trials, two in Europe and one in the United States, that assessed initial weight loss and prevention of weight regain. The first European study was a 2-year multicenter, randomized, double-blind, placebo controlled study [9]. Obese patients were randomized to placebo or orlistat (60 mg or 120 mg, three times a day). During the first year, all participants were on a hypocaloric diet and were on a maintenance diet for the second year. The dosage of drug and assignment of treatment did not change during the second year. Besides body weight, lipid profiles, glycemic control, blood pressure, quality of life, safety, and tolerability were measured. The two groups who were treated with orlistat lost significantly more weight in the first year than the group that was given placebo (8.6% and 9.7% versus 6.6%, respectively). At the end of the second year, less weight regain was seen in the patients who were treated with orlistat compared with placebo. Small, but significant, improvements were also seen in blood pressure, lipid profile, and quality of life.

In a 2-year study that was done in the United States, patients were randomized to orlistat, 120 mg, three times a day versus placebo plus a hypocaloric diet (both groups) for the first year of treatment [8]. At the beginning of the second year, all patients were rerandomized to placebo; orlistat, 60 mg, three times a day; or orlistat, 120 mg, three times a day. After one year of treatment, the group that took orlistat lost an average of 8.7 kg versus 5.8 kg with placebo. At the end of the second year, the group that took 120 mg of orlistat regained 3.2 kg, the group that took 60 mg of orlistat regained 4.2 kg, the and the group that took placebo regained 5.6 kg. Fasting total cholesterol, low-density lipoprotein (LDL) cholesterol, and fasting insulin levels improved.

In the second 2-year European trial, obese patients followed a 4-week hypocaloric diet (-600 calories reduced from regular diet) and were randomized to orlistat, 120 mg, three times a day or placebo for 1 year [10]. At the end of the year, approximately one half of the patients in each group were reassigned to the opposite treatment, which created four treatment groups. All patients were placed on a maintenance diet. During the first year, patients who were treated with orlistat lost on average more weight than the patients who were treated with placebo (10.3 kg versus 6.1 kg). During the second year, patients who continued with orlistat regained half as much weight as those patients who switched to placebo. Patients who switched from placebo to orlistat lost an additional 0.9 kg, compared with a mean regain of 2.5 kg in patients who continued on placebo (Fig. 1). Total cholesterol, LDL cholesterol, and concentration of glucose and insulin improved.

Metabolic syndrome

As shown in the initial 2-year studies, orlistat causes weight loss which as a favorable effect on other cardiovascular risk factors that contribute to the metabolic syndrome, such as lipids, blood pressure, and glucose and insulin levels [25]. Data from 1700 patients who completed 52 weeks of weight loss were analyzed to identify patients who had the metabolic syndrome. One hundred and twenty-eight patients were defined as having syndrome X by being in the quintile with the highest plasma triglyceride levels and lowest high-density lipoprotein (HDL) cholesterol. Initial characteristics of those

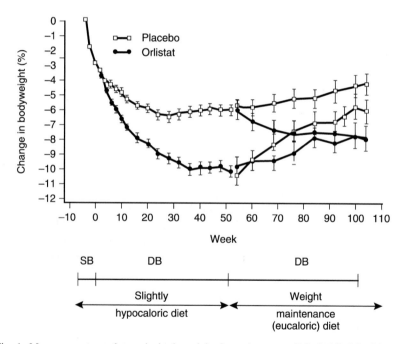

Fig. 1. Mean percentage change in body weight from the start of single-blind lead-in until 2-year examination in orlistat and placebo groups. Initial body weight was close to a mean of 100 kg in both groups. Percentage change, therefore, approximately matches kg lost. DB, double-blind, placebo-controlled treatment during years 1 and 2; Error bars, SB, single-blind lead-in period of 4 weeks. (*From* Sjostrom L, Rissanen A, Andersen T, et al for the European Multicenter Orlistat Study Group. Randomized placebo-controlled trial of orlistat for weight loss and prevention of weight regain in obese patients. Lancet 1998;352:167–72; with permission.)

with syndrome X were similar to characteristic of 119 subjects (without syndrome X) who had the lowest quintile of plasma triglycerides and highest quintile of HDL cholesterol. Although both groups who took orlistat lost equal amounts of weight, there were significantly better effects on lipids and fasting insulin levels in the patients who met the conditions of syndrome X.

Orlistat treatment and its effect on the other multimorbidities that are associated with obesity is highlighted in the results of the Swedish multimorbidity study [26]. In this study, 382 obese adults who were at high coronary risk were placed on a mildly hypocaloric diet and then randomized to double-blind treatment with orlistat or placebo three times a day for 1 year. All patients were required to have one of the following: obesity-associated risk factors, coronary heart disease, type 2 diabetes that was treated by diet or oral agents, hypertension, total cholesterol greater than 250 mg/dL, or LDL greater than 160 mg/dL. At the end of the study, orlistat treatment was associated with significantly greater weight loss than placebo (5.9% versus 4.6% of basal body weight), as well as modest, but significant, improvement in total serum cholesterol, LDL cholesterol, fasting plasma glucose, and HbAlc.

Early responders

Orlistat has been effective in intention-to-treat studies, but not all treated patients in these studies had significant weight loss. A recent study looked at an analysis of early responders to determine which patients may benefit the most from orlistat treatment. Early identification of responders would help to determine who would most benefit from treatment [27]. A retrospective analysis was performed on data from 220 patients who participated in, and completed, one of the 2-year trials of orlistat treatment. The best predictor of good outcome (ie, sustained weight loss and improvement in metabolic factors), was a greater than 5% basal body weight loss after 3 months of orlistat therapy. This group achieved an average weight loss of 11.9% versus 4.7% for patients who did not meet the criteria of initial weight loss. Initial weight loss, therefore, can be a useful criterion to estimate response.

Therapeutic potential in type 2 diabetes and impaired glucose tolerance

During the past 10 years, the incidence of diabetes has increased dramatically in the United States. This epidemic has been fueled by the increase in the prevalence of obesity. Individuals who are at the highest risk for developing type 2 diabetes are those who meet the criteria for impaired glucose tolerance. Two recent studies showed that lifestyle interventions that decrease weight can decrease the risk for development of diabetes by 58% [28,29]. Thus, obese patients who have impaired glucose tolerance may be good candidates for treatment with orlistat. Weight loss that is obtained by treatment with this agent is expected to decrease the risk of developing diabetes.

The results of a retrospective pooled analysis of three double-blind, randomized, placebo-controlled, 2-year trials showed that orlistat-induced weight loss may improve glucose tolerance in obese patients [body mass index (BMI) 30 to 43 kg/m^2] [30]. The studies were 2 years in duration. Patients received orlistat, 120 mg, at each meal, and a hypocaloric diet during the first year and a eucaloric diet during the second year. Baseline and end-of-study oral glucose testing was used to assess glucose status. The patients who were treated with orlistat were more likely to experience an improvement and less likely to experience a deterioration in glucose tolerance status compared with the patients who took placebo. The most significant effect was seen in the patients who took orlistat who had normal or impaired glucose tolerance at baseline. This effect was manifested by a greater reduction in fasting and glucose area under the curve.

The role of orlistat in the prevention of type 2 diabetes was studied in a large, prospective, multi-center, randomized, double-blind, placebo-controlled, 4-year study in Sweden [31]. Approximately 3200 obese patients were enrolled in a lifestyle plus placebo versus orlistat protocol. Twenty-one percent of the patients had impaired glucose tolerance and were randomized equally to orlistat or placebo treatment. Both the patients who were treated with placebo and the patients who were treated with orlistat lost weight: At 1 year, approximately 7.2 kg and 11 kg, respectively, and at the end of study, 4.1 kg and 6.9 kg, respectively. The cumulative incidence of type 2 diabetes was 6.2% in the patients who were treated with orlistat and 9.0% in the patients who were treated with placebo. The difference in rate of development of diabetes between the two groups was seen in the patients who had impaired glucose tolerance. Thus, in patients who have impaired glucose tolerance, the addition of orlistat to lifestyle treatment decreased the risk for diabetes by an additional 37%. Significant improvement also was seen in waist circumference, blood pressure, and LDL cholesterol.

Obese patients who have type 2 diabetes mellitus

Several studies from the past decade showed that glucose control is the key to the prevention of diabetic vascular complications [32,33]. Insulin resistance, an important contributor to the pathophysiology of type 2 diabetes, is closely linked to obesity. Effective weight management is an essential component of the long-term treatment of type 2 diabetes. In overweight and obese patients who have type 2 diabetes, weight loss of 5% to 19% improved glycemic control and may have reduce the requirement for antidiabetic medication [34]. Unfortunately, many of the agents that are used to treat diabetes, such as insulin, the insulin secretagogues, and the thiazolidinediones, are associated with weight gain, and, thus, compound the problem of insulin resistance [35]. After an individual becomes diabetic it is more difficult to lose weight [36]. Therefore, a drug that causes weight loss, and, thereby, an improvement in glycemia would be an attractive agent for the treatment of the obese patient who has type 2 diabetes.

Orlistat has been studied extensively in patients who have type 2 diabetes. Several double-blind, randomized, placebo-controlled studies examined the effects of orlistat in combination with either sulfonylureas, metformin, or insulin.

Sulfonylurea therapy

Sulfonylurea therapy has been associated with weight gain in patients who have diabetes. Therefore, theoretically orlistat would be a logical choice as a partner drug. The first published study of patients who took sulfonylureas was a 52-week study with a 4-week run-in period [11]. All patients were treated with a mildly hypocaloric diet and were randomized to orlistat, 120 mg, three times a day, or placebo. Patients who were treated with orlistat (n = 266) had a significantly greater reduction from baseline in glycosylated hemoglobin levels (−0.28 versus 0.18% for placebo) for an actual difference of 0.46%. The change in HbA1c was associated with a significantly greater reduction from baseline in weight (6.2% versus 4.3%) and in weight circumference. Achieving an early weight loss of more than 3% within the first 12 weeks of orlistat therapy predicted a long-term improvement in glycemic control. After 12 months' treatment, a significantly greater reduction from baseline in glycosylated hemoglobin was seen in the 71% of patients who were treated with orlistat who had lost more than 3.0% of their initial body weight, compared with those who had lost less than 3.0% (0.93 versus 0.25, $P < 0.001$).

Other metabolic parameters also showed improvement. Mild, but significant, changes were seen in total cholesterol and LDL cholesterol, which seemed to be independent of weight change. Further analysis revealed a significant gender effect: Total cholesterol levels were reduced by 8.5% and 4.6%, respectively, in men and women who received orlistat and increased by 0.8% and 2.6%, respectively, in men and women who received placebo.

Metformin therapy

Metformin is known to be a weight-neutral drug when used in therapy for type 2 diabetes. It does have gastrointestinal (GI) side effects, as does orlistat. The combination of metformin and orlistat was evaluated in a 52-week study with no lead-in period [12]. Participants were randomized to orlistat, 120 mg, three times a day, or placebo. Weight loss was significantly higher in the patients who were treated with orlistat compared with placebo (4.6% versus 1.7% of basal body weight). The HbA1c decrease was related to the extent of weight loss and adjustment to medication. In patients in whom the antidiabetic medications were not adjusted, the reduction in HbA1c was significant at 0.73% ± 0.08% versus 0.36% ± 0.09%. Patients who were entered into the study took metformin only (39% placebo, 44% orlistat), or a combination of metformin and sulfonylurea (placebo 60%, orlistat 55%), and on metformin plus acarbose (placebo 1%, orlistat 1%). No difference in weight loss or HbAlc was seen in regard to initial antidiabetic treatment regimen. Modest, but significant, changes in total cholesterol and LDL were seen in the patients who were treated with orlistat compared with placebo. Although more subjects who were treated with orlistat experienced gastrointestinal side effects, more subjects who were taking placebo withdrew prematurely.

Insulin therapy

Insulin treatment has been associated with increase in weight gain. Such weight gain was associated with several factors, including a decrease in glycosuria, an increase in food intake associated with hypoglycemia, and possible stimulation of appetite by insulin. The combination of insulin and orlistat therapy for type 2 diabetes was evaluated in patients in a 52-week study [13]. Participants were randomized to orlistat, 120 mg, three times a day, or placebo. Individuals who were involved in the study were on a stable insulin regimen before randomization. There were no exclusions in terms of type of insulin regimen. Seventy percent of the patients were on insulin only. For the 30% of patients who were on a combination of insulin and oral agent, 54% were on metformin, 36% were on sulfonylurea, and 10% were on metformin and sulfonylurea. Medication changes were made on the basis of excess hypoglycemia and hyperglycemia. Weight loss was significantly higher in the patients who were treated with orlistat compared with placebo (3.89% $\pm$ 0.3% versus 1.27 $\pm$ 0.3% of basal body weight) (Fig. 2). Weight decreased and HbAlc was also significantly improved in the patients who were treated with orlistat compared with placebo (−0.62% $\pm$ 0.08% versus −0.27% $\pm$ 0.08%) (Fig. 3). Rates of hypoglycemia was higher in the group that was treated with orlistat compared with placebo (16.9% versus 9.7%).

Other studies

Seven studies have evaluated the effect of orlistat on glycemic control in overweight and obese patients who have type 2 diabetes. Three of the studies were described earlier in detail. The other four studies were all randomized, placebo-controlled trials in which all patients were placed on a hypocaloric diet deficit of 500 to 600 calories. A total of 1162 patients were randomized in a 4-year trial in Germany and trials of 6 months' duration in Spain, South Africa, and Thailand [37]. All patients were on oral antidiabetic agents. Average weight loss was significantly greater in the treated patients, as was a decrease in HbA1c. The results were similar to those that were seen in the three described studies.

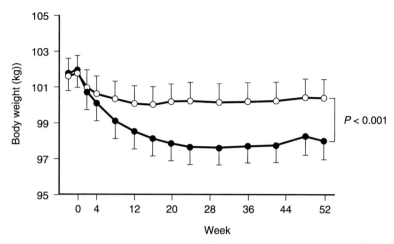

Fig. 2. Mean body weight change (± SE) during 1 year of double-blind treatment with placebo (open circle) or 120 mg, orlistat (closed circle) in patients with type 2 diabetes treated with insulin. $P < 0.001$, least-squares mean difference from placebo in the change from baseline over 52 weeks. (*From* Kelly D, Bray G, Pi-Sunyer X, et al. Clinical efficacy of orlistat therapy in overweight and obese patients with insulin-treated type 2 diabetes: a 1-year randomized controlled trial. Diabetes Care 2002;25(6):1033–41; with permission.)

Responder criteria

Not all patients, whether diabetic or nondiabetic, will respond favorably to a particular weight loss agent or program. To establish the best predictor

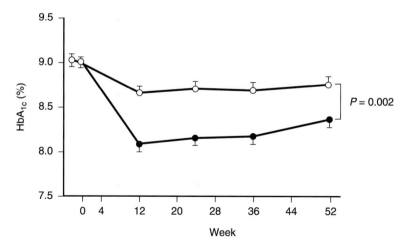

Fig. 3. HbA1c change over 1 year with placebo (open circle) 120 mg, orlistat (closed circle) in patients with type 2 diabetes treated with insulin. $P = 0.02$, least-squares mean difference from placebo in the change from baseline over 52 weeks. (*From* Kelley D, Bray G, Pi-Sunyer X, et al. Clinical efficacy of orlistat therapy in overweight and obese patients with insulin-treated type-2 diabetes: a 1-year randomized controlled trial. Diabetes Care 2002;25(6):1033–41.)

criteria for response to orlistat treatment in patients who had diabetes, a retrospective analysis of pooled data from the seven diabetes studies (2479 patients) was done [38]. HbA1c decrease and weight loss at 3 months were examined. A decrease in HbA1c of atleast 0.6% at 3 months of treatment was the best predictor of HbA1c decrease at the end of a study. A weight loss of 3.0% of basal body weight at 3 months was as good a predictor of best HbAlc decrease and ultimate weight loss, as a loss of 5.0% basal body weight at 3 months. Thus, early response, defined as modest improvements in HbAlc and body weight at week 12, can be used to successfully predict those patients who will achieve better outcomes during treatment with orlistat. If little or no response is seen at 12 weeks, further treatment with orlistat may not be helpful.

Mechanism of action

Orlistat-induced weight loss was shown to have a direct effect on insulin resistance. A retrospective analysis looked at the effect of orlistat on insulin resistance in overweight patients who had type 2 diabetes and a baseline HbA1c that was greater than 8% [39]. The insulin resistance index was calculated by the homeostatic model assessment (HOMA) method. Four hundred and eighty-three patients who were treated with orlistat with a mean baseline HOMA of 8.39 were compared with 435 patients who took placebo with a mean HOMA of 8.39. A significant improvement was seen in the group that was treated with orlistat compared with placebo, with a HOMA decrease of 1.61 versus 0.41.

The question has been raised whether the effect of orlistat on HbAlc is entirely the result of weight loss. Because the drug is not systemically active, the mechanism may be indirect. Orlistat does inhibit cholesterol absorption and was shown to do so independent of weight loss. The role of fatty acids and lipids on insulin resistance, and, therefore, on glucose control in type 2 diabetes is currently being explored. In the trial of insulin-treated patients who had type 2 diabetes, the initial decrease in plasma glucose was greater with orlistat than with placebo, even when matching groups for the amounts of initial weight that was lost [13]. It was shown that orlistat inhibits cholesterol absorption, and, thereby, could lower cholesterol independent of weight loss [40]. The decrease in LDL cholesterol was greater in patients who were treated with orlistat compared with placebo, although both groups lost the same amount of weight [11].

Cost analysis

Orlistat has been studied mainly in combination therapy with traditional antidiabetic agents in patients who have type 2 diabetes. It was shown to have an effect on body weight, glucose, and other comorbidities. A cost analysis, that used pooled data from four randomized, placebo-controlled,

1-year trials of orlistat in overweight or obese patients who had type 2 diabetes, was performed [41]. In all trials, patients were on an antihyperglycemic medication (two trials with sulfonylureas, one trial with metformin, one trial with insulin). A Markov state-transition model, that simulated diabetes-related complications in a population of 52-year-old males with a BMI of 35 and an HbAlc of 8.5%, was developed. The resultant data found that the addition of orlistat translated into a cost-effectiveness of $18,800 per event-free, life-year that is gained.

There is an impressive amount of data that support the use of orlistat as a partner with traditional antihyperglycemic drugs in the treatment of type 2 diabetes. Several diabetic drugs cause weight gain, in particular the insulin secretagogues and insulin. Orlistat was tested extensively in patients who were treated with either of those therapies and was shown to mitigate weight gain, and, in fact, caused weight loss. Moreover, a significant improvement in glucose levels is also seen. The use of orlistat in conjunction with thiazolidinediones (a drug class that is often associated with weight gain) has not been examined. Metformin therapy has been associated with mild weight loss or weight neutrality; however, in combination with orlistat, further significant weight loss is seen with glucose improvement in responders.

Safety/tolerability profile

The safety profile of orlistat is excellent. Over the past several years, millions of individuals have been exposed to orlistat; it has not been associated with a serious event profile. Thus, its safety record is based on extensive clinical trials and widespread commercial exposure. No monitoring requirements are necessary for treatment with the drug.

As would be expected, the tolerability of orlistat relates to its mechanism of action and is manifested in the GI system [42]. The percentage of patients who experienced GI events was consistent across the clinical studies. The GI effects that were noted more frequently in patients who were treated with orlistat included: flatus with discharge, oily spotting, fecal urgency, flatulence, and fatty/oily stools [11]. In general, these events were of mild to moderate intensity, occurred early during treatment, were transient in nature, and resolved spontaneously. In many cases, patients had no more than one event.

Because of its mechanism of action, interference with the absorption of the fat-soluble vitamins was studied closely. In healthy volunteers, the absorption of retinol was not altered by coadministration of orlistat; however, the absorption of vitamin E and beta-carotene was compromised [43]. In some of the studies, a decrease was seen in the fat-soluble vitamin levels in patients who were treated with orlistat, although the levels remained within the reference range [11].

Other drug-to-drug interactions have been studied extensively. Administration of orlistat, up to 360 mg/day, did not alter the pharmacodynamics or pharmacokinetics of glyburide, metformin, phentermine, sibutramine, atorvstatin, amitriptyline orlosartan, warfarin, pravastatin, digoxin, nifedipine, captorpril, atenolol, or furosemide, or combined oral contraceptives [37,44]. No problems were seen in regard to the ingestion of alcohol [45]. There is evidence that orlistat may affect the absorption of cyclosporine [46].

Summary

Orlistat has been well studied in several populations, including patients who do and do not have type 2 diabetes and in patients who have impaired glucose tolerance. Overall, modest, but significant, weight loss was seen in all three groups of patients with favorable effects on the comorbidities of obesity. Orlistat has not been associated with a serious adverse event profile, and the mild GI effects that are seen in some patients are well tolerated. In obese patients who do not have diabetes, weight loss is achieved and maintained as shown in the 2-year studies. Moreover, as was well documented in the Swedish multi-morbidity study, favorable treatment effects on the constituents of the metabolic syndrome are seen. Orlistat, together with a hypocaloric diet, was proven to be effective in preventing diabetes in patients who had impaired glucose tolerance. The addition of orlistat resulted in significant weight loss and significance decreases in levels of HbA1c in patients who had type 2 diabetes who were treated with antihyperglycemic drugs. Studies showed that it is possible to identify early which patients may respond best to treatment. Orlistat offers an attractive treatment option for obese patients who do and do not have diabetes and as a combination drug for treatment of obese patients who have type 2 diabetes.

References

[1] National Institutes of Health. National Heart, Lung and blood Institute. Clinical guidelines on the identification, evaluation, and treatment of overweight and obesity in adults. Bethesda (MD): Department of Health and Human Services; 1998.
[2] Connolly HM, Crary JL, McGoon M, et al. Valvular heart disease associated with fenfluramine-phentermine. N Engl J Med 1997;337:581–6.
[3] Goldstein DJ. Beneficial health effects of modest weight loss. Int J Obes Relat Metab Disord 1992;16:397–401.
[4] Foster G, Wadden T, Vogt R, et al. What is reasonable weight loss? Patients expectations and evaluation of obesity. J Consult Clin Psychol 1997;65:79–85.
[5] Mokdad A, Serdula M, Dietz W, et al. The spread of the obesity epidemic in the United States, 1991–1998. JAMA 1999;282:1519–24.
[6] National Center for Health Statistics, Centers for Disease Control and Prevention. Available at: www.cdc.gov/nchs/products/;ubs/pubd/hestats/obese/obse99.htm. Accessed August 30, 2002.
[7] James W, Astrup A, Finere N, et al for the Storm Study Group. Effect of sibutramine on weight maintenance after weight loss: a randomized trial. Lancet 2000;356: 2119–25.
[8] Davidson M, Hauptman J, Digirolamo M, et al. Weight control and risk factor reduction in obese subjects treated for 2 years with orlistat: a randomized controlled trial. JAMA 1999;281(3):235–42.

[9] Rossner S, Sjostrom L, Noack R, et al for the European Orlistat Obesity Study Group. Weight loss, weight maintenance, and improved cardiovascular risk factors after 2 years treatment with orlistat for obesity. Obes Res 2000;8(1):49–61.

[10] Sjostrom L, Rissanen A, Andersen T, et al for the European Multicenter Orlistat Study Group. Randomized placebo-controlled trial of orlistat for weight loss and prevention of weight regain in obese patients. Lancet 1998;352:167–72.

[11] Hollander P, Elbein S, Hirsch I, et al. Role of orlistat in the treatment of obese patients with type 2 diabetes. A 1-year randomized double-blind study. Diabetes Care 1998; 21(8):1288–94.

[12] Miles J, Leiter L, Hollander P, et al. Effect of orlistat in overweight and obese patients with type 2 diabetes treated with metformin. Diabetes Care 2002;25(7):1123–8.

[13] Kelley D, Bray G, Pi-Sunyer X, et al. Clinical efficacy of orlistat therapy in overweight and obese patients with insulin-treated type 2 diabetes: a 1-year randomized controlled trial. Diabetes Care 2002;25(6):1033–41.

[14] Guerciolini R. Mode of action of orlistat. Int J Obes 1997;(Suppl 3):12–23.

[15] Borovicka J, Schwizer W, Guttmann G, et al. Role of lipase in the regulation of postprandial gastric acid secretion and emptying of fat in humans: a study with orlistat, a highly specific lipase inhibitor. Gut 2000;46:774–81.

[16] Zhi J, Melia A, Guerciolini R, et al. Retrospective population–based analysis of the dose-response (fecal fat excretion) relationship of orlistat in normal and obese volunteers. Clin Pharmacol Ther 1994;56:82–5.

[17] Zhi J, Melia A, Funk C, et al. Metabolic profiles of minimally absorbed Orlistat in obese/overweight volunteers. J Clin Pharmacol 1996;36:1006–11.

[18] Roche Xenical (orlistat). Capsule prescribing information. Nutley (NJ): Roche Pharmaceutical.

[19] Suter P, Mrnier G, Veya-Linder C, et al. Effect of orlistat on postprandial metabolism in healthy subjects. J Obes Res 2001;9(Suppl 3):A68.

[20] Bachmann O, Dahl D, Brechtel K, et al. Orlistat improves insulin sensitivity in obese intentionally weight maintaining subjects. Diabets Res Clin Pract 2000;50(Suppl 1):A70.

[21] Khaodhiar L, Blackburn G. Health benefits and risks of weight loss. In: Bjorntrop L, editor. International textbook of obesity. Chichester (UK): John Wiley and Sons; 2001. p. 413–39.

[22] Rimm EB, Stampfer MJ, Giovanucci E, et al. Body size and fat distribution as predictors of coronary heart disease among middle-aged and older US men. Am J Epidemiol 1995;141:1117–27.

[23] Hu F, Manson J, Stampfer M, et al. Diet, lifestyle, and the risk for type 2 diabetes in women. N Engl J Med 2001;345:970–7.

[24] Wilson PW, Kannel WB, Silbershatz B, et al. Clustering of metabolic factors and coronary heart disease. Arch Intern Med 1999;159:1104–9.

[25] Reaven G, Segal K, Hauptman J, et al. Effect of orlistat-assisted weight loss in decreasing coronary heart disease risk in patients with syndrome X. Amer J Cardio 2001;87:827–31.

[26] Lindgarde F. The effect of orlistat on body weight and coronary heart disease risk profile in obese patients: the Swedish Multimorbidity study. J Intern Med 2000;248:245–54.

[27] Rissiann A. Int J Obes Relat Metab Disord 2002, in press.

[28] Tuomilethto J, Lindstrom J, Eriksson J, et al. Finnish Diabetes Prevention Study Group. Prevention of type 2 diabetes mellitus by changes in lifestyle among subjects with impaired glucose tolerance. N Engl J Med 2001;344:1343–50.

[29] Knowler W, Barrentt-Connor E, Fowler SE, et al. Diabetes prevention program research group. Reduction in the incidence of type 2 diabetes with lifestyle intervention or metformin. N Engl J Med 2002;346:393–403.

[30] Heymsfield S, Segal K, Hauptman J, et al. Effects of weight loss with orlistat on glucose tolerance and progression to type 2 diabetes in obese adults. Arch Intern Med 2000; 160:1321–6.

[31] Sjostrom L, Torgenson J, Hauptman J, et al. Xendos (xenical) in the prevention of diabetes in obese subjects: a landmark study. Presented at the International Conference of Obesity, San Paulo, Brazil, August 2002.

[32] UK Prospective Diabetes Study Group. Intensive blood-glucose control with sulfonylureas or insulin compared with conventional treatment and risk of complications in patients with type 2 diabetes (UKPDS). Lancet 1998;352:857–953.

[33] Ohkubo Y, Kishinkawa H, Araki E, et al. Intensive insulin therapy prevents the progression of diabetic microvascular complications in Japanese patients with non-insulin-dependent mellitus: a randomized prospective 6-year study. Diabetes Res Clin Pract 1995;28:103–17.

[34] Kelley D. Effects of weight loss on glucose homeostasis in NIDDM. Diabetes Review 1995;3:366–7.

[35] Yki-Jarvinen H. Combination therapies with insulin in type 2 diabetes. Diabetes Care 2001;24:758–67.

[36] Wing RR, Marcus MD, Epstein LH, et al. Type II diabetic subjects lose less weight than their overweight nondiabetic spouses. Diabetes Care 1987;10:563–6.

[37] Keating G, Blair J. Orlistat in the prevention and treatment of type 2 diabetes mellitus. Drugs 2001;61:2107–19.

[38] Hollander P, Ruof J. HbAlc reduction at week 12 predicts treatment outcome with orlistat in patients with type 2 diabetes who are overweight/obese. Diabetalogica 2002;45(Suppl 2):A685.

[39] Rissanen A, Hollander P. Effect of orlistat on insulin resistance in patients with type 2 diabetes with baseline HbAlc levels >8%. Diabetes 2002;51(Suppl 2):A413.

[40] Mittendorfer B, Patterson B, Klein S. Orlistat inhibits dietary cholesterol absorption. Obes Res 2001;19(Suppl 3):188S.

[41] Maetzel A, Ruof J, Covington M, et al. Cost effectiveness of treatment of overweight and obese diabetic patients with orlistat. Diabetes 2002;51(Suppl 2):A276.

[42] Van Gaal LF, Broom JI, Enzi G, et al. Efficacy and tolerability of orlistat in the treatment of obesity: a 6-month dose-ranging study. Eur J Clin Pharmacol 1998;54:125–32.

[43] Zhi J, Melia A, Koss-Twardy SG, et al. The effect of orlistat, an inhibitor of dietary fat absorption, on the pharmacokinetics of B-carotene in healthy volunteers. J Clin Pharmacol 1996;36:152–9.

[44] Hartmann D, Guzelhan C, Zuiderwijk P. Lack of interaction between orlistat and oral contraceptives. Eur J Clin Pharmacol 1996;50:421–4.

[45] Melia A, Zhi J, Zelasko R, et al. The interaction of the lipase inhibitor orlistat with ethanol in healthy volunteers. Eur J Clin Parmacol 1998;54:773–7.

[46] Schnetzler B, Konondo-Oestreicher M, Vaala D, et al. Orlistat decreases the plasma level of cyclosporine and maybe responsible for the development of acute rejection episodes [letter]. Transplantation 2000;27:70:1540–1.

14

Use of Sibutramine to Treat Obesity

Donna H. Ryan

Obesity pharmacotherapy comes of age

The negative impact of obesity on the public health of Americans has been reinforced powerfully in a study [1] notable for its size and prospective nature. More than 1 million US adults were followed up for 14 years, demonstrating increased risk from all-cause mortality and from death due to cancer, cardiovascular disease, and other causes associated with elevated body mass index (BMI, the weight in kilograms divided by the square of the height in meters). Increased risk became apparent for BMI greater than or equal to 25 kg/m^2 in men and 23.5 kg/m^2 in women, a category occupied by more than half of Americans [2]. Those risks rose dramatically as BMI exceeded 30 kg/m^2. According to the latest National Health and Nutrition Examination Survey (NHANES), the prevalence of BMI greater than or equal to 30 kg/m^2 for adults in 1999 exceeded 30.5% [3]. Even more alarming results come from an analysis [4] of the 1988 to 1994 NHANES survey showing that more than 24% of American adults meet Adult Treatment Panel III criteria [5] for metabolic syndrome. This astonishingly high prevalence of metabolic syndrome is a harbinger of the type 2 diabetes and cardiovascular disease epidemics that will follow.

Physicians must play a role in stemming the tide, and the National Institutes of Health has published a report fostering this approach, "Clinical guidelines on the identification, evaluation, and treatment of overweight and obesity in adults—the evidence report" [6]. These clinical guidelines emphasize the need for physicians to incorporate lifestyle change into their prescriptions and sanction the clinical use of weight-loss drugs approved by the Food and Drug Administration for long-term use, along with concomitant lifestyle modifications in selected patients (those whose BMI exceeds 27 kg/m^2, who have comorbid conditions, or whose BMI exceeds 30 kg/m^2 with no comorbid conditions and who have been unsuccessful in previous weight-loss attempts). A recent review in a prestigious journal [7] also legitimizes obesity pharmacotherapy. Additionally, primary care approaches to office-based obesity management are targeted in a document cosponsored by the National Institutes of Health and the North American Association for the Study of Obesity, *The Practical Guide to the Identification, Evaluation and Treatment of Overweight and Obesity in Adults* [8].

Still, for many physicians, treatment of obesity is not a routine part of practice, in part because of the stigma associated with "diet pills" [9]. The most recent blow to legitimizing pharmacotherapy for obesity came after the enormously popular "phen-fen" regimen was associated with unforeseen toxicity. Significant (16%) long-term weight loss and maintenance for 3.5 years were demonstrated with the use of fenfluramine and phentermine combined with lifestyle intervention [10–14]. Although a small (n = 121) set of patients formed this study population, the regimen was used widely in clinical practices for 5 years after the trial was published until 1997, when fenfluramine and dexfenfluramine were associated with the previously unsuspected complication of cardiac valvulopathy [15]. The extent of the problem has not proven to be as great as first suspected [16]. It is now recognized that risk for valvulopathy associated with fenfluramines is associated with duration of exposure to the medication [16] and that the lesions are likely to remit once the patient is no longer taking the medication [17]. Still, this experience provides a cautionary example to underscore the need for safety in prescribing for obesity.

The importance of safety in medicating for obesity

Obesity is a chronic disease in which health risks are usually remote rather than immediate. It has been compared with hypertension as a treatment paradigm [18], in that blood pressure is controlled so long as medication is continued. Similarly, treatments, including medication, do not cure obesity but must be maintained to maintain weight reduction. The requirement for long-term treatment and the relative remoteness of risk make safety a prime consideration in evaluating medication (or any treatment, for that matter) for obesity. An additional consideration is that for less severe degrees of overweight in which short-term pharmacotherapy might play a role in preventing more severe weight gain, the risk:benefit equation is an even more important consideration.

Sibutramine—pharmacology and mechanism of action

Sibutramine (marketed as Meridia in the United States and Reductil in Europe) is a selective reuptake inhibitor for norepinephrine, serotonin, and dopamine. The chemical structure of sibutramine and its two active metabolites is illustrated in Fig. 1. The drug is rapidly metabolized to two active metabolites, the half-life of which is 14 to 16 hours, with the peak

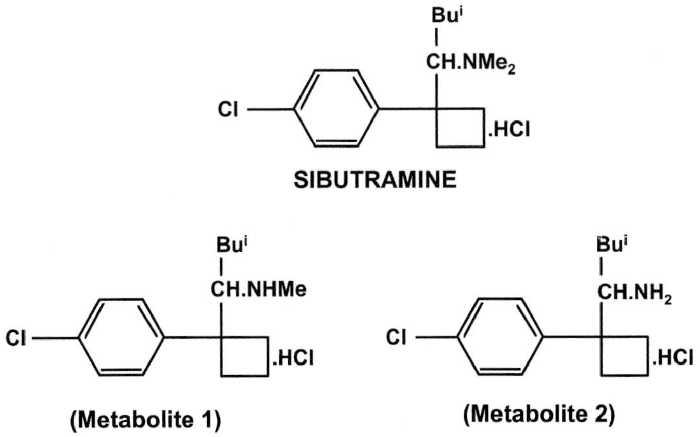

Bu^i
|
CH.NMe$_2$

Cl —⟨ ⟩— ⬛ .HCl

SIBUTRAMINE

Bu^i
|
CH.NHMe

Cl —⟨ ⟩— ⬛ .HCl

(Metabolite 1)

Bu^i
|
CH.NH$_2$

Cl —⟨ ⟩— ⬛ .HCl

(Metabolite 2)

Fig. 1. Chemical structure formulas for sibutramine and the two active metabolites. (*From* Ryan DH, et al. Sibutramine: a novel new agent for obesity treatment. Obes Res 1995;3(Suppl 4):553S–9S with permission.)

concentration at 3 to 4 hours and a plateau from 3 to 7 hours [19]. This pharmacologic profile allows for once-a-day dosing, an advantage when appetite regulation is the aim. The drug first was evaluated as a potential antidepressant in three phase II clinical trials, with disappointing results in depression [20]. Striking weight loss was observed in the enrolled depressed patients [20], however, and the drug has been developed and marketed for weight loss.

The mechanisms by which sibutramine produces its pharmacologic effects are believed to be through the actions of serotonin and norepinephrine in combination, acting within the central nervous system [21]. Sibutramine's dopaminergic action is minimal [21]. When administered to experimental animals, sibutramine has dual mechanisms to induce weight reduction: a decrease in food intake and an increase in energy expenditure [22]. The increase in energy expenditure is prominent in rodents, with sustained (>6 hours) increase in metabolic rate up to 30%, and is based on sympathetic activation of thermogenesis in brown adipose tissue [22,23].

In clinical trials with human beings, sibutramine decreases food intake in nondieting men [24] and women [25] by increasing meal-induced satiety [24–26]. Sibutramine also affects energy expenditure in humans, but the effect on thermogenesis is not as great as that seen in rodents; the thermogenic effect of sibutramine in humans is rather on the order of a 2% to 4% increase in metabolic rate beginning 3 hours from ingestion and lasting less than 24 hours. It takes a well-designed study to detect the increase in energy expenditure with the drug, because of its pharmacologic profile and the inherent variability of human metabolic rate measurements. Two studies document sibutramine's enhancement of metabolic rate. In a study of the acute effects of sibutramine on energy expenditure, Hansen et al [26] measured energy expenditure for 5.5 hours after a dose of 30 mg of sibutramine compared with placebo in fed and fasted men. There was a sibutramine-induced increase in energy expenditure of approximately 3% to 5%. In a study of the thermogenic effects of sibutramine when taken over a longer course, Walsh et al [27] studied obese women receiving 12 weeks of a calorie-reduced diet and either 15 mg/d of sibutramine or placebo. The expected decline in resting energy expenditure usually observed with weight loss and documented in the placebo-treated participants was blunted in the sibutramine-treated patients. The authors suggest that the sibutramine effect is equivalent to 100 kcal/d and might be enough to promote weight-loss maintenance over the long term.

Sibutramine—clinical efficacy

The amount of weight loss with sibutramine is dependent on the dose of the drug and related to the "dose" of the diet and exercise behaviors that are used in conjunction with the drug. One of the advantages of sibutramine is its efficacy in maintaining weight loss. This section reviews examples of these efficacy issues.

The dose-response relationship between sibutramine at 1, 5, 10, 15, 20, and 30 mg and weight loss is illustrated by Figs. 2 and 3, which show the

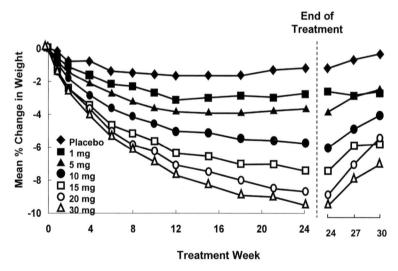

Fig. 2. Weight loss in patients completing 24 weeks of treatment. ♦ = placebo; ■ = 1 mg of sibutramine; ▲ = 5 mg of sibutramine; ● = 10 mg of sibutramine; □ = 15 mg of sibutramine; ○ = 20 mg of sibutramine; △ = 30 mg of sibutramine. $P < 0.05$ versus placebo for all time points for sibutramine doses 5 mg to 30 mg, nonparametric Williams' test. N = 87 to 107 per group. Post-treatment follow-up data also are shown for those patients in whom it was available (N = 50–61 per group). (*From* Bray GA, Blackburn GL, Ferguson JM, Greenway FL, Jain AK, Mendel CM, et al. Sibutramine produces dose-related weight loss. Obes Res 1999;7:189–98; with permission.)

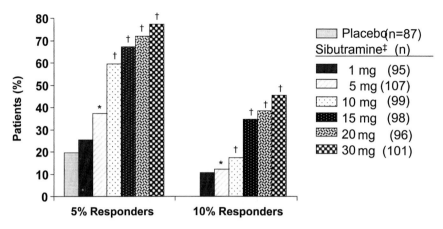

Fig. 3. Percentage of patients losing at least 5% or 10% of baseline weight after 24 weeks of treatment. (*Adapted from* Bray GA, Blackburn GL, Ferguson JM, Greenway FL, Jain AK, Mendel CM, et al. Sibutramine produces dose-related weight loss. Obes Res 1999;7:189–98; with permission.)
*$P < 0.01$ versus placebo, pairwise Fisher's exact test.
†$P < 0.001$.

results of a double-blind, placebo-controlled study conducted in seven centers and enrolling 1047 subjects [28]. The recommended dose levels for use in clinical practice are 5 to 15 mg/d, and these doses produced -3.9%, -6.1%, and -7.4% loss from baseline at week 24. As can be observed in Figs. 2 and 3, the behavioral approach used with pharmacotherapy in this study was relatively weak, because the mean weight loss associated with placebo was only 1.2% from baseline at 24 weeks, and less than 20% of patients on placebo achieved 5% weight loss or greater from baseline. Mean weight loss is useful information, but another way of analyzing results is particularly appropriate for primary care reference. Physicians should find it useful to evaluate the chances of an individual patient achieving significant weight loss. Weight losses of 5% and 10% from baseline are useful benchmarks, because they are associated with significant health benefits. Fig. 3 illustrates that 37.4%, 59.5%, and 63.7% of persons taking sibutramine in 5-, 10-, and 15-mg doses, respectively, achieved 5% weight loss from baseline compared with only 19.5% of those taking placebo. Other placebo-controlled studies of 24 weeks' duration or longer using sibutramine in healthy obese individuals are presented in Table 1, and these studies add additional evidence for the sibutramine dose–weight-loss response relationship.

The intensity of the behavioral component of the weight-loss program also influences the amount of weight loss with sibutramine. Because sibutramine enhances satiety, a dietary program that takes advantage of this mechanism is likely to produce greater weight loss. Wadden et al [29] illustrate the advantage of a highly structured dietary intervention in combination with sibutramine. In that study, 53 women were randomly

Use of Sibutramine to Treat Obesity

Table 1
Sibutramine: randomized, placebo-controlled-double-blind studies $\geq$24 weeks' duration

Authors	Duration	Dose (mg/d)	N	Sibutramine weight loss	>5%	N	Placebo weight loss	>5%
Bray et al, 1999 [28]	24 weeks	5	107/151 (71%)	−3.1%	37.4%[a]	87/148 (59%)	−0.9%	19.5%[a]
		10	99/150 (66%)	−4.7%	59.6%[a]			
		15	98/152 (64%)	−5.8%	67.3%[a]			
Cuellar et al, 2000 [46]	24 weeks	15	22/35 (63%)	−10.4%	76.5%	9/34 (26%)	−1.4%	21%
Smith and Goulder, 2001 [47]	52 weeks	10	94/161 (58%)	−5.0%	39%	80/163 (49%)	−1.8%	20%
		15	82/161 (51%)	−7.3%	52%			
Fanghanel et al, 2001 [48]	6 months	10	40/55 (73%)	−8.7%	72.6%	44/54 (81%)	−4.2%	40.4%
Dujovne et al, 2001 [44]	24 weeks	20	48/162 (29.6%)	−4.9%	42%	54/160 (33.8%)	−0.6%	8%

[a] Completers' analysis.

assigned 'to receive sibutramine, 10 to 15 mg daily, versus the same dosing scheme with a group lifestyle-modification program, versus the same dosing scheme with a highly structured portion-controlled diet included in the first 4 months of the lifestyle-modification program. As can be observed in Fig. 4, the group that received an initial 4 months of a highly structured diet (4 servings of nutritional supplements and an evening meal of a frozen entrée, fruit, and salad) lost the greatest amount (16.5% from baseline) compared with the other two groups, who lost 4.1% (drug alone) and 10.8% (drug plus lifestyle).

Another advantage of sibutramine is its efficacy in weight-loss maintenance. The three trials that have been designed to address this issue are listed in Table 2. After inducing weight loss with a very low-calorie liquid diet [30] or with sibutramine [31,32], patients were randomly assigned to placebo or sibutramine for maintenance of weight loss for up to 18 months. The STORM trial [31] illustrates that sibutramine is quite effective for inducing and maintaining weight loss for up to 2 years and provides a number of lessons for primary care practitioners (Fig. 5). In this multicenter European study, patients received sibutramine (10 mg) and

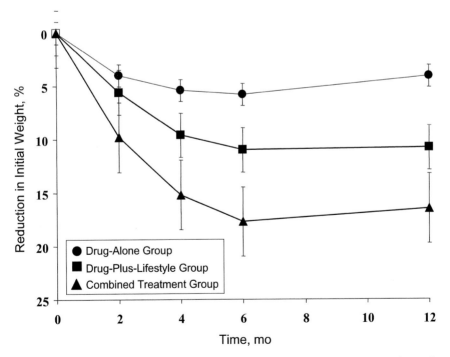

Fig. 4. Percentage of weight changes for patients receiving sibutramine; sibutramine and lifestyle modification; and sibutramine, lifestyle modification, and structured diet. (*From* Wadden TA, Berkowitz RI, Sarwer DB, Prus-Wisniewski R, Steinberg C. Benefits of lifestyle modification in the pharmacologic treatment of obesity. Arch Intern Med 2001;161:218–27; with permission.)

Table 2
Sibutramine: trials of weight-loss maintenance

Authors	Run-in	Duration	Dose (mg/d)	Sibutramine			Placebo			Notes
				N	>5%	Efficacy	N	>5%	Efficacy	
Apfelbaum et al, 1999 [30]	≥6-kg loss with 4-week VLCD; 160/250 completed	1 year	10	53/82 (65%)	86%	75% maintained 100% of weight lost during VLCD	45/78 (58%)	55%	42% maintained 100% of weight lost during VLCD	At 1 year, mean weight change from end of VLCD was −5.4% for sibutramine versus +1% for placebo
James et al, 2000 [31]	≥5% weight loss with 6 months of sibutramine 10 mg/d; 467/605 (77%)	18 months	10–20	204/352 69% (58%)		After 18 months, 43% maintained at least 80% of initial weight lost	57/115 (50%)	~42%	After 18 months, 16% maintained at least 80% of initial weight lost	4% of individuals on sibutramine and 2% on placebo achieved BMI <25 kg/m²
Wirth and Krause, 2001 [32]	≥2% weight loss after 4 weeks treatment with sibutramine (15 mg/d)	44 weeks	15	325/405 65% (80%)		−8.2% loss from pretreatment at 48 weeks	146/201 (73%)	35%	−3.9% loss from pretreatment at 48 weeks	No changes in blood pressure were observed for any groups, so no benefits of intermittent therapy observed
			15*	315/395 63% (80%)		−8.1% loss from pretreatment at 48 weeks				

Abbreviation: VLCD, very low-calorie (liquid) diet.
* 15 mg given intermittently weeks 1–12, 19–30 and 37–48.

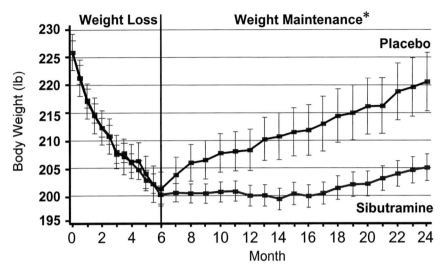

Fig. 5. Mean body weight change during weight-loss and weight-maintenance phases of the STORM trial. (*Adapted from* James WPT, Astrup A, Finer N, Hilsted J, Kopelman P, Rossner S, et al, for the STORM Study Group. Effect of sibutramine on weight maintenance after weight loss: a randomised trial. Lancet 2000;356:2119–25; with permission.)
* Same diet, exercise for sibutramine, placebo. $P \leq 0.001$, sibutramine vs placebo for weight maintenance.

a calorie-deficit diet for 6 months. Of the 605 obese patients who entered the trial, 467 (77%) achieved weight loss of at least 5% from baseline. Those patients were then randomly assigned to receive sibutramine (doses could be titrated from 10–20 mg daily) or placebo. After 24 months of observation, the weight loss of the sibutramine-treated group averaged 10.2 kg from baseline compared with 4.7 kg for placebo. Primary care practitioners might infer from this study that approximately three quarters of obese patients who are prescribed sibutramine (10 mg/d) with a diet program will achieve meaningful weight loss. If medication is continued, almost half of those patients maintain 80% of the weight loss.

Fig. 6 shows the results of an interesting study by Wirth and Krause [32] evaluating an intermittent-therapy approach. In that study, patients who had lost 2% of body weight or 2 kg after 4 weeks of treatment with sibutramine (15 mg/d) were randomly assigned to placebo, versus continued sibutramine, versus sibutramine prescribed intermittently (weeks 1–12, 19–30, and 37–48). Both sibutramine treatment regimens gave equivalent results and were significantly better than placebo. The effect of stopping sibutramine is illustrated in Fig. 6 by a small increase in weight, which then is reversed when the medication is restarted. In clinical practice, it is difficult to obtain long-term medication compliance for weight-loss agents. Patients report that "The medication is not working, since I am no longer losing weight." Patients discontinue weight-loss medications, with subsequent

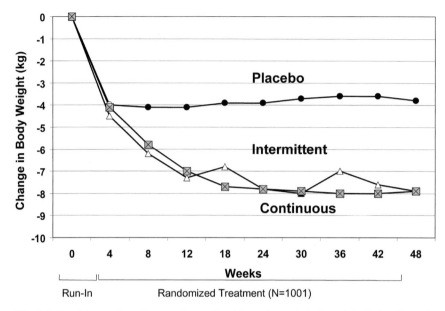

Fig. 6. Intermittent and continuous sibutramine. Mean change in body weight during the study period. Patients (n = 1102) received sibutramine (15 mg/d). Those who lost 2% of body weight or 2 kg in 4 weeks were randomly assigned to placebo (n = 395) versus continued sibutramine (n = 405) versus intermittent sibutramine (weeks 1–12, 19–30, and 37–48) (n = 395). (*From* Wirth A, Krause J. Long-term weight loss with sibutramine. JAMA 2001;286:1331–9; with permission.)

weight regain. This study emphasizes the value of restarting medications before weight regain is advanced.

Apfelbaum et al [30] treated 159 obese subjects with a very low-calorie diet to induce a 7.2% weight loss and then randomly assigned them to receive placebo or sibutramine (10 mg/d). After treatment for 1 year, subjects receiving sibutramine lost a total of 13.5% of their weight compared with 6.7% for the placebo group. The mean reduction in weight from baseline in sibutramine-treated patients is impressive, but the percentage of patients who received significant benefit is even more so. At least 5% reduction from baseline was achieved by 86% in the sibutramine group (55% in the placebo group). Similarly, at month 12, 75% of subjects in the sibutramine group maintained at least 100% of the weight loss achieved with the very low-calorie diet, compared with 42% in the placebo group.

Sibutramine safety and tolerability

The side effects of sibutramine (insomnia, asthenia, dry mouth, and constipation) are generally mild and transient. Sibutramine is not associated with valvulopathy [33]. Although the drug is scheduled as a Class IV substance, there is no evidence for abuse potential, as demonstrated in a study of 31 male recreational stimulant users [34]. In that study, the volunteers were questioned about "street value," and dextroamphetamine 20 mg and 30 mg had higher street values ($2.80 and $3.30, respectively) than sibutramine 20 mg and 30 mg ($0.50 and $0.70, respectively) or placebo ($0.20). The P value was significant ($P < 0.001$) for dextroamphetamine doses compared with placebo or sibutramine doses, but there was no significant difference between placebo and both sibutramine doses. There is no evidence for a clinically relevant interaction of sibutramine with alcohol in impairment of cognitive function [35].

If sibutramine acts by way of central nervous system stimulation of norepinephrine and serotonin and through the sympathetic nervous system to increase thermogenesis, then cardiostimulatory effects are to be expected. The principal concerns with sibutramine safety have been the increase in blood pressure and pulse rate that averages 1 to 3 mm Hg for blood pressure and a 4- to 6-beat-per-minute increase in pulse [28,36,37]. The mean increases do not tell the whole story. Some patients are sensitive to sibutramine and experience blood pressure and pulse increases to unacceptable levels. In the clinical trials reviewed in this chapter, that population usually represents less than 2% of patients exposed to sibutramine. There is one published [38] composite of data from clinical trials describing withdrawals for cardiovascular events, which is shown in Table 3. There is no difference in withdrawals for hypertension between placebo and sibutramine according to this analysis, but there is a significant difference in withdrawals for tachycardia and for palpitations in the overall integrated database. The drug should not be used in patients with a history of cardiac arrhythmias, in patients with uncontrolled hypertension, or in those individuals with cardiovascular disease who would be at health risk because of blood pressure or pulse elevations. It is recommended in the prescribing information that patients be monitored for blood pressure and pulse changes at 2 to 4 weeks after initiating the medication. If blood pressure is in the hypertensive range or pulse is greater than 100 beats per minute, the

Table 3
Patient withdrawals from sibutramine clinical studies show no differences between placebo and sibutramine for the incidence of cardiovascular events

| COSTART-preferred term | Overall integrated database | | | Long-term studies | | |
	Placebo (%) (n = 2335)	Sibutramine (%) (n = 4748)	P <	Placebo (%) (n = 770)	Sibutramine (%) (n = 1741)	P <
Hypertension	0.6	1.1	0.21	0.6	1.1	0.21
Palpitations	0.04	0.3	0.02	0.0	0.2	0.22
Tachycardia	0.04	0.5	0.02	0.0	0.6	0.048
Vasodilation	0.0	0.04	0.32	0.0	0.1	0.48
Total	6.4	8.9		8.7	9.0	

Data from Sharma AM. Sibutramine in overweight/obese hypertensive patients. Int J Obes Relat Metal Disord 1998;22(Suppl 1):S38–S40.

drug should be stopped. Less severe increases in blood pressure and heart rate should prompt consideration of dose reduction.

The mean increases in blood pressure and pulse are problematic on another level other than just the tendency to cause clinically significant changes in some patients and represent a therapeutic dilemma when viewed from a population perspective. Weight loss usually is associated with beneficial effects on risk factors such as lipids, indices of glycemic control, waist circumference, and blood pressure. If sibutramine has mixed effects on risk factors, increasing blood pressure while producing the decreases in cholesterol and improvement in other risk factors associated with weight reduction, how is one to judge the net result?

It has been suggested that the blood pressure effects of sibutramine are mitigated by greater weight loss [38]. That is, with increasing amounts of weight loss, the blood pressure change actually may be a net decrease, albeit less than that observed with similar nonpharmacologic weight loss. For an individual patient who has achieved weight loss successfully with sibutramine, the blood pressure may be reduced from baseline, although the blood pressure reduction may not be as great as that associated with the same degree of weight lost without medications. One strategy for managing the blood pressure effect with sibutramine is described later, and it relies on a treatment algorithm for sibutramine in which weight loss is associated with no adverse blood pressure profile. This author believes in a conservative approach to acceptable blood pressure response while a patient is taking sibutramine.

Another strategy to deal with the cardiostimulatory effects of sibutramine has been described by Berube-Parent et al [39]. In this intervention, an aerobic exercise program was added to a weight-loss program that combined diet and sibutramine (10 mg). This small (n = 8 men), observational study should not be extrapolated to a larger, more diverse population; however, the study did show promise in terms of enhanced weight loss (10.7 kg in 12 weeks) and a benefit in mitigating the blood pressure and pulse side effects of sibutramine with the aerobic exercise component.

Sibutramine efficacy in special populations (diabetes and hypertension)

Obesity is associated with increased risk for type 2 diabetes and for hypertension, and in clinical practice, these comorbidities are encountered frequently. The experience with sibutramine in obese patients with hypertension is presented in Table 4 and with diabetes in Table 5.

In the case of patients with hypertension, there are 4 reports [49,51] documenting the use of sibutramine in hypertension; there are two [49,51] in which the drug was given for 52 weeks. In all instances, the weight-loss pattern favors sibutramine; however, except for one study, mean weight loss was associated with mean blood pressure increases. On average, the blood pressure effect with sibutramine compared with placebo is +2 to +3 increase in mm Hg diastolic blood pressure and +1 to +3 increase in mm

Table 4
Sibutramine: trials in patients with hypertension

Authors	Duration	Population	Dose (mg/d)	Sibutramine			Placebo			Notes
				N	DBP[a]	SBP[b]	N	DBP	SBP	
McMohan et al, 2000 [49]	52 weeks	Calcium channel blocker ± diuretic ± β-blocker medications	20	NR	+2.0	+2.7	NR	-1.3	+1.5	Weight loss favoring sibutramine: -4.7% versus -0.7% for placebo; 40% achieved >5% weight loss with sibutramine versus 8.7% with placebo
Hazenberg, 2000 [50]	12 weeks	All hypertension medications permitted	10	50/62	-3.7	-4.1	56/65	-5.2	-4.2	Weight loss favoring sibutramine, -4.7% versus -2.3% at 12 weeks
Sramek et al, 2002 [40]	12 weeks	β-blocker medications	20	27/29	+1.8	+1.5	28/32	-0.8	+0.3	Weight loss favoring sibutramine: -4.5% versus +0.4%
McMahon et al, 2002 [51]	52 weeks	Ace-inhibitor ± diuretic medications	20	84/146 (58%)	+3.0	+3.8	36/74 (49%)	-0.1	+1.1	Weight loss favoring sibutramine: -4.8% versus -0.3%; 42.8% versus 8.3% achieved 5% response

Abbreviation: NR, not reported.
[a] Diastolic blood pressure.
[b] Systolic blood pressure.

Table 5
Sibutramine: trials in patients with diabetes

Authors	Population run-in	Duration	Dose (mg/d)	Sibutramine N	>5%	Efficacy	Placebo N	>5%	Efficacy	Notes
Fujioka et al, 2000 [52]	Obese patients with poorly controlled diabetes; 5-week placebo run-in period	24 weeks	20	60/89 (67%)	33%	5% responders had HbA$_{1c}$ −0.53%; HbA$_{1c}$ for all patients was +0.17	61/86 (71%)	0%	HbAb$_{1c}$ for all patients was +0.27	Mean weight change was −4.5% for sibutramine versus −0.1% for placebo
Finer et al, 2000 [53]	Obese with diabetes	12 weeks	15	43/47 (91%)	19%	Mean HbA$_{1c}$ −0.3%; 33% of patients achieved decrease in HbA$_{1c}$	40/44 (91%)	0%	Mean HbA$_{1c}$ unchanged; 5% achieved decrease in HbA$_{1c}$	Mean weight change −2.4 kg for sibutramine versus −0.1 kg for placebo
Gokcel et al, 2001 [54]	Obese women with poorly controlled diabetes	6 months	20	29/30 (97%)	NR	Mean HbA$_{1c}$ −2.73%; fasting glucose −124.9 mg/dL	25/30 (83%)	NR	Mean HbA$_{1c}$ unchanged, fasting glucose −15.8 mg/dL	Mean weight change −9.6 kg for sibutramine versus −0.9 kg for placebo
Serrano-Rios et al, 2002 [55]	Obese with diabetes, stable on sulphonylurea therapy	6 months	15	53/69 (77%)	49%	Mean HbA$_{1c}$ −0.78%;	57/65 (88%)	29%	Mean HbA$_{1c}$ −0.68%	Mean weight change −4.5 kg for sibutramine versus −1.7 kg for placebo

Abbreviation: NR, not reported.

Hg systolic blood pressure compared with placebo. Interestingly, the study using β-blocker therapy for hypertension [40] showed no attenuation of the blood pressure or pulse increase with sibutramine, suggesting the effect is not mediated through the β-adrenergic system.

In the case of diabetes, weight loss is expected to improve indices of glycemic control; the expected changes are a reduction in fasting insulin, glucose, and HbA_{1c}. There are 4 published studies using sibutramine in obese patients with type 2 diabetes. With the exception of the study by Gokcel et al [41], the weight loss observed is somewhat disappointing. In most of the studies, less than 50% of the patients achieved a reduction of 5% body weight, reflecting the difficulty in managing complicated obesity. Still, in all of the studies, the percentage of patients on sibutramine who achieved meaningful weight loss was significantly greater than those on placebo, and the analysis of glycemic control showed benefit corresponding to the degree of weight loss. In the study by Gokcel et al, 60 female patients with diabetes who had poorly controlled glucose levels ($HbA_{1c} > 8\%$) on maximal doses of sulfonylureas and metformin were randomly assigned to sibutramine (10 mg twice daily) or placebo. The weight loss at 24 weeks was striking, with -9.6 kg in sibutramine-treated patients compared with -0.9 kg with placebo. The improvements in glycemic control were equally striking. In the sibutramine-treated patients, HbA_{1c} fell -2.73%, compared with -0.53% with placebo. Insulin levels fell 5.66 μU/mL compared with 0.68 for placebo, and fasting glucose fell -124.88 mg/dL compared with -15.76 for placebo.

Sibutramine effect on obesity-related risk factors

With the exception of blood pressure and pulse, the weight loss induced with sibutramine is associated with improvement in all other obesity-related risk factors, including lipids, uric acid, indices of glycemic control, and waist circumference. These positive changes are related to weight loss; the drug does not have an independent effect on these factors. Fig. 7 demonstrates a meta-analysis of 4 long-term obesity studies [42] and shows significant improvement in waist circumference with sibutramine use. The lipid profile improvement with sibutramine is related to the amount of weight lost. Table 6 is a combined analysis of 11 placebo-controlled trials with sibutramine. The degree of improvement in lipids is proportional to the amount of weight lost [43]. Sibutramine has been used in obese patients with hyperlipidemia. In a study [44] of 322 obese men and women with triglyceride levels greater than or equal to 250 and less than or equal to 1000 mg/dL and serum high-density lipoprotein cholesterol levels less than 40 mg/dL (men) or less than or equal to 45 mg/dL (women), patients were put on a Step 1 American Heart Association diet and randomly assigned to sibutramine at a dosage of 20 mg (n = 162) or placebo (n = 160). The mean weight loss at 24 weeks favored sibutramine (-4.9 kg versus -0.6 kg), and 42% of sibutramine-treated patients achieved 5% or greater reduction in weight, compared with

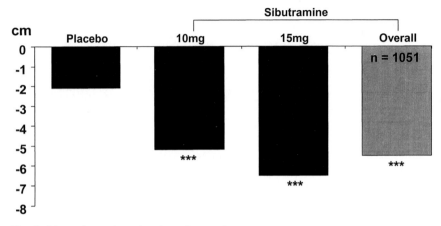

Fig. 7. Mean change in waist circumference from baseline to endpoint in a meta-analysis of four long-term obesity studies involving sibutramine.
(*From* Van Gaal LF, Wauters MA, Peiffer FW, De Leeuw IH. Sibutramine and fat distribution: is there a role for pharmacotherapy in abdominal/visceral fat reduction? Int J Obes Relat Metab Disord 1998;22[Suppl 1]:S38–40; with permission.)
*** $P < 0.001$ versus placebo; n = number of patients.

only 8% of those receiving placebo. For those patients taking sibutramine who achieved 5% or greater loss from baseline weight, serum triglyceride levels decreased 33.4 mg/dL, and high-density lipoprotein cholesterol increased 4.9 mg/dL.

In addition to improvement in obesity-related risk factors, weight loss with sibutramine can produce improvements in health-related quality of life. Samsa et al [45] combined data from four double-blind, randomized, controlled trials of sibutramine at a dosage of 20 mg/dL versus placebo. Moderate weight loss (5.01%–10%) was associated with a statistically significant improvement in health-related quality of life.

Table 6
Changes in serum lipids: combined analysis of 11 placebo-controlled sibutramine studies

		Sibutramine		
Lipids	Placebo (mg/dL)	Total weight loss (mg/dL)	< 5% Weight loss (mg/dL)	≥5% Weight loss (mg/dL)
Triglycerides	+0.53	−8.75*	−0.54	−16.59*
Total cholesterol	−1.53	−2.21	−0.17	−4.87*
LDL cholesterol	−0.09	−1.85	−0.37	−4.56**
HDL cholesterol	−0.56	+4.13*	+3.19	+4.68*

Abbreviations: HDL, high density lipoprotein; LDL, low density lipoprotein. Pooled trial data. Sibutramine package insert. Knoll Pharmaceutical Co, 1997.
  * $P \leq 0.001$ versus placebo.
  ** $P \leq 0.05$ versus placebo.
  Adapted from Aronne LJ. Treating obesity: a new target of prevention of coronary heart disease. Prog Cardiovasc Nurs 2001;16:98–106, 115.

Predicting response to sibutramine

Not all patients experience weight loss with sibutramine. It is important to recognize "nonresponders" and "responders" early, before prolonged exposure to an ineffective drug. A useful benchmark is to use "4 pounds lost in 4 weeks" as a criterion for predicting ultimate successful weight loss. Fig. 8 shows the chances of achieving 5% or greater weight loss with sibutramine rather than placebo. Early weight loss (4 pounds in the first 4 weeks) was predictive of success at 6 months for all doses (including placebo).

Putting it all together: an algorithm for clinical practice

The primary care physician faces great challenges in today's practice environment. Time is at a premium, and patient encounters must be brief. Counseling with an emphasis on health promotion and prevention of chronic diseases is not always reimbursed in a fair manner. The burden of managing obesity (27% of Americans in 1999) [2] and metabolic syndrome (24% of Americans in an analysis of the 1996 NHANES survey) [4] can be daunting to physicians who are not compensated adequately for the time they take counseling for lifestyle change. It is possible to help patients lose weight and improve their health-risk profile by judicious use of medications for obesity, and the investment in physician time need not be lengthy.

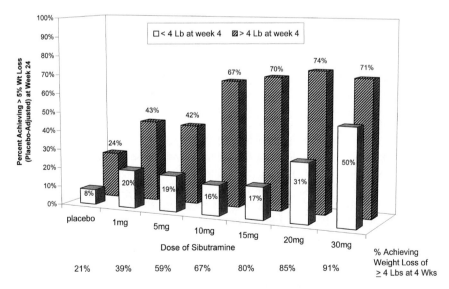

Fig. 8. Weight loss at 24 weeks in patients losing more or less than 4 pounds in the first 4 weeks of treatment. Because mean weight loss in the placebo group was 1.2%, 5% placebo-adjusted weight loss = 6.2% total weight loss. (*From* Bray GA, Blackburn GL, Ferguson JM, Greenway FL, Jain AK, Mendel CM, et al. Sibutramine produces dose-related weight loss. Obes Res 1999;7:189–98; with permission.)

The treatment algorithm in Fig. 9 is meant to guide the busy primary care practitioner through the use of sibutramine in aiding a diet-and-exercise program. Obese patients have usually had multiple weight-loss attempts. They know that reducing food intake and increasing energy expenditure will result in weight loss. Medications can help by reinforcing the behavioral (diet) approach. If sibutramine is prescribed with a reduced-calorie diet plan, satiety is aided and the patient is more likely to comply with the plan. The studies discussed in this chapter demonstrate that when sibutramine is used with a more structured, portion-controlled diet plan, there is likely to be greater weight loss than when the drug is used with a less-structured diet. If the patient is motivated and ready to embark on a program of lifestyle change, the physician can "coach" the patient to the more successful diet plan. The physician also should coach the patient to set an achievable goal (5%–10% weight loss in 6 months).

If the patient meets prescribing guidelines (BMI ≥ 30 or ≥ 27 with a comorbidity), is motivated and ready to make reasonable lifestyle modifications, and if there are no contraindications, sibutramine can be prescribed, starting at a dose of 10 mg daily. Then the patient should be seen at 4 weeks to check for safety, tolerability, and efficacy. At the 4-week visit, the physician will want to see 4 pounds lost as a reasonable criterion to predict ultimate efficacy. There also should be acceptable safety. The author has chosen to recommend conservative blood pressure and pulse limits with sibutramine prescription. If the blood pressure is less than 130/80 mm Hg, the pulse is less than 100 beats per minute, and there has not been an increase in pulse of more than 15 beats per minute in blood pressure of 15 mm Hg, then continued use of the medication would be acceptable, providing weight loss is adequate. If any one of these criteria is exceeded, sibutramine should be reduced or discontinued. Patients should be followed up monthly for the first 6 months and then should be followed up at least every 6 months so long as the medication is continued. Should there be tolerability issues, the dose could be reduced to 5 mg and if there is weight gain, the dose could be increased to 15 mg. So long as weight maintenance continues and so long as blood pressure and pulse meet the preceding guidelines, sibutramine may be continued. If lack of efficacy appears with pronounced weight gain, if blood pressure or pulse exceeds the previously mentioned guidelines, or if other tolerability issues become a problem, then sibutramine should be discontinued.

Patients often discontinue weight-loss medications on their own, without seeking physician advice. Physicians should caution patients regarding the weight gain that occurs when sibutramine is discontinued. Because the nature of obesity is such that relapse is frequent, physicians need to counsel patients to seek medical advice early in a relapse cycle, rather than later, so that appropriate interventions can be discussed.

Obesity is a chronic, incurable condition. The primary care physician can help patients manage their condition by acting as a coach in the patient's

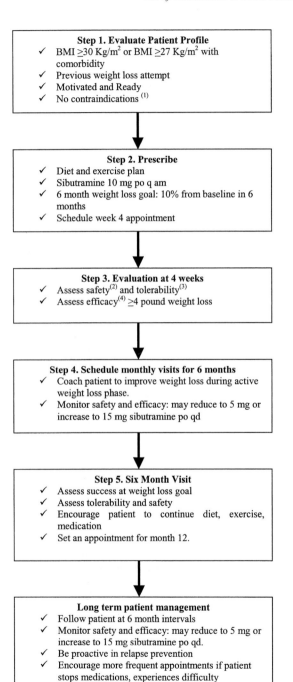

Step 1. Evaluate Patient Profile
✓ BMI $\geq$30 Kg/m^2 or BMI $\geq$27 Kg/m^2 with comorbidity
✓ Previous weight loss attempt
✓ Motivated and Ready
✓ No contraindications [1]

Step 2. Prescribe
✓ Diet and exercise plan
✓ Sibutramine 10 mg po q am
✓ 6 month weight loss goal: 10% from baseline in 6 months
✓ Schedule week 4 appointment

Step 3. Evaluation at 4 weeks
✓ Assess safety[2] and tolerability[3]
✓ Assess efficacy[4] $\geq$4 pound weight loss

Step 4. Schedule monthly visits for 6 months
✓ Coach patient to improve weight loss during active weight loss phase.
✓ Monitor safety and efficacy: may reduce to 5 mg or increase to 15 mg sibutramine po qd

Step 5. Six Month Visit
✓ Assess success at weight loss goal
✓ Assess tolerability and safety
✓ Encourage patient to continue diet, exercise, medication
✓ Set an appointment for month 12.

Long term patient management
✓ Follow patient at 6 month intervals
✓ Monitor safety and efficacy: may reduce to 5 mg or increase to 15 mg sibutramine po qd.
✓ Be proactive in relapse prevention
✓ Encourage more frequent appointments if patient stops medications, experiences difficulty

[1] Contraindications: cardiovascular disease, seizures, use of MAOI or other medications that are serotonergic or noradrenergic
[2] Acceptible BP and pulse limits: BP $\leq$135/80 or increase from baseline $\leq$20 mm Hg; Pulse $\leq$100 or increase from baseline $\leq$20 beats/minute.
[3] Acceptable efficacy profile at 4 weeks: $\geq$4 pound weight loss
[4] Acceptable 6 month efficacy: $\geq$ 5% loss from baseline.

Fig. 9. Treatment algorithm for using sibutramine in weight management. *Abbreviations*: BP, blood pressure; MAOI, monoamine oxidase inhibitor.

obesity management attempts. Physicians should take their prescribing responsibility seriously and address the patient's need for assistance in aiding behavioral weight-loss approaches. Sibutramine plays a role in promoting satiety and in blunting the reduction of metabolic rate that occurs with weight loss. Sibutramine can help selected patients achieve and maintain meaningful weight loss with the attendant improvement in certain obesity-related health risk factors. If a conservative approach is used, blood pressure elevation need not be a barrier to successful weight management with sibutramine.

References

[1] Calle E, Thun MJ, Petrelli JM, Rodriguez C, Heath CS. Body mass index and mortality in a prospective cohort of US adults. N Engl J Med 1999;344:1097–105.

[2] Flegal KM, Carroll MD, Kuczmarski RJ, Johnson CL. Overweight and obesity in the United States: prevalence and trends, 1960–1994. Int J Obes Relat Metab Disord 1998; 22:39–47.

[3] Flegal KM, Carroll MD, Ogden CL, et al. Prevalence and trends in obesity among US adults, 1999–2000. JAMA 2002;288:1723–7.

[4] Ford ES, Giles WH, Dietz WH. Prevalence of the metabolic syndrome among US adults: findings from the third National Health and Nutrition Examination Survey. JAMA 2002;287:356–9.

[5] National Institutes of Health. Third Report of the National Cholesterol Education Program Expert Panel on Detection, Evaluation, and Treatment of High Blood Cholesterol in Adults (Adult Treatment Panel III). NIH publication 01–3670. Bethesda (MD): National Institutes of Health; 2001.

[6] National Institutes of Health. National Heart, Lung, and Blood Institute. Clinical guidelines on the identification, evaluation, and treatment of overweight and obesity in adults—the evidence report. Obes Res 1998;6(Suppl 2):51S–210S.

[7] Yanovski SZ, Yanovski JA. Obesity. N Engl J Med 2002;346:591–602.

[8] National Institutes of Health, National Heart, Lung, and Blood Institute, North American Association for the Study of Obesity. The practical guide to the identification, evaluation, and treatment of overweight and obesity in adults. NIH publication number 00–4084. October 2000.

[9] Bray GA. Uses and misuses of the new pharmacotherapy of obesity [editorial]. Ann Med 1999;31:1–3.

[10] Weintraub M, Sundaresan PR, Madan M, Schuster B, Balder A, Lasagna L, et al. Long-term weight control study. I (weeks 0 to 34). The enhancement of behavior modification, caloric restriction, and exercise by fenfluramine plus phentermine versus placebo. Clin Pharmacol Ther 1992;51:586–94.

[11] Weintraub M, Sundaresan PR, Schuster B, Ginsberg G, Madan M, Balder A, et al. Long-term weight control study. II (weeks 34 to 104). An open-label study of continuous fenfluramine plus phentermine versus targeted intermittent medication as adjuncts to behavior modification, caloric restriction, and exercise. Clin Pharmacol Ther 1992; 51:595–601.

[12] Weintraub M, Sundaresan PR, Schuster B, Moscucci M, Stein EC. Long-term weight control study. III (weeks 104 to 156). An open-label study of dose adjustment of fenfluramine and phentermine. Clin Pharmacol Ther 1992;51:602–7.

[13] Weintraub M, Sundaresan PR, Schuster B, Averbuch M, Stein EC, Cox C, et al. Long-term weight control study. IV (weeks 156 to 190). The second double-blind phase. Clin Pharmacol Ther 1992;51:608–14.

[14] Weintraub M, Sundaresan PR, Schuster B, Averbuch M, Stein EC, Byrne L. Long-term weight control study. V (weeks 190 to 120). Follow-up of participants after cessation of medication. Clin Pharmacol Ther 1992;51:615–8.

[15] Connolly HM, Crary JL, McGoon MD, Hensrud DD, Edwards BS, Edwards WD, et al. Valvular heart disease associated with fenfluramine-phentermine. N Engl J Med 1997; 337:581–8.

[16] Jick H. Heart valve disorders and appetite-suppressant drugs. JAMA 2000;283:1738–40.

[17] Hensrud DD, Connolly HM, Grogan M, Miller FA, Bailey KR, Jensen MD. Echocardiographic improvement over time after cessation of use of fenfluramine and phentermine. Mayo Clin Proc 1999;74:1191–7.

[18] Bray GA. Barriers to the treatment of obesity [editorial]. Ann Intern Med 1991;115:152–3.

[19] Luque CA, Rey JA. Sibutramine: a serotonin-norepinephrine reuptake-inhibitor for the treatment of obesity. Ann Pharmacother 1999;33:968–78.

[20] Kelly F, Jones SP, Lee JK. Sibutramine weight loss in depressed patients [abstract]. Int J Obes 1995;19(Suppl 2):145.

[21] Heal DJ, Aspley S, Prow MR, Jackson HC, Martin KF, Cheetham SC. Sibutramine: a novel anti-obesity drug. A review of the pharmacological evidence to differentiate it from d-amphetamine and d-fenfluramine. Int J Obes Relat Metab Disord 1998;22(Suppl 1):S19–28.

[22] Stock MJ. Sibutramine: a review of the pharmacology of a novel antiobesity agent. Int J Obes 1997;21:S25–9.

[23] Connoley IP, Liu YL, Frost I. Thermogenic effects of sibutramine and its metabolites. Br J Pharmacol 1999;126:1487–95.

[24] Chapelot D, Marmonier C, Thomas F, Hanotin C. Modalities of the food intake-reducing effect of sibutramine in humans. Physiol Behav 2000;68:299–308.

[25] Rolls BJ, Shide DJ, Thorwart ML, Ulbrecht JS. Sibutramine reduces food intake in non-dieting women with obesity. Obes Res 1998;6:1–11.

[26] Hansen DL, Toubro S, Stock MJ, Macdonald IA, Astrup A. Thermogenic effects of sibutramine in humans. Am J Clin Nutr 1998;6:1180–6.

[27] Walsh KM, Leen E, Lean MEJ. The effect of sibutramine on resting energy expenditure and adrenaline-induced thermogenesis in obese females. Int J Obes Relat Metab Disord 1999;23:1009–15.

[28] Bray GA, Blackburn GL, Ferguson JM, Greenway FL, Jain AK, Mendel CM, et al. Sibutramine produces dose-related weight loss. Obes Res 1999;7:189–98.

[29] Wadden TA, Berkowitz RI, Sarwer DB, Prus-Wisniewski R, Steinberg C. Benefits of lifestyle modification in the pharmacologic treatment of obesity. Arch Intern Med 2001; 161:218–27.

[30] Apfelbaum M, Vague P, Ziegler O, Hanotin C, Thomas F, Leutenegger E. Long-term maintenance of weight loss after a very-low-calorie diet: a randomized blinded trial of the efficacy and tolerability of sibutramine. Am J Med 1999;106:179–84.

[31] James WPT, Astrup A, Finer N, Hilsted J, Kopelman P, Rossner S, et al. for the STORM Study Group. Effect of sibutramine on weight maintenance after weight loss: a randomised trial. Lancet 2000;356:2119–25.

[32] Wirth A, Krause J. Long-term weight loss with sibutramine. JAMA 2001;286:1331–9.

[33] Bach DS, Rissanen AM, Mendel CM, Shepherd G, Weinstein S, Kelly F. Absence of cardiac valve dysfunction in obese patients treated with sibutramine. Obes Res 1999;7:363–9.

[34] Cole JO, Levin A, Beake B, Kaiser PE, Scheinbaum ML. Sibutramine: a new weight loss agent without evidence of the abuse potential associated with amphetamines. J Clin Psychopharmacol 1998;18:231–6.

[35] Wesnes KA, Garratt C, Wickens M, Gudgeon A, Oliver S. Effects of sibutramine alone and with alcohol on cognitive function in healthy volunteers. Br J Clin Pharmacol 2000;49:110–7.

[36] Bray GA, Ryan DH, Gordon D, Heidingsfelder S, Cerise F, Wilson K. A double-blind randomized placebo-controlled trial of sibutramine. Obes Res 1996;4:263–70.

[37] Lean ME. Sibutramine: a review of clinical efficacy. Int J Obes 1997;21:S30–6.

[38] Sharma AM. Sibutramine in overweight/obese hypertensive patients. Int J Obes Relat Metab Disord 2001;25(Suppl 4):S20–3.

[39] Berube-Parent S, Prud-homme D, St-Pierre S, Doucet E, Tremblay A. Obesity treatment with a progressive clinical tri-therapy combining sibutramine and a supervised diet-exercise intervention. Int J Obes Relat Metab Disord 2001;25:1144–53.

[40] Sramek JJ, Leibowitz MT, Weinstein SP, Rowe ED, Mendel CM, Levy B, et al. Efficacy and safety of sibutramine for weight loss in obese patients with hypertension well controlled by beta-adrenergic blocking agents: a placebo-controlled, double-blind, randomised trial. J Hum Hypertens 2002;16:13–9.

[41] Gokcel A, Bumurdulu Y, Karakose H, Melek Ertorer E, Tanaci N, BascilTutuncu N, et al. Evaluation of the safety and efficacy of sibutramine, orlistat and metformin in the treatment of obesity. Diabetes Obes Metab 2002;4:49–55.

[42] Van Gaal LF, Wauters MA, Peiffer FW, De Leeuw IH. Sibutramine and fat distribution: is there a role for pharmacotherapy in abdominal/visceral fat reduction? Int J Obes Relat Metab Disord 1998;22(Suppl 1):S38–40.

[43] Aronne LJ. Treating obesity: a new target of prevention of coronary heart disease. Prog Cardiovasc Nurs 2001;16:98–106,115.

[44] Dujovne CA, Zavoral JH, Rowe E, Mendel CM. Effects of sibutramine on body weight and serum lipids: a double-blind, randomized, placebo-controlled study in 322 overweight and obese patients with dyslipidemia. Am Heart J 2001;142:489–97.

[45] Samsa GP, Kolotkin RL, Williams GR, Nguyen MH, Mendel CM. Effect of moderate weight loss on health-related quality of life: an analysis of combined data from 4 randomized trials of sibutramine vs. placebo. Am J Manag Care 2001;7:875–83.

[46] Cuellar GEM, Ruiz AM, Monsalve MCR, Berber A. Six-month treatment of obesity with sibutramine 15 mg: a double-blind, placebo-controlled monocenter clinical trial in a Hispanic population. Obes Res 2000;8:71–82.

[47] Smith IG, Goulder MA. Randomized placebo-controlled trial of long-term treatment with sibutramine in mild to moderate obesity. J Fam Pract 2001;50:505–12.

[48] Fanghanel G, Cortinas L, Sanchez-Reyes L, Berber A. A clinical trial of the use of sibutramine for the treatment of patients suffering essential obesity. Int J Obes Relat Metab Disord 2001;24:144–50.

[49] McMahon FG, Fujioka K, Singh BN, Mendel CM, Rowe E, Rolston K, et al. Efficacy and safety of sibutramine in obese white and African American patients with hypertension. Arch Intern Med 2000;160:2185–91.

[50] Hazenberg BP. Randomized, double-blind, placebo-controlled, multicenter study of sibutramine in obese hypertensive patients. Cardiology 2000;94:152–8.

[51] McMahon FG, Weinstein SP, Rowe E, Ernst KR, Johnson F, Fujioka K. Sibutramine is safe and effective for weight loss in obese patients whose hypertension is well controlled with angiotensin-converting enzyme inhibitors. J Hum Hypertens 2002;16:5–11.

[52] Fujioka K, Seaton TB, Rowe E, Jelinek CA, Raskin P, Lebovitz HE, et al. Weight loss with sibutramine improves glycaemic control and other metabolic parameters in obese patients with type 2 diabetes mellitus. Diabetes, Obesity, and Metabolism 2000;2:175–87.

[53] Finer N, Bloom SR, Frost GS, Banks LM, Griffiths J. Sibutramine is effective for weight loss and diabetic control in obesity with type 2 diabetes: a randomised, double-blind, placebo-controlled study. Diabetes, Obesity, and Metabolism 2000;2:105–12.

[54] Gokcel A, Karakose H, Ertorer EM, Tanaci N, Tutuncu NB, Guvener N. Effects of sibutramine in obese female subjects with type 2 diabetes and poor blood glucose control. Diabetes Care 2001;24:1957–60.

[55] Serrano-Rios M, Melchionda N, Moreno-Carretero E. Spanish Investigators. Role of sibutramine in the treatment of obese Type 2 diabetic patients receiving sulphonylurea therapy. Diabet Med 2002;19:119–24.

15

Herbal Preparations for Obesity: Are They Useful?

David Heber

Herbal products for weight reduction may ultimately prove to be helpful in overcoming clinically significant obesity when combined with healthy diet and lifestyle changes. The safety of available herbal products for weight reduction, as well as their efficacy, remain major issues that need to be resolved through research and education, as well as better regulation of the manufacture and sale of these products. These surmountable problems severely limit current enthusiasm of the medical community for the use of any herbal supplements. Physicians, outside of the small number of researchers who are familiar with the potential of botanical dietary supplements, have received little or no education on the safety or efficacy of using any herbal products in primary care practice, including those botanical dietary supplements that are used for weight reduction.

Despite the negative view of herbs held by the mainstream medical community, botanical dietary supplements for weight loss remain extremely popular with the general public. In fact, the use of herbal and alternative medicines has increased in the last decade in the United States. In response to public demands for these products, the U.S. Congress passed the Dietary Supplements Health Education Act (DSHEA) in 1994, which enables manufacturers to market these products without the extensive previous proof of efficacy and safety that is required of prescription drug manufacturers. Although this law has made these products available for purchase without a prescription, the law also prohibited any claim that such products could cure, prevent, or mitigate a disease. Another provision of the law established Centers for Dietary Supplement Research in Botanicals supported by the National Institutes of Health through the Office of Dietary Supplements and the National Center for Complementary and Alternative Medicine (currently at UCLA, University of Illinois, Purdue University, University of Alabama, Birmingham, University of Arizona, University of Missouri, and Iowa State University) to conduct clinical and basic research investigations on botanical dietary supplements for the prevention of chronic diseases. This effort is aimed at building the science base for the use of dietary supplements so that the potential public health benefits of botanical dietary supplements can be realized. Herbal supplements have unique characteristics that differentiate them from prescription drugs, and which may make them more appropriate than drugs for the prevention and treatment of many common chronic diseases, including obesity.

Obesity is not universally classified as a disease; under the DSHEA law, herbal products for weight reduction use a structure-function claim for "achieving and maintaining a healthy body weight" to be considered botanical dietary supplements that are approved for sale to the general public. Contrary to a widely held public opinion, the DSHEA law does not remove the responsibility for appropriate oversight and regulation of product labeling, good manufacturing practices, and other quality control measures that could reassure the public of the safety and usefulness of these products from government agencies. The Food and Drug Administration (FDA) is still responsible for issuing good manufacturing processes as required under the DSHEA legislation and has not issued these regulations almost 10 years after the law was passed. Given these considerations, it is vital that obese patients who plan to use supplements choose products from reliable manufacturers, carefully read labels, and obtain knowledge about which products are efficacious. The advice and supervision of an informed primary care physician can certainly minimize the risk of adverse side effects and maximize the chances for benefit.

To monitor safety retrospectively, the FDA relies on reports of adverse effects as part of a program called Medwatch, which was originally designed for postmarketing surveillance of prescription drugs. Unfortunately, this method has significant drawbacks when it comes to scientifically examining the causal relationship between the use of a particular botanical dietary supplement and a reported side effect. This can be especially difficult when the reported side effects are comorbid diseases, such as heart disease or hypertension, that are associated with obesity, even in the absence of using a dietary supplement. Authors of articles in major medical journals, such as the New England Journal of Medicine, assume that all reported side effects that can be related to supplement use are, in fact, related to supplement use. Also, because there is no population reference for adverse side effects, actual incidence per 100,000 population cannot be determined to weigh risks and benefits.

The Federal Trade Commission has the responsibility to monitor advertising claims that incorporate some elements of proof of efficacy. These supplements are often advertised on the radio, rather than the television, because the standards for radio advertising are less stringent than those for television advertising. Furthermore, gray areas exist in broadcast advertising that relate to constitutional protections of free speech; this limits the effective regulation of some outlandish claims about weight loss products. Some of these claims clearly violate the Laws of Thermodynamics, but are legal under current laws that regulate advertising. This atmosphere also makes it difficult for manufacturers who wish to adhere to higher standards to compete with the companies that make outrageous and unsubstantiated claims for their products. This chapter provides information on the most commonly used herbal weight loss preparations so that you can communicate the risks and benefits to your obese patients and encourage them to use safe and effective products within an overall approach of diet and lifestyle for the achievement and maintenance of healthy body weight.

Herbal preparations containing ephedra alkaloids and herbal caffeine

Herbal caffeine and ephedrine

The most widely used herbal supplements for weight loss contain ephedra alkaloids and herbal forms of caffeine (guarana or gotu kola). The use of these ingredients is derived from recipes that are used in Traditional Chinese Medicine (TCM) that include an herb called "ma huang." In TCM, ma huang is one of several herbs that are combined in recipes that also sometimes include guarana or other caffeine-equivalent herbs, such as gotu-kola.

Much of the biological rationale for the use of this combination comes from clinical research that was conducted using ephedrine and caffeine as purified compounds. These compounds have been extensively studied, beginning with pioneering work in Denmark. This research, that used modern scientific methods, provides strong evidence for a synergistic interaction of ephedrine and caffeine; this is one of the basic features that distinguishes complex herbal mixtures from purified crystallized chemicals that are used in drugs. Another difference is that ephedra is made up of a family of related compounds, among which ephedrine is the most active. A question about ephedra and other botanical dietary supplements is whether these related families of compounds contribute in a unique way to the action, metabolism, or safety profile of botanical dietary supplements compared with purified preparations of the putative, most active ingredients, such as caffeine and ephedrine. Herbal ephedrine has four isomers, whereas pharmaceutical grade ephedrine contains only the most potent member of the family of related compounds [1]. Theoretically, the herbal form of ephedrine should be safer than equivalent doses of the pharmaceutical grade product because it contains less of the most potent isomer. Although not proven, it is possible that the multiple related compounds in herbal ephedra may be metabolized differently than a single, purified pharmaceutical, such as ephedrine.

Supplements that contain ma huang, guarana, and multiple other herbs in combination may be based on TCM recipes and are widely promoted and used in the United States. The many individuals who purchase and use these products have stymied efforts to remove these products from the marketplace. The FDA proposed limits on the dose and duration of use of such supplements, but the proposals have not been issued as formal regulations.

Recently, an 8-week randomized, double-blind, placebo-controlled study of a botanical dietary supplement that provides 72 mg/day of ephedrine alkaloids and 240 mg/day caffeine of was conducted with 67 overweight men and women with a body mass index between 29 kg/m^2 and 35 kg/m^2 [2]. Patients were randomized to placebo (n = 32) or active ma huang/guarana (n = 35); 24 subjects in each group completed the study. The botanical dietary supplement produced significantly greater loss of weight compared with placebo treatment (4.0 ± 3.4 kg versus 0.8 ± 2.4 kg) over the 8-week treatment period ($P < 0.006$). Body fat was also significantly decreased. Eight of the 35 (23%) subjects who were treated with the supplement withdrew from the protocol because of potential treatment-related effects that included dry mouth, insomnia, and headache. The popular herbal mixture of ma huang and guarana effectively promoted short-term weight and fat loss in this study. Clearly, long-term studies are required to assess safety and efficacy.

The FDA requested an independent review of reports of adverse events that were related to the use of supplements that contained ephedra alkaloids to assess causation and to estimate the level of risk that the use of these supplements poses to consumers. This report was published in the New England Journal of Medicine and widely publicized [3]. A total of 140 reports of adverse events that were associated with the use of dietary supplements that contained ephedra alkaloids that were submitted to the FDA between June 1, 1997, and March 31, 1999 were reviewed. A standardized rating system for assessing causation was applied to each adverse event. Thirty-one percent of cases were judged by the investigators to be "related" to the use of supplements that contained ephedra alkaloids; 31% were deemed to be "possibly related" to the use of supplements. Among the adverse events that were deemed "definitely, probably, or possibly" related to the use of supplements that contained ephedra alkaloids, 47% involved cardiovascular symptoms and 18% involved the central nervous system. Hypertension was the most frequent adverse effect (17 reports), followed by palpitations, tachycardia, or both (13 reports), stroke (10 reports), and seizures (seven reports). Ten events were associated with deaths, and 13 associated events resulted in permanent disability; these represented 26% of the "definite, probable, and possible" cases. Although these reports possibly associate the use of herbal dietary supplements that contain ephedra with side effects, they do not in any way prove a causative relationship between herbal use and these problems.

Two recent, randomized, controlled trials by Boozer et al [2,4] examine efficacy and side effects of a combination of ma huang and guarana versus placebo. In the first study, subjects were randomized to a combination ma huang/guarana supplement or placebo and were followed for 6 months. Active treatment produced greater weight loss and fat loss. In this study, 8 of the 35 subjects who took the supplement withdrew because of side effects of dry mouth, insomnia, or headache. Over the short-term, the combination supplement resulted in greater weight loss for the subjects who completed the trial. In a more recent, randomized, placebo-controlled study, Boozer et al [2] conducted a 6-month study of an herbal/ephedra combination (92 mg/day of ephedra alkaloids and 192 mg/day of caffeine) in 167 patients at two outpatient weight control clinics. The group that took the supplement had greater weight loss (5.3 ± 5.0 kg versus 2.6 ± 3.2 kg, $P < 0.001$) and greater fat loss. By self-report, dry mouth ($P < 0.01$), heartburn ($P < 0.05$), and insomnia ($P < 0.01$) were more frequent among supplement-treated patients. Incidence of irritability, nausea, chest pain, and palpitations did not differ between the two groups, nor did the number of patients who withdrew from the study. In this study, the ephedra/caffeine combination produced more weight loss without significant, adverse effects. These studies were conducted under careful observation by professional staff, and it is not clear that the same results would occur in a free-living population of supplement users.

Nonetheless, there is significant scientific support for an herbal formulation that combines ephedra and caffeine. Although the combination, as a botanical dietary supplement, has its origins in traditional Chinese medicine, Western medicine has studied the pharmaceutical combination of ephedrine and caffeine. In 1972, Dr. Erikson, a Danish general practitioner in Elsinore, Denmark, noted unintentional weight loss when he prescribed a compound that contained ephedrine, caffeine, and phenobarbital to patients that he was treating for asthma. As he pursued his observation, rumor spread from his patients to the rest of the country. By 1977, more than 70,000 patients were taking the "Elsinore Pill," and one Danish pharmaceutical house was producing one million tablets a week.

During the time that the "Elsinore Pill" was used for the treatment of obesity, there were more skin rashes reported, some serious. These were most likely caused by the phenobarbital in the "Elsinore Pill." In 1977, the Danish Institute of Health issued a warning to doctors not to prescribe the compound because of the increased incidence of skin rashes, and Dr. Erikson was harshly criticized in the public and scientific press. The "Elsinore Pill" without phenobarbital was compared with the appetite suppressant, diethylpropion, and to placebo in 132 subjects in a 12-week, double-blind trial. Diethylpropion, 25 mg, three times a day and the "Elsinore Pill" without phenobarbital (caffeine, 100 mg and ephedrine, 40 mg, three times a day) resulted in 8.4 kg and 8.1 kg weight loss, respectively, which were not different from each other, but were greater than the weight loss of 4.1 kg that was experienced by the subjects who took placebo ($P < 0.01$). Tremor and agitation were more frequent on the "Elsinore Pill," but were transient and the withdrawal for side effects was equal in the groups that took diethylpropion and the "Elsinore Pill." There was no increase in blood pressure, pulse rate, or laboratory parameters. The investigators concluded that the ephedrine and caffeine combination had advantages over diethylpropion because of its lower cost with equivalent safety and efficacy [5].

Other early studies of ephedrine and caffeine also used commercial asthma preparations. Theophylline and caffeine are methylxanthines and have the same pharmacologic actions. One milligram of theophylline is equivalent to 2 milligrams of caffeine [6]. Miller [7] used the "Do-Do" pill that was manufactured by Ciba-Geigy (Basel, Switzerland) in the United Kingdom that contained 22 mg of ephedrine, 30 mg of caffeine, and 50 mg of theophylline per pill. Each pill, therefore, contained the equivalent of 22 mg of ephedrine and 130 mg of caffeine. The ephedrine/methylxanthines mixture was twice as effective as ephedrine alone in increasing the resting metabolic rate. Ephedrine with theophylline was the primary treatment for asthma in the 1960s and 1970s and ephedrine is still sold in the United States without a prescription for the treatment of asthma [8]. Ephedrine with caffeine is still the most widely sold prescription weight loss medication in Denmark and held 80% of the market share, even when dexfenfluramine was available.

Caffeine has been studied separately in animals and humans, because it can increase sympathetic nervous system activity, and obesity has been associated with low sympathetic activity [9]. In genetically obese mice without endogenous leptin production (ob/ob mice), caffeine decreased body fat and improved sympathetic activity; this suggested a possible role in the treatment of human obesity [10]. Caffeine in an oral dose of 250 mg increased free fatty acids and glucose, but not cortisol levels, in obese and lean humans compared with a water placebo with each subject acting as his own control [11]. Oxygen consumption, fat oxidation, and serum free fatty acids were increased in six normal subjects who were given caffeine 8 mg/kg orally compared with 0.5 gram glucose. Oxygen consumption and fat oxidation were also increased in seven normal and six obese subjects after ingesting 4 mg/kg of caffeinated coffee compared with a decaffeinated control after fasting and after a mixed meal [12].

In small studies, the administration of caffeine was shown to increase lipolysis, circulating fatty acid levels, and oxygen consumption [13–16]. In one study, caffeine administration significantly elevated systolic blood pressure from 4.5 to 6.6 mm Hg, but there was no change in diastolic blood pressure or pulse rate [15]. Subjects reported no symptoms or side effects. The caffeine-induced increase in thermogenesis is dissipated through an increase in skin temperature [17], a reaction that is familiar to anyone who has consumed several cups of coffee at one sitting. The increase in resting metabolic rate that was induced by 4 mg/kg of caffeine predicted the amount of weight lost in response to a diet and exercise program; the dose-response characteristics were carefully documented [18–21]. Therefore, the scientific evidence in animals and humans supports a potential role for caffeine in weight reduction through increases in oxygen consumption and fat oxidation.

Several epidemiologic studies addressed the safety of caffeine. The positive correlation found between heavy coffee drinking and elevated cholesterol is believed to be caused by factors other than the caffeine in coffee, because caffeine consumption in the form of tea or cola has no effect on cholesterol [22,23]. A clinical trial with 288 healthy subjects evaluated the effects of a single 200 mg/day dose of caffeine compared with placebo. Caffeine caused a 2.2 mm Hg increase in diastolic blood pressure, which was believed to be clinically insignificant. There was no change in pulse rate or systolic blood pressure [24]. Similarly, the negative effects of drinking more than two cups of coffee per day on osteoporosis in women is associated with factors other than the caffeine in coffee [25]. The FDA approved caffeine for sale without a prescription for use as a stimulant [26] by persons 12 years of age or older at a dose up to 200 mg every 3 hours (1600 mg/d) and as an ingredient in pain medications, which gives further support to its safety.

Ephedrine elevates oxygen consumption without increasing food intake in animals while causing weight and fat loss [27–29]. Ephedrine was one of the two most efficient compounds in comprehensive studies of several putative weight loss compounds in animal models of obesity; this led to its proposed use in the treatment of obesity [30,31].

Ephedrine stimulates brown adipose tissue thermogenesis through the activation of beta-receptors. It was estimated that 40% of the acute rise in oxygen consumption in response to ephedrine is due to activation of the beta-3 adrenergic receptor [32]; ephedrine was the most potent of the four isomers in ephedra when tested in this assay [33]. Propranalol prevents the weight loss that is induced in ob/ob mice by ephedrine [34] which demonstrated its action through the beta-receptors. Animal studies also showed the potentiation of ephedrine activity when used with aspirin [35].

Concerns with the potential side effects of ephedrine [36–38] stimulated a 3-month trial that compared ephedrine, 25 mg, three times a day (13 subjects), ephedrine, 50 mg three times a day (17 subjects), and placebo (16 subjects). There were similar weight losses in all groups with significantly more side effects (blood pressure elevation, pulse elevation, agitation, insomnia, headache, weakness, palpitations, giddiness, euphoria, tremor, and diarrhea) in the group that took ephedrine, 50 mg, three times a day compared with those who took placebo [39]. There was more weight loss in the groups that took ephedrine, however, at the end of the first and second months, a difference that was lost by the end of the third month [40].

A second trial compared ephedrine, 50 mg, three times a day, with placebo over 8 weeks in 10 low-energy adapted women who had already lost weight. The study used a crossover design. Weight loss was greater during the 2-month period while the subjects took ephedrine (2.4 kg versus 0.6 kg with placebo). Side effects were uncommon and included, agitation (two subjects), insomnia (three subjects), giddiness (two subjects), and palpitations (two subjects); none required withdrawal of medication [41].

Ephedrine was also evaluated in conjunction with a very low calorie diet. Ephedrine decreased urinary nitrogen and blunted the fall in resting metabolic rate [42]. With the administration of ephedrine at the dose of 1 mg/kg body weight, oxygen consumption was increased by 5 weeks of exercise training for 1 hour per day on a bicycle at a heart rate of 140 to 160 beats per minute [43].

In another study, 180 obese subjects were randomized to ephedrine, 20 mg, three times a day; caffeine, 200 mg, three times a day; ephedrine, 20 mg, with caffeine, 200 mg, three times a day; or placebo for a 24-week, double blind trial. Weight loss with the caffeine and ephedrine combination was greater than with placebo after 8 weeks until the end of the trial. Ephedrine and caffeine alone were not different than placebo. The group that took caffeine with ephedrine lost 17.5% of their body weight during the 24-week trial. Side effects of tremor, insomnia, and dizziness reached the levels of placebo by 8 weeks and blood pressure fell similarly in all four groups. Heart rate rose in a statistically significant manner in the group that took ephedrine compared with placebo, but fell below the baseline value in the group that took caffeine and ephedrine [44]. Two weeks after cessation of the 24-week trial, headache and tiredness were more frequent in the group that had taken caffeine with ephedrine. At the end of the 2-week washout period, all subjects were given the opportunity to participate in an additional 24-week, open-label trial that used caffeine with ephedrine. The subjects who remained on caffeine with ephedrine maintained their weight loss to the end of trial at week 50 [45]. Seventy-five percent of the weight loss was explained by anorexia and 25% was explained by increased thermogenesis [46]. Because acute treatment with caffeine, 200 mg and ephedrine, 20 mg, three times a day, had cardiovascular and metabolic effects, the chronic effects were evaluated in the 24-week trial. By week 12, the blood pressure had dropped 4 to 11 mm Hg below baseline and remained similar to the placebo group. The pulse rate dropped 1 to 2 bpm from baseline during the trial, and reductions in plasma glucose, cholesterol, and triglycerides were not different between the groups at the end of the 24-week, double-blind trial [47]. These findings were confirmed in an 8-week, double blind, placebo-controlled trial that used ephedrine, 50 mg; caffeine, 50 mg; and aspirin, 110 mg, given three times a day. There was no significant change in heart rate, blood pressure, blood glucose, insulin, cholesterol, or side effects in the group that took placebo, but weight loss was greater in the group that took ephedrine, caffeine, and aspirin [48].

The effect of caffeine, 200 mg, with ephedrine, 20 mg, three times a day on body composition was studied using bioimpedance analysis. At the end of 8 weeks, weight loss was not different, but the group that took caffeine and ephedrine lost 4.5 kg more fat and 2.5 kg less lean tissue than the placebo group, which was a significant difference. As one might expect, the fall in energy expenditure was 13% in the placebo group and only 8% in the group that was treated with caffeine and ephedrine [49]. Treatment with caffeine and ephedrine over 8 weeks also prevented the expected drop in HDL cholesterol. Because HDL cholesterol protects from atherogenesis, this finding suggested that caffeine and ephedrine may have the potential to reduce atherosclerotic cardiovascular disease. The group that took placebo experienced the drop in HDL cholesterol that is routinely reported with diet-induced weight loss [50].

Ephedrine with or without a methylxanthine was evaluated in adolescents. The effect of ephedrine in stimulating thermogenesis was lost after 1 week of treatment, but was restored by combining it with aminophylline for 1 week [51]. This explains why the trials with ephedrine alone, compared with placebo, led to more weight loss early in the trial that decreased with time, unless combined with a methylxanthine. The same group reported a 20-week, double-blind, placebo-controlled, randomized clinical trial of caffeine and ephedrine in 32 adolescents aged 15 to 17 years years and Tanner stage III–V [52]. Subjects who weighed less than 80 kg were given one tablet that contained 100 mg caffeine and 10 mg ephedrine, three times a day; subjects that weighed more than 80 kg were given two pills, three times a day. The loss of initial body weight was 14.4% and 2.2% in the groups that took caffeine with ephedrine and placebo, respectively ($P < 0.01$). All three subjects who dropped out of the study were in the placebo group; adverse events were described as negligible. After the first 4 weeks, the adverse events were similar in both groups.

Caffeine with ephedrine caused weight loss in the range of 15% to 20% of initial body weight in 6 months; this is comparable to what was seen with phentermine/fenfluramine [53]. Caffeine, 200 mg, with ephedrine, 20 mg, that was given three times a day was compared with dexfenfluramine, 15 mg, twice a day, in a double-blind trial. In subjects with a BMI that was greater than 30 kg/m^2, the weight loss was greater with the caffeine and ephedrine treatment. Blood pressure declined significantly in both groups (7.8/4.6 mm Hg in the group that took dexfenfluramine, 10.6/3.5 mm Hg in the group that took caffeine and ephedrine) but they were not significantly different from each other. Pulse rate declined 1.1 to 2.7 bpm and was not different between the groups. The subjects who were treated with dexfenfluramine had more gastrointestinal symptoms (diarrhea, dry mouth, thirst) whereas the subjects that were treated with caffeine and ephedrine had more symptoms of central nervous system stimulation (tremor, insomnia, agitation). Symptoms in both groups declined by the end of the first month of the 15-week trial [54].

Although dexfenfluramine is no longer available because of cardiac valvular toxicity, caffeine and ephedrine are available without prescription. The cardiac valvular problems that are associated with fenfluramine and dexfenfluramine are believed to be related to serotonin and have not been associated with caffeine and ephedrine, which have a noradrenergic mechanism of action. Fenfluramine with phentermine, fenfluramine with mazindol, caffeine with ephedrine, and mazindol alone were compared in their ability to reduce weight, cardiovascular risk, and LDL cholesterol. Caffeine with ephedrine was found to be the most cost-effective treatment [55].

Concerns have been raised about the safety of caffeine and ephedrine use in subjects with controlled hypertension. One hundred thirty-six overweight normotensive or drug-controlled, hypertensive subjects were randomized to five groups. After 6 weeks of treatment, systolic blood pressure was reduced 5.5 mm Hg more in the group with controlled hypertension who was treated with caffeine, 200 mg, and ephedrine, 20 mg, three times a day, than in the subjects who received placebo and had their hypertension treated with medication other than beta-blockers. The antihypertensive effect of beta-blocker medication was not reduced by caffeine and ephedrine. Normotensive patients who were treated with caffeine and ephedrine had a 4.4/3.9 mm Hg greater drop in blood pressure than those who were treated with placebo. The mean loss of weight of 4 kg was significant for all groups [56].

Caffeine and ephedrine have been included in recent reviews of obesity medication [57–62]. Thermogenic approaches to treat obesity have been reviewed [63]. More specifically, caffeine and ephedrine used for obesity treatment have also been reviewed [64–67]. In a letter to the editor of the journal in which the clinical trial was published, Astrup et al [68] reported that on reanalysis, ephedrine alone actually caused more weight loss than placebo, but less weight loss than ephedrine and caffeine, in the 24-week trial of caffeine, ephedrine, caffeine with ephedrine, and placebo. Caffeine and ephedrine have been used to induce weight loss before comparing different weight maintenance diets [69].

Ephedrine products are sold without a prescription for the treatment of asthma and have a recommended dosage of up to 150 mg per day. Caffeine sold without a prescription has a recommended dose of up to 1600 mg per day. The popular herbal products that contain caffeine and ephedrine that are taken for weight loss have dosage recommendations of up to 100 mg of ephedrine equivalent per day as ephedra. The caffeine content of the herbal products that contain caffeine and ephedrine varies, but is less than 600 mg a day. The most popular and widely sold herbal product that contains caffeine and ephedra provides 240 mg of caffeine per day, less caffeine that is contained in three cups of coffee. Pharmaceutical-grade products have greater potency than herbal products that contain caffeine and ephedrine in equivalent doses because the herbal products contain some of the less active isomers of ephedra. The peer-reviewed literature documented central nervous system stimulation and increases in pulse, blood pressure, and glucose when caffeine and ephedrine were given acutely, either separately or together. The side effects disappear with chronic treatment, and are no longer present after 4 to 12 weeks, depending on the trial. A 24-week trial of caffeine and ephedrine found a decrease in pulse and blood pressure. The pulse rate was no different in those who took caffeine and ephedrine compared with those who took placebo, but was significantly higher in those who took ephedrine alone compared with placebo. There were no differences in serum glucose, serum cholesterol, or symptoms of stimulation between the groups that took caffeine and ephedrine combination and placebo.

Ephedrine and caffeine have each been sold for years without a prescription for the treatment of asthma and to combat drowsiness, respectively. Toxicity has not been a concern, even with doses that are higher than those which are used in herbal products that contain caffeine and ephedrine for weight loss. Overweight and obesity are common problems that affect more than half of the population, yet obesity is stigmatized by society. Therefore, it is not surprising that an effective weight loss product that contains compounds with a long history of safe, nonprescription use would be embraced enthusiastically by the public. When large numbers of the public use any product, adverse events can be associated with its use; establishing a cause and effect relationship should be required before the withdrawal, prohibition, or licensing of such products.

Green tea catechins

Green tea that is prepared by heating or steaming the leaves of *Camelia sinensis* is widely consumed on a regular basis throughout Asia. Black tea is the most widely consumed tea, however, and is drunk by more than 80% of the world's population [70]. Black tea is made by allowing the green tea leaves to auto-oxidize enzymatically, which leads to the conversion of a large percentage of green tea catechins to theaflavins. The catechins are a family of compounds that include epigallocatechin gallate, which is considered to be the most potent antioxidant in the family of compounds. Drinking one cup of tea per day was reported to decrease the odds ratio of suffering a myocardial infarction to 0.56 compared with nontea drinkers [71]. These compounds are flavonoids in the class of polyphenols and have many activities, that include inhibition of the catechol-O-methyl transferase enzyme, which degrades norepinephrine [72]. The catechins seem to be able to enhance sympathetic nervous system activity at the level of the fat cell adrenoreceptor. In vitro, a green tea extract that contains catechins and caffeine was more potent in stimulating brown adipose tissue thermogenesis than equimolar concentrations of caffeine alone [73]. The use of ephedrine to release norepinephrine increased the thermogenic effect that was noted with green tea catechins. Oolong tea or placebo was orally administered to mice over a 10-week period during high-fat feeding. Mean food consumption was not different between the groups, but oolong tea prevented the obesity and fatty liver that was induced by the high-fat diet. Noradrenaline-induced lipolysis increased and pancreatic lipase activity was inhibited by the oolong tea [74]. Because caffeine occurs naturally in green tea extract, it has been difficult to separate the effects of green tea from caffeine in humans. Dulloo et al [65] gave subjects green tea extract capsules three times per day which provided a total of 150 mg caffeine, and 375 mg total catechins, of which 270 mg was epigallocatechin gallate. Each subject acted as their own control and spent three 24-hour periods in an energy chamber, during which they received the green tea extract, 150 mg of caffeine, or placebo. Urinary excretion of norepinephrine, but not epinephrine, was noted in the 24 hours when green tea was administered compared with the caffeine or placebo-treatment periods. Energy expenditure was higher by 4.5% during the green tea period compared with placebo and 3.2% higher than when the same dose of caffeine was given alone. In addition, fat oxidation was increased. The net effect that was attributable to green tea could be estimated at 328 kJ/d or approximately 80 cal/d. Clearly, it is difficult to demonstrate the effects of green tea catechins alone, but there is the possibility of a synergistic interaction with ephedrine, independent of the caffeine content of green tea, that should be evaluated.

Synephrine from Citrus aurantium

Bitter orange (*Citrus aurantium*) contains small amounts of alkaloids, such as synephrine and octopamine, that are direct and indirect sympathomimetic agonists. These substances occur in minute concentrations in orange juice on the order of parts per million. In one placebo-controlled study [75], 23 subjects with body mass index of higher than 25 kg/m^2 were randomly assigned to receive a maltose placebo, nothing, or 975 mg of a *Citrus aurantium* extract with 528 mg of caffeine and 900 mg of St. John's Wort daily. Subjects in the treated group lost 1.4 kg more weight than those in the placebo groups and also lost a significant amount of body fat (2.9%), whereas there was no fat loss in the placebo groups. It is claimed that these alkaloids act in a similar, but milder, fashion than the ephedra alkaloids, but this has not been carefully studied in a bioequivalence trial.

Capsaicin from chili peppers

Capsaicin from chili peppers and red peppers was shown to stimulate fat oxidation and thermogenesis [76,77]. The exact mechanism for this effect is not known, but the constituents seem to activate neural signals that result in vasodilation and endorphin release. There are also reports of modest weight loss in subjects who consume chili peppers regularly.

Fat metabolism and nutrient partitioning

Conjugated linoleic acid

The cis-9, trans-11 isomer of conjugated linoleic acid [78] is formed naturally in the rumen of cattle [79]; supplementation of cattle feed with linoleic or linolenic acids increases the amount of conjugated linoleic acid in milk [80]. Synthetic conjugated linoleic acid is a mixture of the cis-9, trans-11 isomer, and trans-10, cis-12 isomer [81]. The 9–11 isomer is believed to be responsible for the anticancer activity of conjugated linoleic acid [82], whereas the 10–12 isomer is believed to be responsible for the body compositional changes that are observed in animals [83,84].

Mice who were fed a diet that was supplemented with 0.5% conjugated linoleic acid at constant calories developed 60% less body fat than animals who were fed a control diet [85]. This decrease in body fat is most likely the result of a combination of reduced fat deposition, increased lipolysis, and increased fat oxidation. These findings were confirmed by West et al [86] who demonstrated that conjugated linoleic acid reduced energy intake, growth rate, carcass lipid, and carcass protein in mice. Metabolic rate was increased and nocturnal respiratory quotient was decreased in these mice. DeLany et al [87] showed that conjugated linoleic acid decreased body fat without suppressing energy intake in mice on a high-fat diet [87]. In this study, there was a marked decrease in body fat and increase in body protein without changes in food intake. Rats also responded to conjugated linoleic acid with a decrease in body fat [88].

Conjugated linoleic acid induces apoptosis of adipocytes and results in a form of lipodystrophy in which there is a decrease in white adipose tissue with the development of insulin resistance and enlargement of the liver [89]. The mechanism is uncertain, however. Satory and Smith [90] postulated a reduction in fat accumulation in growing animals by inhibition of stromal vascular preadiposite hyperplasia. Azain et al [91] found a reduction in fat cell size rather than a change in fat cell number [91]. Initial studies in humans to treat obesity, presented in abstract form, suggested a lack of efficacy of conjugated linoleic acid. Increases in insulin resistance in animals treated with conjugated linoleic acid raised safety concerns, as well.

Garcinia cambogia (hydroxycitric acid)

Garcinia cambogia contains hydroxycitric acid (HCA), which is extracted from the rind of the brindall berry. HCA is one of 16 isomers of citric acid and is the only one that inhibits citrate lyase, the enzyme that catalyzes the first step in fatty acid synthesis outside the mitochondrion. HCA was studied by Roche Pharmaceuticals in the 1970s in rodents. Those studies, that used the sodium salt of HCA, demonstrated weight reduction in three rodent models of obesity, that included the mature rat; the gold thioglucose-induced, obese mouse; and the ventromedial hypothalamic-lesioned, obese rat. Food intake, body weight gain, and body lipid content were all reduced with no change in body protein [92]. Three clinical trials evaluated the efficacy and safety of HCA. The first trial evaluated a product that contained HCA from *Garcinia cambogia* and chromium picolinate. In this single-arm, open-label, 8-week trial in 77 adults, 500 mg of *Garcinia cambogia* extract was combined with 100 micrograms of chromium picolinate taken 3 times per day. A 5.5% weight loss was seen in women and a 4.9% weight loss was seen in men [93]. HCA is also sold as an herbal supplement that contains the calcium salt for which the dose is 3 g/d as a treatment for obesity. Two human clinical trials evaluated the safety and efficacy of this marketed product. The first trial used 10 males who acted as their own controls in a crossover trial that evaluated energy expenditure and substrate oxidation. There was no difference in respiratory quotient, energy expenditure, glucose, insulin, glucagon, lactate, or beta-hydroxybutyrate at rest or during exercise [94]. The second trial randomized 135 obese adults using a double-blind, placebo-controlled design. HCA, 1500 mg/d, was administered for 12 weeks; both groups were given a low-fat, high-fiber diet. In this trial, there was no significant difference in the weight loss observed in both groups (3.2 ± 3.3 kg for HCA versus 4.1 ± 3.9 kg for placebo, $P = 0.14$) [95]. It is unclear whether the insolubility of the calcium salt or a species difference between rodents and humans is responsible for the lack of efficacy in humans. Further trials with measures of bioavailability are needed to resolve this issue, but the HCA herbal dietary supplements that are presently available seem to have no effect in human obesity.

Fibers

Soluble and insoluble dietary fibers

It was suggested that the increase in obesity in Western countries since 1900 may be related to changes in dietary fiber. The fiber content of starchy foods in the diet has decreased whereas the fiber that is associated with fruits and vegetables has increased [96]. Ludwig et al [97] enrolled 578 children from public schools and studied them from 1995 to 1997. The investigators examined the change in intake of sugar-sweetened drinks and difference in measures of obesity using linear and logistic regression to adjust for potentially confounding variables. Baseline consumption of soft drinks was associated with obesity in this study after adjustment for anthropometric, demographic, dietary, and lifestyle variables. Each additional serving of sugar-sweetened drinks was associated with a body mass index increase of 0.24 kg/m^2 on average.

Efforts to evaluate the association of dietary fiber with body weight regulation began in the 1980s. Guar gum, a water-soluble fiber, was shown to reduce hunger and weight more effectively than water-insoluble bran fiber in the absence of a prescribed diet [98].

When glucomannan, another water-soluble fiber, was supplemented at 20 g/d over 8 weeks it resulted in a 2.5 kg weight loss with no prescribed diet [99]. These results were confirmed in a 2-month study that used the same fiber with a calorie-restricted diet [100]. In a 2-week trial, 45 subjects on psyllium, a third water-soluble fiber, were compared with 40 subjects on bran, a water-insoluble fiber, and a control group without a specific diet. There was no difference in weight, but hunger was reduced in both of the fiber groups [101].

In an effort to further define the physiology of fiber, 31 normal males and 19 overweight males were given a 5.2 gram or 0.2 gram fiber preload. The high fiber preload increased fullness in normal and overweight subjects, but only overweight subjects decreased food intake at the subsequent meal [102]. Another study confirmed fiber's ability to decrease appetite [103]. The relationship between appetite and fiber was further defined by a study that used two doses of water-soluble fiber. During 1 week of supplementation (40 g/d) without calorie restriction, food intake was reduced without a change in appetite. During 1 week of supplementation (20 g/d) with calorie restriction, hunger was suppressed without a change in food intake [104].

Baron et al [105] compared two 1000 kcal/d diets in 135 subjects; one diet was lower in carbohydrate and fiber. In contrast with subsequent studies, there was significantly more weight loss (5.0 kg versus 3.7 kg) over 3 months on the lower fiber diet [105]. In a trial of 52 overweight subjects who were randomized to 7 grams of fiber per day or a placebo with a calorie restricted diet for 6 months, the group that had the fiber supplement lost more weight (5.5 kg versus 3.0 kg) and had less hunger [106].

Solum et al [107] randomized 60 overweight women to dietary fiber tablets or placebo and a weight-reducing diet for 12 weeks. The group on fiber lost more weight (8.5 kg vs. 6.7 kg) than those who were on placebo. An 8-week study compared fiber tablets (5 g/d) with placebo and a calorie-restricted diet in 60 obese females. The group that took fiber lost significantly more weight (7.0 kg versus 6.0 kg). This finding was confirmed in a second study of 45 obese females. The group that took 7 grams of fiber per day lost more weight than the group that took placebo (6.2 kg versus 4.1 kg) [108].

Because of its safety, dietary fiber supplementation was evaluated in obese children. There was no difference between children who took 15 g/d fiber supplement and controls during a 4-week trial [109]. Longer term trials in adults were conducted as well. Ninety obese females were randomly assigned to a 6 to 7 g/d dietary supplement or placebo and a 1200 to 1600 kcal/d diet in 1-year, double-blind trial. The group that took fiber lost 3.8 kg (4.9% of initial body weight) compared with 2.8 kg (3.6% of initial body weight) that was lost by the group that took placebo; this was a statistically significant difference [110].

Fiber, 30 g/d, was supplemented in a very low calorie diet in a 4-week, crossover trial. Weight loss was not different, but hunger was less during the supplementation with fiber [111]. In a 14 month study with a two-month very low calorie intervention followed by a 12-month maintenance phase that involved 20 obese subjects and 11 obese controls, there was no difference in weight loss between the groups that were supplemented with 20 grams guar gum per day during the 14 months or placebo [112].

The relationship between obesity and fiber has also been evaluated epidemiologically. Using food frequency questionnaires, obese men and women had significantly more fat and less fiber in their diets than lean men and women [113]. These findings were confirmed with the use of 3-day food diaries. Total fiber intake was higher in the lean group than in the obese group and the grams of fiber/1000 kcal was inversely related to BMI [114].

In summary, the bulk of evidence suggests that dietary fiber decreases food intake and decreases hunger; water-soluble fiber may be more efficient than water-insoluble fiber. Dietary fiber supplements (5–40 g/d) lead to small (1–3 kg) weight losses greater than that produced by placebo. Although the weight loss that was obtained with dietary fiber is less than the 5% of initial body weight that is believed to confer clinically significant health benefits, the safety of dietary fiber and its potential benefits on cardiovascular risk factors recommend its inclusion in weight reduction diets.

Chitosan

Chitosan is acetylated chitin from the exoskeletons of crustaceans, such as shrimp. The product has a molecular weight of more than a million Daltons, and is designed to bind to intestinal lipids, including cholesterol and tri-glycerides. Chitosan was originally developed as a lipid-binding resin in the 1970s, based on its properties as a charged, nonabsorbable carbohydrate. It has received a great deal of attention as a potential weight loss aid working through a "fat blocker" mechanism. In public demonstrations, chitosan is mixed with corn oil in a glass; the precipitation of the oil and clarification of the solution is emphasized as a mechanism that would result in fat malabsorption and weight loss in humans. This promises individuals that they can eat the fatty foods that they desire without gaining weight.

Mice who were fed a high-fat diet with 3% to 15% chitosan for 9 weeks had less weight gain, hyperlipidemia, fatty liver, and higher fecal fat excretion than control mice who were fed high-fat diets. These changes were the result of chitosan-binding of dietary fat, rather than through the inhibition of fat digestion [115].

Two double-blind, clinical trials were performed to evaluate the effect of chitosan, 1200 to 1600 mg orally, twice a day. One trial included 51 obese women who were treated for 8 weeks without any reduction in weight [116]. The second trial included 34 overweight men and women who were treated for 28 days without any weight reduction relative to controls [117]. There were no serious adverse events or changes in safety laboratory in either trial, and no changes in fat-soluble vitamins or iron metabolism were seen. In a more recent, randomized, open-label, two-period, sequential study that compared orlistat (Xenical), a lipase inhibitor, and chitosan in 12 healthy volunteers, Guerciolini et al [118] found that orlistat increased fecal fat loss (16.13 ± 7.27 g/d) and there was no significant effect with chitosan (-0.27 ± 1.02 g/d). Taken together with the other studies that have been conducted with this supplement, one would have to conclude that although chitosan can bind fat in "in vitro" demonstrations, this does not translate into fat binding that is significant in the human. It is highly unlikely that this supplement will be effective for weight loss based on its putative fat binding effects. Chitosan has the potential for weight reduction by binding dietary fat, but is not effective in the doses that are presently used in humans.

Efficacy and safety assessment

Although many of the studies that were presented in this chapter are not conclusive, and others are incomplete or poorly-controlled, there are some general conclusions that can be drawn about the safety and efficacy of the herbal and alternative approaches.

One of the key problems in this assessment is that only agents that were found to be effective had adequate clinical studies performed to begin to look at safety. Even in these cases, it is possible that the adverse effects reports will be obtained in the field. It is sometimes difficult to assess whether the agent being used causes the effects. This problem will require careful documentation, but this work is only likely to be done with the most effective agents that become widely used.

Summary

The opportunities for additional research in this area are plentiful. Unfortunately, there has been relatively limited funding for research on herbal supplements compared with the amount of funding that is available for research on pharmaceuticals. Botanical dietary supplements often contain complex mixtures of phytochemicals that have additive or synergistic interactions. For example, the tea catechins include a group of related compounds with effects that are demonstrable beyond those that are seen with epigallocatechin gallate, the most potent catechin. The metabolism of families of related compounds may be different than the metabolism of purified crystallized compounds. In some cases, herbal medicines may simply be less purified forms of single active ingredients, but in other cases they represent unique formulations of multiple, related compounds that may have superior safety and efficacy compared with single ingredients.

Obesity is a global epidemic, and traditional herbal medicines may have more acceptance than prescription drugs in many cultures with emerging epidemics of obesity. Several ethnobotanical studies found herbal treatments for diabetes, and similar surveys, termed bioprospecting, for obesity treatments may be productive.

Beyond increasing thermogenesis, there are other biological rationales for the actions of several different alternative medical and herbal approaches to weight loss. For example, several supplements and herbs claim to result in nutrient partitioning so that ingested calories will be directed to muscle, rather than fat. These include an herb (*Garcinia cambogia*), and a lipid which is the product of bacterial metabolism (conjugated linoleic acid). Moreover, a series of approaches attempt to physically affect gastric satiety by filling the stomach. Fiber swells after ingestion and has was found to result in increased satiety. A binding resin (Chitosan) has the ability to precipitate fat in the laboratory and is touted for its ability to bind fat in the intestines so that it is not absorbed. In double-blind studies, however, this approach was found to be ineffective.

There are two key attractions of alternative treatments to obese patients. First, they are viewed as being natural and are assumed by patients to be safer than prescription drugs. Second, there is no perceived need for professional assistance with these approaches. For obese individuals who cannot afford to see a physician, these approaches often represent a more accessible solution. Finally, for many others, these approaches represent alternatives to failed attempts at weight loss with the use of more conventional approaches. These consumers are often discouraged by previous failures, and are likely to combine approaches or use these supplements at doses higher than are recommended. It is vital that the primary care physician is aware of the herbal preparations that are being used by patients so that any potential interaction with prescription drugs or underlying medical conditions can be anticipated.

Unfortunately, there have been several instances where unscrupulous profiteers have plundered the resources of the obese public. Although Americans spend $30 billion per year on weight loss aids, our regulatory and monitoring capability as a society are woefully inadequate. Without adequate resources, the FDA resorted to "guilt by association" adverse events reporting, which often results in the loss of potentially helpful therapies without adequate investigation of the real causes of the adverse events that are reported. Scientific investigations of herbal and alternative therapies represent a potentially important source for new discoveries in obesity treatment and prevention. Cooperative interactions in research between the Office of Dietary Supplements, the National Center for Complementary and Alternative Medicine, and the FDA could lead to major advances in research on the efficacy and safety of the most promising of these alternative approaches.

References

[1] Vansal SS, Feller DR. Direct effects of ephedrine isomers on human beta-adrenergic receptor subtypes. Biochem Pharmacol 1999;58:807–10.
[2] Boozer CN, Nasser JA, Heymsfield SB, et al. An herbal supplement containing Ma Huang-Guarana for weight loss: a randomized, double-blind trial. Int J Obes Relat Metab Disord 2001;25:316–24.
[3] Haller CA, Benowitz NL. Adverse cardiovascular and central nervous system events associated with dietary supplements containing ephedra alkaloids. N Engl J Med 2000;343:1833–8.
[4] Boozer CN, Daly PA, Homel P, et al. Herbal ephedra/caffeine for weight loss: a 6-month randomized safety and efficacy trial. Int J Obes 2002;26:593–604.

[5] Malchow-Moller A, Larsen S, Hey H, et al. Ephedrine as an anorectic: the story of the "Elsinore pill". Int J Obes 1981;5:183–7.

[6] Goodman L, Gilman A. The pharmacological basis of therapeutics. 7th edition. New York: Macmillan Publishing Company; 1985.

[7] Miller DS. A controlled trial using ephedrine in the treatment of obesity [letter]. Int J Obes 1986;10:159–60.

[8] Drug topics red book. Montvale (NJ): Medical Economics Company, Inc.; 2000.

[9] Macdonald IA. Advances in our understanding of the role of the sympathetic nervous system in obesity. Int J Obes Relat Metab Disord 1995;19(Suppl 7):S2–7.

[10] Chen MD, Lin WH, Song YM, et al. Effect of caffeine on the levels of brain serotonin and catecholamine in the genetically obese mice. Chung Hua I Hsueh Tsa Chih 1994;53:257–61.

[11] Oberman Z, Herzberg M, Jaskolka H, et al. Changes in plasma cortisol, glucose and free fatty acids after caffeine ingestion in obese women. Isr J Med Sci 1975;11:33–6.

[12] Acheson KJ, Zahorska-Markiewicz B, Pittet P, et al. Caffeine and coffee: their influence on metabolic rate and substrate utilization in normal weight and obese individuals. Am J Clin Nutr 1980;33:989–97.

[13] Jung RT, Shetty PS, James WP, et al. Caffeine: its effect on catecholamines and metabolism in lean and obese humans. Clin Sci 1981;60:527–35.

[14] Dulloo AG, Geissler CA, Horton T, et al. Normal caffeine consumption: influence on thermogenesis and daily energy expenditure in lean and postobese human volunteers. Am J Clin Nutr 1989;49:44–50.

[15] Bracco D, Ferrarra JM, Arnaud MJ, et al. Effects of caffeine on energy metabolism, heart rate, and methylxanthine metabolism in lean and obese women. Am J Physiol 1995; 269:E671–8.

[16] Bondi M, Grugni G, Velardo A, et al. Adrenomedullary response to caffeine in prepubertal and pubertal obese subjects. Int J Obes Relat Metab Disord 1999;23:992–6.

[17] Tagliabue A, Terracina D, Cena H, et al. Coffee induced thermogenesis and skin temperature. Int J Obes Relat Metab Disord 1994;18:537–41.

[18] Yoshida T, Sakane N, Umekawa T, et al. Relationship between basal metabolic rate, thermogenic response to caffeine, and body weight loss following combined low calorie and exercise treatment in obese women. Int J Obes Relat Metab Disord 1994; 18:345–50.

[19] Abernethy DR, Todd EL, Schwartz JB. Caffeine disposition in obesity. Br J Clin Pharmacol 1985;20:61–6.

[20] Cheymol G. Clinical pharmacokinetics of drugs in obesity. An update. Clin Pharmacokinet 1993;25:103–14.

[21] Caraco Y, Zylber-Katz E, Berry EM, et al. Caffeine pharmacokinetics in obesity and following significant weight reduction. Int J Obes Relat Metab Disord 1995;19:234–9.

[22] Haffner SM, Knapp JA, Stern MP, et al. Coffee consumption, diet, and lipids. Am J Epidemiol 1985;122:1–12.

[23] La Vecchia C, Franceschi S, Decarli A, et al. Risk factors for myocardial infarction in young women. Am J Epidemiol 1987;125:832–43.

[24] Noble R. A controlled clinical trial of the cardiovascular and psychological effects of phenylpropanolamine and caffeine. Drug Intell Clin Pharm 1988;22:296–9.

[25] Barrett-Connor E, Chang JC, Edelstein SL. Coffee-associated osteoporosis offset by daily milk consumption. The Rancho Bernardo Study. JAMA 1994;271:280–3.

[26] Sawynok J. Pharmacological rationale for the clinical use of caffeine. Drugs 1995;49:37–50.

[27] Massoudi M, Miller DS. Ephedrine, a thermogenic and potential slimming drug. Proc Nutr Soc 1977;36:135A.

[28] Yen TT, McKee MM, Bemis KG. Ephedrine reduces weight of viable yellow obese mice (Avy/a). Life Sci 1981;28:119–28.

[29] Wilson S, Arch JR, Thurlby PL. Genetically obese C57BL/6 ob/ob mice respond normally to sympathomimetic compounds. Life Sci 1984;35:1301–9.

[30] Massoudi M, Evans E, Miller DS. Thermogenic drugs for the treatment of obesity: screening using obese rats and mice. Ann Nutr Metab 1983;27:26–37.

[31] Dulloo AG, Miller DS. Thermogenic drugs for the treatment of obesity: sympathetic stimulants in animal models. Br J Nutr 1984;52:179–96.

[32] Liu YL, Toubro S, Astrup A, et al. Contribution of beta 3-adrenoceptor activation to ephedrine-induced thermogenesis in humans. Int J Obes Relat Metab Disord 1995;19: 678–85.

[33] Bukowiecki L, Jahjah L, Follea N. Ephedrine, a potential slimming drug, directly stimulates thermogenesis in brown adipocytes via beta-adrenoreceptors. Int J Obes 1982;6:343–50.

[34] Bailey CJ, Thornburn CC, Flatt PR. Effects of ephedrine and atenolol on the development of obesity and diabetes in ob/ob mice. Gen Pharmacol 1986;17:243–6.

[35] Dulloo AG, Miller DS. Aspirin as a promoter of ephedrine-induced thermogenesis: potential use in the treatment of obesity. Am J Clin Nutr 1987;45:564–9.

[36] Sapeika N. Drugs in obesity. S Afr Med J 1974;48:2027–30.

[37] Astrup A, Lundsgaard C, Madsen J, et al. Enhanced thermogenic responsiveness during chronic ephedrine treatment in man. Am J Clin Nutr 1985;42:83–94.

[38] Astrup A, Madsen J, Holst JJ, et al. The effect of chronic ephedrine treatment on substrate utilization, the sympathoadrenal activity, and energy expenditure during glucose-induced thermogenesis in man. Metabolism 1986;35:260–5.

[39] Pasquali R, Baraldi G, Cesari MP, et al. A controlled trial using ephedrine in the treatment of obesity. Int J Obes 1985;9:93–8.

[40] Pasquali R, Cesari MP, Besteghi L, et al. Thermogenic agents in the treatment of human obesity: preliminary results. Int J Obes 1987;11:23–6.

[41] Pasquali R, Cesari MP, Melchionda N, et al. Does ephedrine promote weight loss in low-energy-adapted obese women? Int J Obes 1987;11:163–8.

[42] Pasquali R, Casimirri F, Melchionda N, et al. Effects of chronic administration of ephedrine during very-low-calorie diets on energy expenditure, protein metabolism and hormone levels in obese subjects. Clin Sci (Colch) 1992;82:85–92.

[43] Nielsen B, Astrup A, Samuelsen P, et al. Effect of physical training on thermogenic responses to cold and ephedrine in obesity. Int J Obes Relat Metab Disord 1993;17:383–90.

[44] Astrup A, Breum L, Toubro S, et al. The effect and safety of an ephedrine/caffeine compound compared to ephedrine, caffeine and placebo in obese subjects on an energy restricted diet. A double blind trial. Int J Obes Relat Metab Disord 1992;16:269–77.

[45] Toubro S, Astrup A, Breum L, et al. The acute and chronic effects of ephedrine/caffeine mixtures on energy expenditure and glucose metabolism in humans. Int J Obes Relat Metab Disord 1993;17(Suppl 3):S73–7; discussion, S82.

[46] Astrup A, Toubro S, Christensen NJ, et al. Pharmacology of thermogenic drugs. Am J Clin Nutr 1992;55:246S–8.

[47] Astrup A, Toubro S. Thermogenic, metabolic, and cardiovascular responses to ephedrine and caffeine in man. Int J Obes Relat Metab Disord 1993;17(Suppl 1):S41–3.

[48] Daly PA, Krieger DR, Dulloo AG, et al. Ephedrine, caffeine and aspirin: safety and efficacy for treatment of human obesity. Int J Obes Relat Metab Disord 1993;17(Suppl 1):S73–8.

[49] Astrup A, Buemann B, Christensen NJ, et al. The effect of ephedrine/caffeine mixture on energy expenditure and body composition in obese women. Metabolism 1992;41:686–8.

[50] Buemann B, Marckmann P, Christensen NJ, et al. The effect of ephedrine plus caffeine on plasma lipids and lipoproteins during a 4.2 MJ/day diet. Int J Obes Relat Metab Disord 1994;18:329–32.

[51] Molnar D. Effects of ephedrine and aminophylline on resting energy expenditure in obese adolescents. Int J Obes Relat Metab Disord 1993;17(Suppl 1):S49–2.

[52] Molnar D, Torok K, Erhardt E, et al. Safety and efficacy of treatment with an ephedrine/caffeine mixture. The first double-blind placebo-controlled pilot study in adolescents. Int J Obes Relat Metab Disord 2000;24:1573–8.

[53] Atkinson RL, Blank RC, Loper JF, et al. Combined drug treatment of obesity. Obes Res 1995;3(Suppl 4):497S–500.

[54] Breum L, Pedersen JK, Ahlstrom F, et al. Comparison of an ephedrine/caffeine combination and dexfenfluramine in the treatment of obesity. A double-blind multi-centre trial in general practice. Int J Obes Relat Metab Disord 1994;18:99–103.

[55] Greenway FL, Ryan DH, Bray GA, et al. Pharmaceutical cost savings of treating obesity with weight loss medications. Obes Res 1999;7:523–31.

[56] Svendsen TL, Ingerslev J, Mork A. Is Letigen contraindicated in hypertension? A double-blind, placebo controlled multipractice study of Letigen administered to normotensive and adequately treated patients with hypersensitivity. Ugeskr Laeger 1998;160:4073–5.

[57] Ryan DH. Medicating the obese patient. Endocrinol Metab Clin North Am 1996;25: 989–1004.

[58] Davis R, Faulds D. Dexfenfluramine. An updated review of its therapeutic use in the management of obesity. Drugs 1996;52:696–724.

[59] Finer N. Present and future pharmacological approaches. Br Med Bull 1997;53:409–32.

[60] Carek PJ, Dickerson LM. Current concepts in the pharmacological management of obesity. Drugs 1999;57:883–904.

[61] Bray GA, Greenway FL. Current and potential drugs for treatment of obesity. Endocr Rev 1999;20:805–75.

[62] Bray GA. Drug treatment of obesity. Baillieres Best Pract Res Clin Endocrinol Metab 1999;13:131–48.

[63] Astrup A, Lundsgaard C. What do pharmacological approaches to obesity management offer? Linking pharmacological mechanisms of obesity management agents to clinical practice. Exp Clin Endocrinol Diabetes 1998;106:29–34.

[64] Astrup AV. Treatment of obesity with thermogenic agents [editorial]. Nutrition 1989; 5:70.

[65] Dulloo AG, Miller DS. Ephedrine, caffeine and aspirin: "over-the-counter" drugs that interact to stimulate thermogenesis in the obese. Nutrition 1989;5:7–9.

[66] Dulloo AG. Ephedrine, xanthines and prostaglandin-inhibitors: actions and interactions in the stimulation of thermogenesis. Int J Obes Relat Metab Disord 1993;17(Suppl 1): S35–40.

[67] Astrup A, Breum L, Toubro S. Pharmacological and clinical studies of ephedrine and other thermogenic agonists. Obes Res 1995;3(Suppl 4):537S–40S.

[68] Astrup A, Breum L, Toubro S, et al. Ephedrine and weight loss. Int J Obes Relat Metab Disord 1992;16:715.

[69] Toubro S, Astrup A. Randomised comparison of diets for maintaining obese subjects' weight after major weight loss: ad lib, low fat, high carbohydrate diet v fixed energy intake. BMJ 1997;314:29–34.

[70] Steele VE, Kelloff GJ, Balentine D, et al. Comparative chemopreventive mechanisms of green tea, black tea and selected polyphenol extracts measured by in vitro bioassays. Carcinogenesis 2000;21:63–7.

[71] Sesso HD, Gaziano JM, Buring JE, et al. Coffee and tea intake and the risk of myocardial infarction. Am J Epidemiol 1999;149:162–7.

[72] Borchardt RT, Huber JA. Catechol O-methyltransferase. 5. Structure-activity relationships for inhibition by flavonoids. J Med Chem 1975;18:120–2.

[73] Dulloo AG, Seydoux J, Giradier L. Tealine and thermogenesis: interactions between polyphenols caffeine and sympathetic activity. Int J Obes Relat Metab Disord 1996;20(Suppl 4):71.

[74] Han LK, Takaku T, Li J, et al. Anti-obesity action of oolong tea. Int J Obes Relat Metab Disord 1999;23:98–105.

[75] Colker C, Kalman D, Torina G, et al. Effects of *Citrus aurantium* extract, caffeine and St. John's wort on body fat loss, lipid levels and mood state in overweight healthy adults. Curr Ther Res 1999;60:145–53.

[76] Henry CJ, Emery B. Effect of spiced food on metabolic rate. Hum Nutr Clin Nutr 1986;40:165–8.

[77] Yoshioka M, St-Pierre S, Suzuki M, et al. Effects of red pepper added to high-fat and high-carbohydrate meals on energy metabolism and substrate utilization in Japanese women. Br J Nutr 1998;80:503–10.

[78] Choi Y, Kim YC, Han YB, et al. The trans-10,cis-12 isomer of conjugated linoleic acid downregulates stearoyl-CoA desaturase 1 gene expression in 3T3–L1 adipocytes. J Nutr 2000;130:1920–4.

[79] Griinari JM, Corl BA, Lacy SH, et al. Conjugated linoleic acid is synthesized endogenously in lactating dairy cows by Delta(9)-desaturase. J Nutr 2000;130:2285–91.

[80] Dhiman TR, Satter LD, Pariza MW, et al. Conjugated linoleic acid (CLA) content of milk from cows offered diets rich in linoleic and linolenic acid. J Dairy Sci 2000;83:1016–27.

[81] Kritchevsky D. Antimutagenic and some other effects of conjugated linoleic acid. Br J Nutr 2000;83:459–65.

[82] MacDonald HB. Conjugated linoleic acid and disease prevention: a review of current knowledge. J Am Coll Nutr 2000;19:111S–8S.

[83] Pariza MW, Park Y, Cook ME. Conjugated linoleic acid and the control of cancer and obesity. Toxicol Sci 1999;52:107–10.

[84] Park Y, Storkson JM, Albright KJ, et al. Evidence that the trans-10, cis-12 isomer of conjugated linoleic acid induces body composition changes in mice. Lipids 1999;34:235–41.

[85] Park Y, Albright KJ, Liu W, et al. Effect of conjugated linoleic acid on body composition in mice. Lipids 1997;32:853–8.

[86] West DB, Delany JP, Camet PM, et al. Effects of conjugated linoleic acid on body fat and energy metabolism in the mouse. Am J Physiol 1998;275:R667–72.

[87] DeLany JP, Blohm F, Truett AA, et al. Conjugated linoleic acid rapidly reduces body fat content in mice without affecting energy intake. Am J Physiol 1999;276:R1172–79.

[88] Yamasaki M, Mansho K, Mishima H, et al. Dietary effect of conjugated linoleic acid on lipid levels in white adipose tissue of Sprague-Dawley rats. Biosci Biotechnol Biochem 1999;63:1104–6.

[89] Tsuboyama-Kasaoka N, Takahashi M, Tanemura K, et al. Conjugated linoleic acid supplementation reduces adipose tissue by apoptosis and develops lipodystrophy in mice. Diabetes 2000;49:1534–42.

[90] Satory DL, Smith SB. Conjugated linoleic acid inhibits proliferation but stimulates lipid filling of murine 3T3–L1 preadipocytes. J Nutr 1999;129:92–7.

[91] Azain MJ, Hausman DB, Sisk MB, et al. Dietary conjugated linoleic acid reduces rat adipose tissue cell size rather than cell number. J Nutr 2000;130:1548–54.

[92] Sullivan C, Triscari J. Metabolic regulation as a control for lipid disorders. I. Influence of (−)-hydroxycitrate on experimentally induced obesity in the rodent. Am J Clin Nutr 1977;30:767–76.

[93] Badmaev V, Majeed M. Open field, physician-controlled clinical evaluation of botanical weight loss formula citrin. Nutracon: Nutraceuticals, dietary supplements and functional foods. [Abstract] Las Vegas: Nutracon; 1995.

[94] Kriketos AD, Thompson HR, Greene H, et al. Hydroxycitric acid does not affect energy expenditure and substrate oxidation in adult males in a post-absorptive state. Int J Obes Relat Metab Disord 1999;23:867–73.

[95] Heymsfield SB, Allison DB, Vasselli JR, et al. *Garcinia cambogia* (hydroxycitric acid) as a potential antiobesity agent: a randomized controlled trial. JAMA 1998;280:1596–600.

[96] Van Itallie TB. Dietary fiber and obesity. Am J Clin Nutr 1978;31:S43–2.

[97] Ludwig DS, Peterson KE, Gortmaker SL. Relation between consumption of sugar-sweetened drinks and childhood obesity: a prospective, observational analysis. Lancet 2001;357:505–8.

[98] Krotkiewski M. Effect of guar gum on body-weight, hunger ratings and metabolism in obese subjects. Br J Nutr 1984;52:97–105.

[99] Walsh DE, Yaghoubian V, Behforooz A. Effect of glucomannan on obese patients: a clinical study. Int J Obes 1984;8:289–93.

[100] Cairella M, Marchini G. Evaluation of the action of glucomannan on metabolic parameters and on the sensation of satiation in overweight and obese patients. Clin Ter 1995;146:269–74.

[101] Hylander B, Rossner S. Effects of dietary fiber intake before meals on weight loss and hunger in a weight-reducing club. Acta Med Scand 1983;213:217–20.

[102] Porikos K, Hagamen S. Is fiber satiating? Effects of a high fiber preload on subsequent food intake of normal-weight and obese young men. Appetite 1986;7:153–62.

[103] Witkowska A, Borawska MH. The role of dietary fiber and its preparations in the protection and treatment of overweight. Pol Merkuriusz Lek 1999;6:224–6.

[104] Pasman WJ, Saris WH, Wauters MA, et al. Effect of one week of fibre supplementation on hunger and satiety ratings and energy intake. Appetite 1997;29:77–87.

[105] Baron JA, Schori A, Crow B, et al. A randomized controlled trial of low carbohydrate and low fat/high fiber diets for weight loss. Am J Public Health 1986;76:1293–6.

[106] Rigaud D, Ryttig KR, Angel LA, et al. Overweight treated with energy restriction and a dietary fibre supplement: a 6-month randomized, double-blind, placebo-controlled trial. Int J Obes 1990;14:763–9.

[107] Solum TT, Ryttig KR, Solum E, et al. The influence of a high-fibre diet on body weight, serum lipids and blood pressure in slightly overweight persons. A randomized, double-blind, placebo-controlled investigation with diet and fibre tablets (DumoVital). Int J Obes 1987;11:67–71.

[108] Rossner S, von Zweigbergk D, Ohlin A, et al. Weight reduction with dietary fibre supplements. Results of two double- blind randomized studies. Acta Med Scand 1987; 222:83–8.

[109] Gropper SS, Acosta PB. The therapeutic effect of fiber in treating obesity. J Am Coll Nutr 1987;6:533–5.

[110] Ryttig KR, Tellnes G, Haegh L, et al. A dietary fibre supplement and weight maintenance after weight reduction: a randomized, double-blind, placebo-controlled long-term trial. Int J Obes 1989;13:165–71.

[111] Quaade F, Vrist E, Astrup A. Dietary fiber added to a very-low caloric diet reduces hunger and alleviates constipation. Ugeskr Laeger 1990;152:95–8.

[112] Pasman WJ, Westerterp-Plantenga MS, Muls E, et al. The effectiveness of long-term fibre supplementation on weight maintenance in weight-reduced women. Int J Obes Relat Metab Disord 1997;21:548–55.

[113] Miller WC, Niederpruem MG, Wallace JP, et al. Dietary fat, sugar, and fiber predict body fat content. J Am Diet Assoc 1994;94:612–5.

[114] Alfieri MA, Pomerleau J, Grace DM, et al. Fiber intake of normal weight, moderately obese and severely obese subjects. Obes Res 1995;3:541–7.

[115] Han LK, Kimura Y, Okuda H. Reduction in fat storage during chitin-chitosan treatment in mice fed a high-fat diet. Int J Obes Relat Metab Disord 1999;23:174–9.

[116] Wuolijoki E, Hirvela T, Ylitalo P. Decrease in serum LDL cholesterol with microcrystalline chitosan. Methods Find Exp Clin Pharmacol 1999;21:357–61.

[117] Pittler MH, Abbot NC, Harkness EF, et al. Randomized, double-blind trial of chitosan for body weight reduction. Eur J Clin Nutr 1999;53:379–81.

[118] Guerciolini R, Radu-Radulescu L, Boldrin M, et al. Comparative evaluation of fecal fat excretion induced by orlistat and chitosan. Obes Res 2001;9(6):364–7.

16

The Management of the Obese Diabetic Patient

Jeanine Albu

Nazia Raja-Khan

Obesity is a major worldwide epidemic that is associated with a significantly increased risk of type 2 diabetes, cardiovascular disease, and premature death [1,2]. Obesity is associated with increased mortality, especially when it coexists with diabetes. In a 12-year follow-up study of more than 700,000 patients, a weight of more than 50% above average was associated with a twofold increase in mortality. The presence of diabetes, in addition to obesity, raised mortality by five to eight fold [3]. In the past few decades, the prevalence of obesity in the United States and worldwide has increased dramatically. Approximately 60% of Americans are overweight or obese with a body mass index (BMI) of 25 kg/m^2 or higher [4].

Overweight and obese individuals are at increased risk for developing type 2 diabetes [5–7]. In fact, there is an inverse relationship between BMI and the age of diabetes onset in obese adults who are younger than 70 years old [8]. The duration and degree of obesity, central distribution of weight, and recent weight gain are all independent risk factors for type 2 diabetes [3]. Studies have shown that weight loss by caloric restriction and exercise could prevent type 2 diabetes in overweight and obese individuals. The Finnish Diabetes Prevention Study showed that a weight loss of at least 5% of initial body weight reduced the risk of progression to diabetes in high-risk, overweight patients with impaired glucose tolerance [9]. In the United States, the Diabetes Prevention Program Research Group showed that life-style changes (caloric restriction and exercise) or treatment with metformin reduced the incidence of diabetes in persons at high risk; the lifestyle intervention was more effective than metformin [10]. These effective interventions are slow to be implemented into the daily life of Americans. Over the next decade this dual epidemic is predicted to grow because the number of people who are afflicted with obesity and diabetes continues to rise at an alarming rate.

Currently, 17 million Americans are estimated to have diabetes mellitus (DM). Type 2 diabetes accounts for most (about 95%) of these patients. Diabetes is the leading cause of renal failure, blindness, and amputations in adults. It is a major risk factor for heart disease, stroke, and birth defects. Diabetes decreases the average life expectancy, independently of the degree of overweight, and costs the nation $98 billion annually in health-related expenditures [11]. The United Kingdom Prospective Diabetes Study (UKPDS), the Diabetes Control and Complications Trial (DCCT), and the Japanese Kumamoto study showed that aggressive glycemic control in diabetes slowed the progression of microvascular disease, including retinopathy, nephropathy, and neuropathy [12–15]. For every 1% decrease in hemoglobinAic [HgbA$_{1C}$ (glycosylated hemoglobin)], microvascular complications decreased 35%, diabetes-related mortality decreased 25%, and all-cause mortality decreased 7% [13]. A continuous, positive relationship exists between HgbA$_{1C}$ level and the risk of complications. As diabetic control worsens, diabetic complications increase.

In the National Health and Nutrition Examination Survey III (NHANES III), only 50% of diabetics were able to achieve a HgbA$_{1C}$ of 7% or less with available aggressive management [16]. Data from NHANES III showed that less than one third of patients who have diabetes have their HgbA$_{1C}$ measured more than once a year; nearly 20% of patients who are being treated for diabetes have a HgbA$_{1C}$ that is greater than 9.5% [16].

Obesity is present in most patients who have type 2 DM. When present, obesity complicates the management of diabetes, especially the goal of achieving tight glycemic control [17,18]. First, tight glycemic control should be achieved, but not at the expense of adipose tissue accumulation, especially in the visceral adipose depot. Second, weight control must be achieved without losing sight of the need for tight glycemic control. Moreover, cardiovascular risk factors are likely exacerbated by obesity in type 2 DM. Special attention must be paid to control of cardiovascular risk factors in the obese patient who has type 2 diabetes; treatment and control of obesity by caloric restriction and exercise is likely to result in tighter glycemic control and the reduction of cardiovascular risk factors.

Antidiabetic therapy in obese patients

In the obese diabetic patient, just as is in other diabetic patients, microvascular disease is primarily related to the presence of hyperglycemia [12–15]. Uncontrolled hyperglycemia is also responsible for an unfavorable lipoprotein pattern, an increase in glycosylation end-products in all tissues, and an increased risk of thrombotic events [19]. Therefore, tight glycemic control is warranted in the obese diabetic patient. Goals for glycemic control as recommended by the American Diabetes Association include: a preprandial glucose of 90 to 130 mg/dL, a bedtime glucose of 110 to 150 mg/dL, and a HgbA$_{1C}$ level of less than 7% [20]. The American College of Endocrinology has proposed stricter guidelines which include: a preprandial glucose of less than or equal to 110 mg/dL, postprandial glucose of less than or equal to 140 mg/dL, and HgbA$_{1C}$ level of less than or equal to 6.5% [21].

Diet and exercise are important in maintaining glycemic control in type 2 diabetics. Physical activity, in particular, improves insulin sensitivity, independent of weight loss, and, thus, plays an important role in the strategy of achieving glycemic control in the obese diabetic patient [22]. Supplementation of diet and exercise with oral pharmacotherapy is often needed to maintain glycemic control. Oral agents have been developed that address the two main defects in type 2 diabetes, insulin resistance and β-cell dysfunction [23]. The different classes of hypoglycemic agents, when used to normalize blood glucose, have variable effects on weight gain, the rates of hypoglycemic events, and the degree of hyperinsulinemia [14,24]. These factors are important to consider in the management of the obese patient who has type 2 diabetes (Table 1).

Oral agents for treatment of hyperglycemia

Sulfonylureas (eg, glyburide, glipizide, chlorpropamide, glimepiride) and nonsulfonylurea secretagogues (eg, repaglinide, nateglinide) bind to receptors on the surface of pancreatic β cells and stimulate the release of insulin. Although hyperinsulinemia is believed to be a precursor for cardiovascular disease, the UKPDS showed that sulfonylurea or insulin therapy was not associated with increased cardiovascular mortality [13]. Adverse effects of insulin secretagogues are hypoglycemic episodes and weight gain. Third generation sulfonylurea and nonsulfonylurea secretagogues may be associated with lower rates of hypoglycemia and less weight gain than the older sulfonylurea [27,53–55]. The nonsulfonylurea secretagogues, with a rapid onset of action and short duration of action, are designed for mealtime dosing [28] and significantly reduce postprandial and fasting blood glucose and HgbA$_{1C}$ [27,29]. Increases in fasting insulin levels, mean weight gain, and hypoglycemic events may be similar to those produced by sulfonylurea treatments [27–29]. In general, the more efficacious the treatment in reducing hyperglycemia, the more often weight gain, hyperinsulinemia, and hypoglycemia are seen [27,28].

Insulin sensitizers, in contrast with insulin secretagogues, theoretically should decrease insulin levels without increasing weight or producing hypoglycemia, as long as they are not combined with insulin secretagogues. There are two classes of insulin sensitizers: biguanide and thiazolidinediones.

Metformin, a biguanide, works by improving insulin sensitivity and reducing hepatic glucose output [16]. Metformin is particularly beneficial for the obese diabetic patient, because it reduces hyperinsulinemia and

Table 1
Oral medications and insulin for the treatment of type 2 diabetes: effects on weight and risk of hypoglycemia

Drug class (References)	Sulfonylurea [13,14,25,26]	Nonsulfonylurea Secretagoges [27–32]	Biguanide [14,25–27,33]	α-glucosidase inhibitors [32,34–40]	Thiazolidinediones [41–49]	Insulin [13,14,26,43,47,50–52]
Drug names	Chlorpropamide, Glipizide, Glyburide, Glimepride	Repaglinide, Nateglinide	Metformin	Acarbose, Miglitol	Pioglitazone, Rosiglitazone	NPH, Regular, Lispro, Aspart, Glargine, Lente, Ultralente
Mechanism of action	Stimulates the release of insulin from pancreatic β cells	Stimulates the release of insulin from pancreatic β cells	Decreases hepatic glucose production and improves peripheral insulin sensitivity	Delays intestinal carbohydrate absorption	Enhances insulin sensitivity in muscle, liver, and adipose tissue; decreases hepatic glucose production	Stimulates peripheral glucose uptake by skeletal muscle and fat; inhibits hepatic glucose production and lipolysis
Effects on weight	↑↑	↑	↓(−)	↓(−)	↑	↑↑↑
Risk of hypoglycemia	↑↑	↑	(−)	(−)	(−)	↑↑↑
Hyperinsulinemia	↑	↑	↓	↓	→	↑↑↑
Other adverse effects		Diarrhea, headache	Diarrhea, nausea, rarely lactic acidosis	Diarrhea, flatulence, abdominal cramps and discomfort	Fluid retention, edema, anemia, CHF exacerbation, potential liver toxicity	

Other advantages	Decreases required dose of exogenous insulin; effective in lowering post prandial glucose	Decreases required dose of exogenous insulin	Especially effective in lowering post prandial glucose	May improve lipid profile; effective in lowering post prandial glucose
Contra indications		Creatinine >1.4 in women and >1.5 in men; severe heart failure; hepatic dysfunction	Inflammatory bowel disease, cirrhosis	Use with caution in congestive heart failure

Abbreviations: CHF, congestive heart failure; ↑, ↑↑, ↑↑↑↑, degree of weight change or hypoglycemia; (−), no change in weight or hypoglycemia.

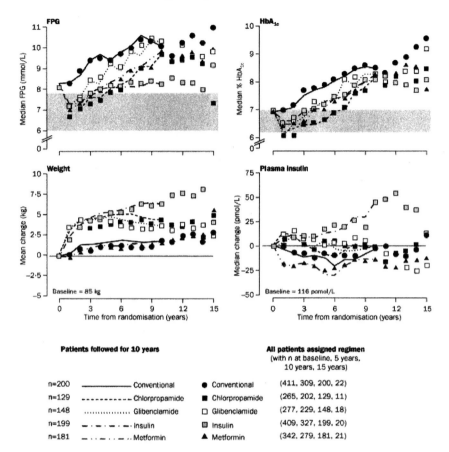

Fig. 1. Changes in fasting plasma glucose (FPG), HgbA$_{1C}$, body weight, and serum insulin levels over 10 years in patients who had type 2 diabetes on various treatment modalities. (*From* U.K. Prospective Diabetes Study Group. Effect of intensive blood glucose control with melformin on complications in overweight patients with type 2 diabetes (UKPDS 34). Lancet 1998;352:854–65; with permission.)

promotes weight loss [14]. In the UKPDS, a 10-year randomized, controlled trial, intensive blood glucose control in overweight type 2 diabetics effectively resulted in risk reductions of 32% for any diabetes-related endpoint, 42% for diabetes-related death, and 36% for all-cause mortality [14]. Although all patients who had type 2 diabetes in the UKPDS experienced weight gain over the 10-year period of follow-up, obese patients who were allocated to metformin gained the least amount of weight and had the fewest hypoglycemic attacks, compared with patients who were treated with insulin or sulfonylurea [14]. Patients who were given or metformin or were treated conventionally with diet, gained 1 kg to 2 kg during the study, whereas those who were given sulfonylurea or insulin had a weight gain of 5 kg to 7 kg (Fig. 1) [14]. There was no significant difference among insulin, sulfonylurea, and metformin in glycemic control and microvascular risk reduction. In another large randomized, controlled study, a mean weight loss of 3.8 kg was observed in obese type 2 diabetic patients who were treated with metformin monotherapy for 29 weeks [25]. The best study that showed metformin, may, in fact, produce weight loss was of the 3234 prediabetic patients of the Diabetes Prevention Program [10]. Over 3 years, the average weight loss was 5.6 kg, 2.1 kg, and 0.1 kg in the patients who were randomized to receive lifestyle changes (caloric restriction and exercise), metformin, or placebo, respectively [10]. Metformin also has beneficial effects on the lipid profile [25]. Thus, metformin is a drug of choice in the treatment of the obese diabetic patient. Side effects of metformin include nausea and diarrhea; however, it is reasonably well tolerated by most patients. Lactic acidosis is a rare, but serious, complication that is more likely to occur in patients who have renal insufficiency, secondary to the accumulation of metformin. Metformin is contraindicated in patients who have renal insufficiency, congestive heart failure, hepatic disease, and alcohol abuse.

A newer class of antidiabetic agents, the thiazolidinediones (glitazones), bind to nuclear peroxisome-proliferator activated receptor-γ (PPAR-γ) that is found in adipose and muscle cells to increase peripheral uptake of glucose by skeletal muscle cells. This enhances insulin sensitivity and decreases serum insulin levels [41,42,56]. The glitazones also reduce lipolysis, and, thus, free fatty acid levels and improve high-density lipoprotein (HDL) and triglyceride levels. Studies in type 2 diabetics showed that the addition of a glitazone to sulfonylurea or insulin monotherapy resulted in better glycemic control, but was associated with hypoglycemia and weight gain [41,43–45]. Hypoglycemia is a common adverse effect of glitazone-insulin combination, but it can be avoided with a gradual reduction of the insulin dosage [43,44]. The significance of weight gain from glitazones is difficult to assess. Despite the weight gain, the glitazones are beneficial because they redistribute fat from visceral to subcutaneous areas [46–48]. In addition, some of the weight gain is the result of peripheral edema and an increase in extracellular fluid [57]. Therefore, these agents must be used with caution in patients who have congestive heart failure. In addition, liver functions tests must be monitored closely.

α-Glucosidase inhibitors, such as acarbose, work by delaying intestinal carbohydrate absorption and reducing postprandial hyperglycemia. Acarbose, when given alone or in combination with sulfonylurea, metformin, or insulin resulted in improvement of glycemic control [34,58,59] and is particularly beneficial for the obese diabetic patient because it reduces hyperinsulinemia and does not produce weight gain [34,35]. One randomized, placebo-controlled trial showed a small, but statistically significant, weight loss of 0.46 kg in obese type 2 diabetic patients who were treated with acarbose for 12 months [36]. Common side effects include diarrhea, flatulence, and abdominal discomfort; slow titration may lessen these effects.

Because of the progressive nature of β-cell dysfunction in type 2 diabetes, monotherapy with oral agents usually fails over time [13,26]. In the UKPDS, the patients who were treated with monotherapy achieved an initial improvement in HgbA$_{1C}$, regardless of the agent used; however, monotherapy failed to maintain HgbA$_{1C}$ at less than 7% over time [60]. Thus, combination therapy often is needed. Combination therapy is generally more effective than monotherapy bercause it yields additive effects on HgbA$_{1C}$ reduction [23] but it may compound the weight gain and the frequency of hypoglycemic events.

Insulin therapy

Because of the progressive loss of β-cell function, eventually the insulin secretory capacity is insufficient to overcome the insulin resistance; a state of relative insulin deficiency develops in patients who have type 2 diabetes. Thus, when other therapeutic measures fail to normalize blood glucose, the initiation of insulin therapy becomes necessary [61]. Edelman and Henry [62] reviewed the use of insulin for the treatment of type 2 DM. They concluded that obese diabetic patients could and should be evaluated for intensive insulin therapy. The candidates should be motivated, compliant, and able to do home glucose monitoring and insulin administration. The adverse effects and potential risks of intensive insulin treatment included weight gain, which was directly associated with increased hyperinsulinemia [18,63–65]. Hyperinsulinemia has been associated with atherosclerotic risk factors, although a cause and effect relationship has not been proven [66]. In the UKPDS, intensive blood glucose control with either insulin or sulfonylurea therapy significantly decreased the progression of microvascular disease and was not associated with increased cardiovascular mortality. Patients who were allocated to insulin gained more weight and had more hypoglycemic events than patients who were allocated to sulfonylurea [16,60]. It is not known if the benefit of glucose control that is achieved with intense insulin therapy offsets the effect of hyperinsulinemia on cardiovascular disease. This is currently being investigated.

The first types of insulin that were used in the treatment of diabetes were bovine and porcine insulin compounds that differ from the human insulin by 1 to 3 amino acid residues [67]. In the 1980s, biosynthetic human insulin became widely available [68] and protein engineering allowed the development of insulin analogs (Table 2). Insulin analogs are molecules that differ from human insulin in amino acid sequence but are capable of binding and activating the human insulin receptor. These include two rapid acting insulins, lispro and aspart, and the long-acting insulin, glargine.

Traditionally, twice daily injections of short-acting (regular) and intermediate acting (NPH) insulin have been used to treat diabetes. This regimen does not accurately reproduce normal physiologic insulin secretion [69]. Subcutaneous injection of regular insulin produces its peak effect in 2 hours

Table 2
Characteristics of insulin preparations

Insulin	Type	Onset (h)	Peak concentration (h)	Effective duration of action (h)	Maximum duration of action (h)
Lispro	Rapid acting	<0.25	0.5–1.5	3–4	4–6
Aspart	Rapid acting	0.17–0.33	0.67–0.83	1–3	3–5
Regular	Short acting	0.5–1.0	2–3	3–6	6–8
Lente	Intermediate acting	3–4	6–12	12–18	16–20
NPH	Intermediate acting	2–4	6–10	10–16	14–18
Glargine	Long acting	2	none	24	24
Ultralente	Long acting	6–10	10–16	18–20	20–24

Adapted from Hirsch IB. Pharmacotherapeautics of insulin therapy. Optimizing insulin therapy in patients with diabetes. Lawrenceville (NJ): Clinical Connexion 2002. p. 7–12.

and lasts 3 to 6 hours, which may lead to inadequate postprandial glucose control, postprandial hyperinsulinemia, and, possibly, late hypoglycemia [69,70]. Intermediate-acting NPH insulin reaches its peak effect at 6 to 10 hours, lasts 10 to 18 hours with considerable inter- and intrasubject variations in bioavailability, and, when given at dinnertime, may cause nocturnal hypoglycemia [70,71]. For obese patients who have type 2 diabetes and require insulin, physiologic regimens, such as basal and bolus therapy with long-acting (glargine) insulin and rapid-acting (lispro or aspart) insulin, may be more beneficial. Unlike regular insulin, lispro and aspart are absorbed more quickly and have a rapid onset of action [69,71,72]; they are ideal for improving postprandial glucose control [73]. Perhaps the greatest advantage of lispro or aspart is that it can be injected at meal time; however, to avoid early postprandial hypoglycemia, patients must be taught to check their glucose levels before meals and to adjust the insulin dose according to their current glucose level and the carbohydrate content of their meal [68].

Insulin glargine is a novel recombinant human insulin analog with low aqueous solubility at neutral pH [74]. Glargine is produced as an injection solution with a pH of 4. When the solution is injected into the subcutaneous tissue, it immediately neutralizes which results in microprecipitates of insulin. The slow release of small amounts of insulin into the bloodstream results in a relatively constant serum level over 24 hours. The advantage of insulin glargine is that it produces less nocturnal hypoglycemia, and, in some studies, less weight gain [75]. The lesser weight gain that was seen with insulin glargine is attributed to the less frequent hypoglycemia, and, thus, the decreased need to increase caloric supplementation [76]. The use of insulin glargine, compared with NPH, is also associated with lower post-dinner glucose levels [76].

The major limitation of insulin is that the standard route of administration is subcutaneous injection. Preliminary studies on inhaled insulin therapy are so far promising. If successful, these agents may revolutionize the treatment of diabetes [77,78].

Combination insulin and oral therapy

Hypoglycemic agents that are not likely to produce weight gain should be used in the obese diabetic patient whenever possible (ie, when endogenous insulin secretion is adequate). If insulin secretagogues or exogenous insulin need to be used, it is beneficial to combine them with either insulin sensitizing agents, carbohydrate blockers, or weight loss-producing agents (eg, sibutramine or orlistat) to minimize weight gain and the amount of insulin that is needed to achieve glycemic control. Metformin, in particular, but also sulfonylureas and acarbose, when combined with insulin, minimize weight gain in type 2 diabetics [57]. The combination of insulin and metformin is used widely and is a successful strategy. Several randomized clinical trials showed that the combination of exogenous insulin with metformin in the treatment of hyperglycemia in the type 2 diabetic patient led to a reduction in the total daily dosage of insulin that was required, improved HgbA$_{1C}$, and minimized weight gain [79–82]. The insulin-sulfonylurea combination reduced the total daily dosage of required insulin to achieve a given level of glycemic control and modestly improved glycemic control. The Veterans Affairs Cooperative Study in Type II Diabetes showed that some patients were able to achieve near-normal glycemic control with Bedtime Insulin and Daytime Sulfonylurea (BIDS therapy) [83]. In a meta-analysis of more than 40 randomized, controlled trials in type 2 diabetics, combination insulin-sulfonylurea therapy was not associated with weight gain [84]. Sulfonylurea may induce a more physiologic release of insulin during the day in response to increased glucose levels with meals. In addition, combining sulfonylurea and insulin resulted in a 30% reduction in the total amount of insulin that was required daily to maintain a certain level of glycemic control [85,86]. Similarly, the addition of repaglinide in patients who had type 2 diabetes that was suboptimally controlled on insulin monotherapy resulted in significant reductions in HgbA$_{1C}$, postprandial glucose levels, and required insulin dosage, with no change in the hypoglycemic risk [30]. The repaglinide-insulin combination therapy, however, was not as effective in reducing HgbA$_{1C}$ and was associated with more weight gain, compared with metformin-insulin therapy (2.7 kg vs. 0.9 kg, respectively) [31]. Adding acarbose to insulin treatment was beneficial in reducing postprandial hyperglycemia, especially in patients who consumed a high carbohydrate diet [87]. Studies showed that this combination moderately reduced the HgbA$_{1C}$ by 0.4% to 0.7% and variably reduced weight, triglyceride levels, and insulin dosage [34,36,59].

Antiobesity therapy in patients who have type 2 diabetes mellitus

Weight control is an important part of diabetes management. Diet and exercise improve glycemic control and weight control. These interventions should be initiated early in the management of diabetes and should continue throughout the duration of the treatment in the obese diabetic patient [88]. The guidelines for the treatment of obesity as published under the sponsorship of National Heart, Lung, and Blood Institute (NHLBI) should be followed for the obese patient who has type 2 diabetes as for other obese patients [89]. Whether some of these guidelines need to be modified specifically for the obese patient with type 2 DM needs to be determined.

Weight loss by caloric restriction

Caloric restriction and consequent weight loss in obese diabetic patients greatly improves their metabolic control because it results in improved insulin action in liver and muscle, and, frequently results in improved β-cell response to insulin secretory stimuli [88]. In addition, weight control improves cardiovascular disease risk factors, such as hypertension and dyslipidemia [88]. Weight control can and must be achieved through a medically supervised, moderately restricted-calorie diet and an exercise program with long-term maintenance goals [90]. Recently studies showed that even moderate weight loss, when sustained, significantly improves the patient's metabolic profile and prolongs their life expectancy [91–94]. Patients who had type 2 DM who underwent a 16-week lifestyle modification program and lost at least 5% of their initial body weight, had a significant improvement in HgbA$_{1C}$ that was sustained at a 1-year follow-up. These patients also had significant reductions in their need for diabetic medications [95]. The effect of weight loss, through a program of diet and exercise, on macrovascular complications in patients who have type 2 DM is the subject of a large, multicenter national study (Look AHEAD study).

Effectiveness of weight-reducing programs for obese patients who have type 2 diabetes may be decreased by treatment with large dosages of insulin. In such instances, the danger of hypoglycemia must be recognized and the blood glucose must be monitored closely with frequent decreases in insulin, as necessary. Some of the postulated reasons for weight gain with insulin therapy are decreased thermogenesis [96,97] and increased appetite [98]. Thus, it may be impossible to achieve weight loss with caloric restriction unless insulin (or oral agents which increase insulin levels) is being adequately adjusted to the lower calorie diet that is prescribed.

Despite good success in the short term, most obese patients are unable to maintain a modest long-term reduction in their weight [96]. Obese patients who have type 2 diabetes may be more resistant to weight loss and its maintenance because antidiabetic drugs, such as insulin and sulfonylurea, often promote weight gain [13,63]. These patients would likely benefit from the addition of weight management drugs, such as sibutramine and orlistat (Table 3), as adjunctive therapy to the traditional interventions of low calorie diet, physical activity, and behavior management [99].

Table 3
Antiobesity medications shown to improve glycemic control in obese patients who have type 2 diabetes

Medication	Mechanism of action	Adverse effects	Recommended dosage	Contraindications
Sibutramine	Selective serotonin and norepinephrine reuptake inhibitor; enhances satiety and increase energy expenditure	Hypertension, tachycardia, headache, insomnia, dry mouth, constipation	Start with 10 mg daily, increase to 15 mg daily after 4 weeks. A maximum daily dosage of 20 mg has been used in type 2 diabetes.	Coronary artery disease, arrythmias, congestive heart failure, stroke, poorly-controlled hypertension, severe hepatic dysfunction, or severe renal impairment
Orlistat	Gastrointestinal lipase inhibitor; decreases the absorption of dietary fat by 30%	Fecal incontinence, flatulence, vitamin malabsorption	120 mg, three times a day, with meals	Acute gastrointestinal illnesses

Sibutramine

Sibutramine is a selective serotonin and noradrenaline reuptake inhibitor. Blocking of serotonin reuptake produces satiety enhancing; inhibition of norepinephrine uptake increases thermogenesis by way of β-3 adreno-receptors [100,101]. Sibutramine is recommended as an adjunct to reduced calorie diet in patients with a BMI of 30 kg/m^2 or higher, or 27 kg/m^2 or higher in the presence of other risk factors, such as diabetes, hypertension, or dyslipidemia. The use of sibutramine has resulted in significant weight loss and the maintenance of this weight loss for up to 2 years.

Sibutramine has been successfully used in obese patients who have type 2 diabetes for the purposes of weight loss, weight loss maintenance, and improvement of glycemic control and cardiovascular risk factors. Sibutramine, 15 mg once daily for 12 weeks, along with a customized reduced calorie diet significantly reduced weight compared with placebo (2.4 kg vs. 0.1 kg, respectively) in obese and overweight patients with type 2 diabetes, who were treated previously with diet alone or stable regimens of insulin or oral agents [100]. This was accompanied by improvements in postprandial glucose, fasting glucose, and glycosylated hemoglobin [100]. Several other studies showed the benefits of combining sibutramine and oral hypoglycemic therapy in patients with type 2 diabetes [101–104]. In obese patients who had type 2 diabetes that was poorly controlled on diet alone or diet plus either a sulfonylurea or metformin, sibutramine produced significantly greater weight loss compared with placebo (4.3 kg or 4.5% vs. 0.4 kg or 0.5%, respectively). The decreases in HgbA$_{1C}$ and fasting plasma glucose correlated with the amount of weight loss [101]. Improvements were also seen in fasting insulin, triglycerides, HDL cholesterol, and quality of life [101]. In obese patients who had poorly controlled type 2 diabetes (HgbA$_{1C}$ of more than 8%) while on maximum doses of sulfonylurea and metformin, the addition of sibutramine 10 mg, twice a day for 6 months, significantly improved glucose levels, insulin resistance, waist circumference, BMI, HgbA$_{1C}$, and lipid profile. Fasting and postprandial glucose levels decreased below baseline. The mean decrease in HgbA$_{1C}$ was 2.73% with sibutramine [104]. Patients who took sibutramine lost an average of 9.61 kg, whereas those who took placebo gained 0.91 kg [104]. Thus, sibutramine is an effective adjunct to oral hypoglycemic therapy in the obese diabetic patient. The longest study of sibutramine therapy in diabetic patients (12 months) reported a weight loss of 7.1 kg with sibutramine, compared with a 2.1 kg weight loss with diet alone. Improvements were also seen in lipid levels [102]. Sibutramine helps obese patients lose weight and it may also prevent relapse after successful weight reduction. This, however was studied only in nondiabetics (Sibutramine Trial of Obesity Reduction and Maintenance). In this study, nearly 70% of patients who took sibutramine were able to maintain a 5% weight loss at 2 years, compared with only 44% of patients with diet and exercise alone [105].

In the aforementioned studies, sibutramine was safe and well tolerated. The safety and efficacy of sibutramine therapy beyond 2 years has not been established. Sibutramine is known to increase blood pressure by 2 to 3 mm Hg on average; therefore, blood pressure should be carefully monitored during treatment. In the long term, weight loss from sibutramine results in a net decrease in blood pressure [106]. Other side effects of sibutramine include headache, dry mouth, anorexia, constipation, and insomnia; however, these are mild to moderate and transient. Sibutramine should not be used in patients who have a history of coronary artery disease, arrhythmias, congestive heart failure, stroke, poorly-controlled hypertension, severe hepatic dysfunction, or severe renal impairment. Sibutramine is contraindicated in patients who take monoamine oxidase inhibitors or other centrally-acting appetite suppressants. Coadministration of sibutramine with other serotoninergic agents is not advised; if this is clinically indicated, however, it requires close monitoring [106].

Orlistat

Orlistat, a specific inhibitor of gastrointestinal (GI) lipases, decreases the absorption of dietary triglycerides from the gastrointestinal tract in a dosage-dependent manner. At the maximum effective dosage of 120 mg, three times a day, orlistat reduced the absorption of dietary fat by 30% [107]. When given in combination with a mild calorie-restricted diet, orlistat produced more significant and long-lasting weight loss than diet alone [106–111]. In addition, a recent epidemiologic prediction model suggested that orlistat is a cost-effective treatment for obese patients who have type 2 diabetes [108].

In obese patients who have type 2 diabetes, orlistat therapy for 24 to 52 weeks, decreased weight, HgbA$_{1C}$, fasting plasma glucose, and low-density lipoprotein (LDL) cholesterol, compared with placebo [109]. Over a 1-year period, orlistat, 120 mg three times a day, given in combination with a low calorie diet [110] to obese patients who had type 2 diabetes that was maintained on oral sulfonylurea, produced a 6.2% decrease in body weight compared with a 4.3% weight loss in the group who took placebo [110]. The improvement in HgbA$_{1C}$ was proportional to the amount of weight lost. Those who lost 5% to 10% of their body weight had a mean decrease in HgbA$_{1C}$ of 0.95%. Those who lost more than 10% of body weight had an average decrease in HgbA$_{1C}$ of 1.53%. In addition, improvements were seen in total cholesterol, LDL, triglycerides, apo-lipoprotein B, the LDL:HDL ratio, and waist circumference. In obese patients who had type 2 diabetes that was poorly controlled by insulin therapy, the addition of orlistat resulted in significant reductions in weight, HgbA$_{1C}$, fasting blood glucose, and LDL cholesterol [111]. Of particular significance for the obese diabetic patient, orlistat therapy reduced the dosage of insulin that was needed to maintain glycemic control. Thus, in the obese type 2 diabetic patient who requires insulin, orlistat may be used to counteract the weight gain. Possible side effects of orlistat include, the reduction of serum levels of fat-soluble vitamins and beta-carotene. GI side effects are mild to moderate and usually transient.

Overall, as part of an integrated program of diet, exercise, and behavior management, nearly one third of obese patients who had type 2 diabetes achieved a weight loss of up to 10% of initial body weight after 1 year of treatment with either sibutramine or orlistat. The weight loss resulted in decreased HgbA$_{1C}$, decreased blood pressure, and improved lipid profiles [100,112,113]. Furthermore, in a short-term study, orlistat improved glucose tolerance and decreased the risk of progression to type 2 diabetes in patients who had impaired glucose tolerance [114]. A combination of sibutramine and orlistat therapy may be beneficial in severely obese patients who have type 2 diabetes, because each drug works differently to induce weight loss; however, this needs to be evaluated in randomized clinical trials. Studies are also needed to assess the long-term efficacy and safety of sibutramine and orlistat therapy on morbidity and mortality in obese patients who have type 2 diabetes.

Other agents

Glucagon-like peptide (GLP-1), is an insulinotropic gut hormone that is released into the bloodstream after eating; abnormalities in GLP-1 function are believed to contribute to the inappropriate insulin secretion that is seen in type 2 diabetes [115–117]. In patients who have type 2 diabetes, the administration of exogenous GLP-1 enhanced the glucose responsiveness of pancreatic β cells, which resulted in increased insulin secretion and decreased plasma glucose [115,118]. In addition, GLP-1 acts on the central nervous system to produce a satiating effect and is believed to improve glycemic control by decreasing the desire for food, delaying gastric emptying, reducing glucagon levels, and enhancing insulin sensitivity [119–121]. Also, stimulation of GLP-1 receptors in certain areas of the brain elicits strong taste aversions [122]. Therefore, GLP-1 and its analogs are promising agents for weight and glycemic control in the obese patient who has type 2 diabetes.

In patients who have type 2 diabetes, GLP-1 infusion significantly enhanced satiety and fullness, reduced energy intake by 27% [123], and produced significant improvement in glucose levels, compared with placebo [124]. A limitation of GLP-1 is its short half-life, as in vivo, it is rapidly inactivated by the protease dipeptidyl peptidase IV (DPP-IV) [125]. Exendin-4, a more potent and longer-acting analog of GLP-1 that originates in the saliva of *Heloderma suspectum* (Gila monster), was shown to induce satiety and weight loss in rats [126]. Exendin-4 binds and activates the human pancreatic GLP-1 receptor, thus exhibiting the same antidiabetic effects as GLP-1. Unlike GLP-1, exendin-4 is not affected by DPP-IV, and, therefore, remains active in plasma for 6 hours after subcutaneous injection. A synthetic exendin-4, called AC2993, was developed by Amylin Pharmaceuticals (San Diego, CA); this drug is now in phase III trials.

Other agents that are presently being studied for weight loss may prove to be beneficial in type 2 DM. Selective β-3 adrenoreceptor agonists induced weight loss and produced a weight-independent improvement in insulin resistance and glucose intolerance in animal studies [99]. When these studies were attempted in humans, however, little benefit was seen. This was attributed to the fact that the agents that were used in the earlier studies were not selective for the human β-3 adrenergic receptor. New β-3 agonists are being developed that have a higher selectivity for humans [99].

Leptin is an adipocyte-derived hormone that is released into the blood stream and acts as a satiety signal in the brain. In the first clinical study in humans, subcutaneous administration of a biosynthetic leptin reduced body fat and decreased weight in a dose-dependent manner [99]. Thus, leptin is another potential weight-reducing agent for obese diabetic patients. Further studies on the safety and efficacy of leptin are needed before it can become an acceptable treatment for weight reduction [99].

Bariatric surgery

In the severely obese patient (BMI > 40 kg/m^2), diet, behavior modification, and drug therapy are often unsuccessful in the long term. Severely obese patients may lose weight initially on these treatments, but may be unable to maintain the weight lost. The cumulative recidivism rate for diet therapy is close to 100% at 5 years [127,128]. Moreover, the limited weight reduction with sibutramine and orlistat may not be acceptable in the long-term in severely obese patients who need to lose and maintain larger amounts of weight [129].

The weight loss that is achieved with bariatric surgery in severely obese patients is significantly larger and longer-lasting than the weight loss that is achieved with diet and pharmacotherapy [130–134]. Within 2 years of gastric bypass, nearly two thirds of excess body weight is lost. Most of this weight loss is maintained for many years after surgery [131,135]. In nearly 600 patients who underwent gastric bypass, the loss of more than 50% of excess body weight was maintained for up to 14 years [135]. A large percentage of patients who had diabetes or glucose intolerance and underwent gastric bypass, developed marked resolution of their glucose intolerance with improvements in hyperglycemia, hyperinsulinemia, insulin resistance, hypertension, dyslipidemia, and other comorbidities [131–133,136–138]. As a result of their improved metabolic profile, most patients were able to significantly reduce the dosage of their antidiabetic medications, especially insulin and sulfonylurea [138,139]. Studies that were done in the United States and Sweden showed that patients who had type 2 diabetes who underwent bariatric gastric surgery developed normal glucose tolerance within months after the surgery [91,140]. Patients who had diabetes were shown to benefit from gastroplasty, gastric bypass, and biliopancreatic diversion [135,138, 141–143]. Thus, in the severely obese diabetic patient (BMI > 30 kg/m^2), bariatric surgery is a successful method of achieving long-term weight loss, glycemic control, and resolution of comorbidities.

The indications for bariatric surgery as defined by the National Institutes of Health (NIH) Consensus Conference in 1991, include BMI of 35 kg/m^2 or higher in patients who have comorbidities, such as diabetes, and BMI of 40 kg/m^2 or higher in patients with or without comorbidities [144]. After bariatric surgery, intensive long-term, postoperative care is needed; therefore, potential candidates should be well informed and motivated to ensure proper long-term follow-up and compliance [3]. Bariatric surgery alone will not guarantee successful long-term weight loss because some patients may slowly regain a tolerance for high-fat foods and carbohydrates [132,145]. Patients need to comply with a diet and exercise program postoperatively. In addition, patients who are unable to cope with the post-operative lifestyle changes may develop major depression, despite successful weight loss after surgery [146].

The three main categories of bariatric surgery are purely malabsorptive, purely restrictive, and mixed malabsorptive/restrictive [137,146,147]. The purely restrictive Vertical Banded Gastroplasty (VBG) and the combined restrictive/malabsorptive Gastric Bypass (GB) are the two most frequently performed bariatric operations in the United States [3]. Both procedures are considered safe with low reported morbidity and mortality [3,132,136].

Of the many variations of gastric bypass, the Roux-en-Y gastric bypass (RYGB) is the most popular [132]. Gastric restriction is achieved by creating a small 5 mL to 15 mL upper gastric pouch with a 1 cm outlet orifice [136]. The pouch empties swallowed food into the small intestine through a Roux limb gastrojejunostomy. The degree of malabsorption depends on the extent of the bypass, which minimally consists of the distal stomach, the duodenum, and the proximal jejunum. Most patients who underwent gastric bypass surgery lost 30 pounds in the first month, 60 pounds in 6 months, and 100 pounds in 1 year [148]. They continued to lose weight for a total of 24 months and were able to maintain a weight that was 20% to 30% above their ideal weight for more than 14 years [148]. In addition, comorbidities, such as diabetes and hypertension, resolved rapidly after surgery [139,148–150].

Pories and his associates [135] performed gastric bypass on more than 600 morbidly obese patients, including 146 patients who had type 2 diabetes and 152 patients who had impaired glucose tolerance. In 82.9% of the patients who had type 2 diabetes and 98.7% of the patients who had impaired glucose tolerance, gastric bypass resulted in normalization of glucose, insulin, and HgbA$_{1C}$ levels. These results were maintained during the 14 years of follow-up. In a retrospective study of 232 morbidly obese patients who had type 2 diabetes, 154 patients underwent gastric bypass and the 78 control patients did not have the surgery because of personal preference or lack of insurance coverage. In the group who underwent surgery, the mean glucose level decreased from 187 mg/dL and remained at less than 140 mg/dL for up to 10 years of follow-up (Figs. 2,3) [151]. More importantly,

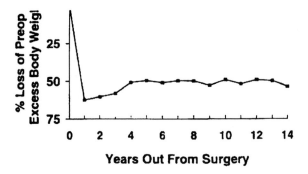

Years Out From Surgery

Fig. 2. Percentage of excess body weight lost in surgical patients (n = 154). The mean percentage loss of excess body weight reached a maximum of 62.4% 1 year after gastric bypass and remained at approximately 50% out to 14 years. (*From* MacDonald KG, Long SD, Swanson MS, et al. The gastric bypass operation reduces the progression and mortality of non-insulin-dependent diabetes mellitus. J Gastrointest Surg 1997;2:213–20; with permission.)

the mortality rate was 28% in the control group but only 9% in the group that underwent surgery. For every year of follow-up, medically-treated patients had a significantly higher chance of dying compared with those who had undergone gastric bypass surgery (4.5% vs. 1.0%, $P<0.0001$) [151]. The improvement in mortality that was seen in the group who underwent surgery was largely the result of a decrease in cardiovascular deaths. The long-term effects of bariatric surgery on the morbidity and mortality of the obese diabetic patient have yet to be elucidated in prospective, controlled trials, such as the ongoing Swedish Obese Study [137,150].

In general, gastric bypass is more effective than VBG in producing weight loss [132,145,152–154]. In the obese diabetic patient, weight loss and glycemic control are better achieved with the gastric bypass than with VBG [131,154]. These results are attributed to the fact that patients with VBG

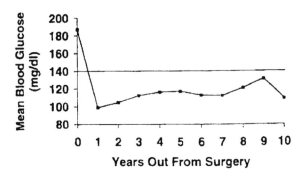

Years Out From Surgery

Fig. 3. The mean fasting blood glucose decreased from 187 mg/dL to a 98.9 mg/dL (combination of random and fasting) at 1 year after gastric bypass surgery and remained less than 140 mg/dL out to 10 years. (*From* MacDonald KG, Long SD, Swanson MS, et al. The gastric bypass operation reduces the progression and mortality of non-insulin-dependent diabetes mellitus. J Gastrointest Surg 1997;2:213–20; with permission.)

often consume excessive amounts of high-calorie liquids and carbohydrates; patients who undergo GB develop an aversion to sweets because of the development of the dumping syndrome [155]. In purely restrictive procedures, such as VBG, ingested food is temporarily retained in an upper gastric pouch to induce satiety. Gastric restriction works by inducing nausea and vomiting when excess food is ingested. On average, maximal weight loss is achieved over 6 to 9 months; half of this maximal weight loss is maintained at 10 years after surgery [156].

Gastric banding is another kind of purely restrictive bariatric surgery, but is less invasive. The Swedish Adjustable Gastric Band (Obtech Medical AG, Baar, Switzerland) and the Lap-Band System laparoscopically placed adjustable gastric band (LAGB; Lap-Band Systems; BioEnterics, Carpinteria, CA) are two commonly used, adjustable band prosthetics [157–159]. Gastric banding, which is popular in Europe, is still in its evolving stages; little is known about its long-term effects. Results of the large, multicenter, United States Lap-Band trial have yet to be published. In the United States, the Lap-Band is approved by the Food and Drug Administration for limited distribution [157]. Several studies, however, showed that laparoscopic adjustable gastric banding could be effective in the management of the obese diabetic patient. In one study, surgical obese patients with a BMI of greater than 35 kg/m^2 who underwent the Lap-Band, had greater decrease in HgbA$_{1C}$, as well as loss of visceral adipose tissue, compared with controls who did not undergo surgery [160]. In another study, diabetes resolved completely in 64% of severely obese diabetic patients, 1 year after undergoing the Lap Band procedure with normalization of fasting plasma glucose and insulin, and of HgbA$_{1C}$ [161].

Every bariatric surgery, even the most complicated, can now be performed laparoscopically. Laparoscopic surgery is often preferred because it is less invasive and decreases the length of hospital stay [3,145,162].

Summary

The prevalence of obesity and diabetes is increasing in the United States and worldwide. These diseases are predicted to explode to epidemic proportions, unless appropriate counteractive measures are taken. Several large studies (DCCT, UKPDS, Kumamoto) clearly showed that intensive glycemic control in the diabetic patient reduced microvascular complications and improved mortality. Despite this, the NHANES III showed that only 50% of diabetics have been able to achieve a HgbA$_{1C}$ level that is less than 7%; this suggests the need for a re-evaluation of our approach to these patients. The management of the obese diabetic patient involves glycemic control and weight reduction. These goals are particularly difficult to achieve in the obese diabetic patient because progressive β-cell dysfunction and increasing insulin resistance necessitates the administration of increasingly higher dosages of insulin, which, in turn, promotes weight gain. A vicious cycle may ensue. Lifestyle modifications with diet and exercise are an essential part of the management of the obese diabetic patient. These measures alone are often insufficient and concomitant pharmacologic therapy is usually required to achieve glycemic and weight control. Oral agents that improve glycemia, decrease insulin resistance, and limit weight gain are desirable. Because of the progressive nature of diabetes, glycemic control with monotherapy often deteriorates over time, which necessitates the addition of other pharmacologic agents, including insulin. When insulin therapy is required in the treatment of the obese diabetic patient, combinations with oral agents that have been shown to minimize the amount of exogenous insulin that is required, may minimize weight gain. In addition, the obese diabetic patient who is poorly controlled with maximum oral hypoglycemic therapy may benefit from weight-reducing agents, such as sibutramine or orlistat. The introduction of these agents at other points in the management of the obese diabetic patients have been successful. Finally, for the severely obese diabetic patient, bariatric surgery may be the only effective treatment. Gastric bypass has been unequivocally shown to produce significant weight loss and improve glycemic control on a long-term basis in the obese diabetic patient. It is recommended that physicians avail themselves of all of these strategies in the management of the obese patient who has type 2 diabetes.

References

[1] Calle EE, Thun MJ, Petrelli JM, et al. Body mass index and mortality in a prospective cohort of US adults. N Engl J Med 1999;341:1097–105.

[2] Stevens J, Cai J, Pamuk ER, et al. The effect of age on the association between body mass index and mortality. N Engl J Med 1998;338:1–7.

[3] American Society for Bariatric Surgery. Rationale for the surgical treatment of morbid obesity. Available at: www.asbs.org/html/rationale.html. Accessed September 25, 2002.

[4] Mokdad AH, Bowman BA, Ford ES, et al. The continuing epidemics of obesity and diabetes in the United States. JAMA 2001;286:1195–200.

[5] Ford ES, Williamson DF, Liu S. Weight change and diabetes incidence: findings from a national cohort of US adults. Am J Epidemiol 1997;146:214–22.

[6] Resnick H, Valsania P, Halter J, Lin X. Relation of weight gain and weight loss on subsequent diabetes risk in overweight adults. J Epidemiol Community Health 2000; 54:596–602.

[7] Harris MI, Flegal KM, Cowie CC, et al. Prevalence of diabetes, impaired fasting glucose, and impaired glucose tolerance in US adults: the Third National Health and Nutrition Examination Survey, 1988–1994. Diabetes Care 1998;21:518–24.

[8] Hillier TA, Pedula KL. Characteristics of an adult population with newly diagnosed type 2 diabetes. Diabetes Care 2001;24:1522–7.

[9] Tuomilehto J, Lindström J, Eriksson JG, et al. Prevention of type 2 diabetes mellitus by changes in lifestyle among subjects with impaired glucose tolerance. N Engl J Med 2001;344:1343–50.

[10] Diabetes Prevention Program Research Group. Reduction in the incidence of type 2 diabetes with lifestyle intervention or metformin. NEJM 2002;346:393–403.

[11] American Diabetes Association. Facts and figures: impact of diabetes. Available at: www.diabetes.org. Accessed September 25, 2002.

[12] The Diabetes Control and Complications Trial Research Group. The effect of intensive treatment of diabetes on the development and the progression of long-term complications in insulin-dependent diabetes mellitus. N Engl J Med 1993;329:977–86.

[13] UK Prospective Diabetes Study Group. Intensive blood glucose control with sulfonyl-ureas or insulin compared with conventional treatment and risk of complications in patients with type 2 diabetes (UKPDS 33). Lancet 1998;352:837–53.

[14] UK Prospective Diabetes Study Group. Effect of intensive blood glucose control with metformin on complications in overweight patients with type 2 diabetes (UKPDS 34). Lancet 1998;352:854–65.

[15] Ohkubo Y, Kishikawa H, Araki E, et al. Intensive insulin therapy prevents the progression of diabetic microvascular complications in Japanese patients with non-insulin-dependent diabetes mellitus: a randomized prospective 6-year study. Diabetes Res Clin Pract 1995;28:103–17.

[16] Harris MI. Frequency of blood glucose monitoring in relation to glycemic control in patients with type 2 diabetes. Diabetes Care 2001;24:979–82.

[17] Galloway JA. Treatment of NIDDM with insulin agonists or substitutes. Diabetes Care 1990;13:1209–39.

[18] Genuth S. Insulin use in NIDDM. Diabetes Care 1990;13:1240–64.

[19] Brownlee M. Glycation products and the pathogenesis of diabetic complications. Diabetes Care 1992;15:1835–43.

[20] American Diabetes Association. Standards of medical care for patients with diabetes mellitus. Diabetes Care 2002;25:213–29.

[21] American Association of Clinical Endocrinologists and the American College of Endocrinology. Medical guidelines for the management of diabetes mellitus: 2002 update. [Suppl]. Endocrine Pract 2002;8:40–82.

[22] Helmrich SP, Ragland DR, Leung RW, et al. Physical activity and reduced occurrence of non-insulin-dependent diabetes mellitus. N Engl J Med 1991;325:147–52.

[23] Inzucchi SE. Oral antihyperglycemic therapy for type 2 diabetes. JAMA 2002;287:360–72.

[24] Bressler R, Johnson D. New pharmacological approaches to therapy of NIDDM. Diabetes Care 1992;15:792–805.

[25] DeFronzo RA, Goodman AM, and the Multicenter Metformin Study Group. Efficacy of metformin in patients with non-insulin dependent diabetes mellitus. N Engl J Med 1995;333:541–9.

[26] United Kingdom Prospective Diabetes Study Group. UKPDS 24: a 6-year, randomized, controlled trial comparing sulfonylurea, insulin, and metformin therapy in patients with newly diagnosed type 2 diabetes that could not be controlled with diet therapy. Ann Intern Med 1998;128:165–75.

[27] Moses R, Slobodniuk R, Boyages S, et al. Effect of repaglinide addition to metformin monotherapy on glycemic control in patients with type 2 diabetes. Diabetes Care 1999;22:119–24.

[28] Raskin P, Jovanovic L, Berger S, et al. Repaglinide/troglitazone combination therapy: improved glycemic control in type 2 diabetes. Diabetes Care 2000;23:979–83.

[29] Schmitz O, Lund S, Andersen PH, et al. Optimizing insulin secretagogue therapy in patients with type 2 diabetes. Diabetes Care 2002;25:342–6.

[30] De Luis DA, Aller R, Cuellar L, et al. Effect of repaglinide addition to NPH insulin monotherapy on glycemic control in patients with type 2 diabetes. Diabetes Care 2001;24:1844–5.

[31] Furlong NJ, Hulme SA, O'Brien SV, et al. Repaglinide versus metformin in combination with bedtime NPH insulin in patients with type 2 diabetes established on insulin/metformin combination therapy. Diabetes Care 2002;25:1685–90.

[32] Hoffmann J, Spengler M. Efficacy of 24-week monotherapy with acarbose, glibenclamide, or placebo in NIDDM patients. The Essen Study. Diabetes Care 1994;17:561–6.

[33] DeFronzo RA. Pharmacologic therapy for type 2 diabetes mellitus. Ann Intern Med 1999;131:281–303.

[34] Chiasson JL, Josse RG, Hunt JA, et al. The efficacy of acarbose in the treatment of patients with non-insulin-dependent diabetes mellitus: a multicenter controlled clinical trial. Ann Intern Med 1994;121:928–35.

[35] Halimi S, Le Berre MA, Grangé V. Efficacy and safety of acarbose add-on therapy in the treatment of overweight patients with type 2 diabetes inadequately controlled with metformin: a double-blind, placebo-controlled study. Diabetes Res Clin Pract 2000;50: 49–56.

[36] Wolever TM, Chiasson JL, Josse RG, et al. Small weight loss on long-term acarbose therapy with no change in dietary pattern or nutrient intake of individuals with non-insulin-dependent diabetes. Int J Obes Relat Metab Disord 1997;21:756–63.

[37] Willms B, Ruge D. Comparison of acarbose and metformin in patients with type 2 diabetes mellitus insufficiently controlled with diet and sulphonylureas: a randomized, placebo-controlled study. Diabet Med 1999;16:755.

[38] Holman RR, Cull CA, Turner RC, UKPDS Study Group. Acarbose in type 2 diabetes shows improved glycemic control over 3 years (UKPDS 44). Diabetes Care 1999;22:960–4.

[39] Hoffmann J, Spengler M. Efficacy of 24-week monotherapy with acarbose, metformin, or placebo in dietary-treated NIDDM patients: the Essen-II Study. Am J Med 1997; 103:483–90.

[40] Mertes G. Safety and efficacy of acarbose in the treatment of type 2 diabetes; data from a 5-year surveillance study. Diabetes Res Clin Pract 2001;52:193–204.

[41] Miyazaki Y, Mahankali A, Matsuda M, et al. Improved glycemic control and enhanced insulin sensitivity in type 2 diabetic subjects treated with pioglitazone. Diabetes Care 2001;24:710–9.

[42] Raskin P, Rappaport EB, Cole ST, et al. Rosiglitazone short-term monotherapy lowers fasting and postprandial glucose in patients with type II diabetes. Diabetologia 2000;43:278–84.

[43] Schwartz S, Raskin P, Fonesca V, et al. Troglitazone and Exogenous Insulin Study Group. Effect of troglitazone in insulin-treated patients with type II diabetes mellitus. N Engl J Med 1998;338:861–6.

[44] Raskin P, Rendell M, Riddle MC, et al. A randomized trial of rosiglitazone therapy in patients with inadequately controlled insulin-treated type 2 diabetes. Diabetes Care 2001;24:1226–32.

[45] Rubin C, Egan J, Schneider R. Pioglitazone 014 Study Group: combination therapy with pioglitazone and insulin in patients with type 2 diabetes [abstract]. Diabetes 1999;48:A110.

[46] Akazawa S, Sun F, Ito M, et al. Efficacy of troglitazone on body fat distribution in type 2 diabetes. Diabetes Care 2000;23:1067–71.

[47] Mori Y, Murakawa Y, Okada K, et al. Effect of troglitazone on body fat distribution in type 2 diabetic patients. Diabetes Care 1999;22:908–12.

[48] Kawai T, Takei I, Oguma Y, et al. Effects of troglitazone on fat distribution in the treatment of male type 2 diabetes. Metabolism 1999;48:1102–7.

[49] Khan MA, St. Peter JV, Xue JL. A prospective, randomized comparison of the metabolic effects of pioglitazone or rosiglitazone in patients with type 2 diabetes who were previously treated with troglitazone. Diabetes Care 2001;25:708–11.

[50] Aviles-Santa L, Sindling J, Raskin P. Effect of metformin in patients with poorly controlled, insulin-treated type 2 diabetes mellitus: a randomized, double-blind, placebo-controlled trial. Ann Intern Med 1999;131:182–8.

[51] Makimattila S, Nikkila K, Yki-Jarvinen H. Causes of weight gain during insulin therapy with and without metformin in patients with type II diabetes mellitus. Diabetologia 1999;42:406–12.

[52] Relimpio F, Pumar A, Losada F, et al. Adding metformin versus insulin dose increase in insulin-treated but poorly controlled type 2 diabetes mellitus: an open-label randomized trial. Diabet Med 1998;15:997–1002.

[53] Hollander PA, Schwartz SL, Gatlin MR, et al. Importance of early insulin secretion: comparison of nateglinide and glyburide in previously diet-treated patients with type 2 diabetes. Diabetes Care 2001;24:983–8.

[54] Horton ES, Clinkingbeard C, Gatlin M, et al. Nateglinide alone and in combination with metformin improves glycemic control by reducing mealtime glucose levels in type 2 diabetes. Diabetes Care 2000;23:1660–5.

[55] Schneider J. An overview of the safety and tolerance of glimepiride. Horm Metab Res 1996;28:413.

[56] Gale EAM. Lessons from the glitazones: a story of drug development. Lancet 2001; 357:1870–5.

[57] Yki-Järvinen H. Combination therapies with insulin in type 2 diabetes. Diabetes Care 2001;24:758–67.

[58] Raptis SA, Dimitriadis GD. Oral hypoglycemic agents: insulin secretagogues, α-glucosidase inhibitors and insulin sensitizers. Exp Clin Endocrinol Diabetes 2001; 109(Suppl 2):S265–87.

[59] Kelly DE, Bidot P, Freedman Z, et al. Efficacy and safety of acarbose in insulin-treated patients with type 2 diabetes. Diabetes Care 1998;21:2056–61.

[60] Turner RC, Cull CA, Frighi V, et al. Glycemic control with diet, sulfonylurea, metformin, or insulin in patients with type 2 diabetes mellitus. Progressive requirement for multiple therapies (UKPDS 49). JAMA 1999;281:2005–12.

[61] American Diabetes Association. The pharmacologic treatment of hyperglycemia in NIDDM. Diabetes Care 1995;18:1510–18.

[62] Edelman SV, Henry RR. Insulin therapy for normalizing glycosylated hemoglobin in type II diabetes. Application, benefits and risks. Diabetes Reviews 1995;3:308–34.

[63] Henry RR, Gumbiner B, Ditzler T, et al. Intensive comventional insulin therapy for type II diabetes: metabolic effects during a 6-month outpatient trial. Diabetes Care 1993;16:21–31.

[64] Yki-Jarvinen H, Kauppila M, Kujansuu E, et al. Comparison of insulin regimens in patients with non-insulin-dependent diabetes mellitus. N Engl J Med 1992;327:1426–33.

[65] Kudlacek S, Schernthaner G. The effect of insulin treatment on HbA1c, body weight and lipids in type 2 diabetic patients with secondary failure to sulfonylureas: a five year follow up study. Horm Metab Res 1992;24:478–83.

[66] Stolar MW. Atherosclerosis in diabetes: the role of hyperinsulinemia. Metabolism 1988;37(Suppl 1):1–9.

[67] Brange J, Owens DR, Kang S, et al. Monomeric insulins and their experimental and clinical implications. Diabetes Care 1990;13:923–54.

[68] Hollerman F, Hoekstra JB. Insulin lispro. NEJM 1997;337:176–83.

[69] Home PD, Lindholm A, Hylleberg B, et al. Improved glycemic control with insulin aspart. Diabetes Care 1998;21:1904–9.

[70] Vajo Z, Fawcett J, Duckworth WC. Recombinant DNA technology in the treatment of diabetes: insulin analogs. Endocr Rev 2001;22:706–17.

[71] Herbst KL, Hirsch IB. Insulin strategies for primary care providers. Clinical Diabetes 2002;20:11–7.

[72] Mudaliar SR, Lindberg FA, Joyce M, et al. Insulin aspart (B28 Asp-Insulin): a fast acting analog of human insulin. Diabetes Care 1999;22:1501–6.

[73] Rosenfalck AM, Thorsby P, Kjems L, et al. Improved postprandial glycemic control with insulin aspart in type 2 diabetic patients treated with insulin. Acta Diabetol 2000;37:41–6.

[74] Lantus [package insert]. Kansas City, (MO); Aventis Pharmaceuticals Inc.; 2000.

[75] Rosenstock J, Schwartz SL, Clark CM Jr, et al. Basal insulin therapy in type 2 diabetes. Diabetes Care 2001;24:631–6.

[76] Yki-Järvinen H, Dressler A, Ziemen M, et al. Less nocturnal hypoglycemia and better post-dinner glucose control with bedtime insulin glargine compared with bedtime NPH insulin during insulin combination therapy in type 2 diabetes. Diabetes Care 2000; 23:1130–6.

[77] White JR, Campbell K. Inhaled insulin: an overview. Clinical Diabetes 2001;19: 13–6.

[78] Gerber RA, Cappelleri JC, Kourides IA, et al. Treatment satisfaction with inhaled insulin in patients with type 1 diabetes. Diabetes Care 2001;24:1556–9.

[79] Chow CC, Tsang LWW, Sorensen JP, et al. Comparison of insulin with or without continuation of oral hypoglycemic agents in the treatment of secondary failure in NIDDM patients. Diabetes Care 1995;18:307–14.

[80] Bergenstal R, Johnson M, Whipple D, et al. Adavantages of adding metformin to multiple dose insulin therapy in type 2 diabetes [abstract]. Diabetes 1998;47(Suppl 1):A89.

[81] Yki-Jarvinen H, Ryysy L, Nikkika K, et al. Comparison of bedtime insulin regimens in patients with type 2 diabetes mellitus: a randomized controlled trial. Ann Intern Med 1999;130:389–96.

[82] Hermann LS, Kalen J, Katzman P, et al. Long-term glycemic improvement after addition of metformin to insulin in insulin-treated obese type 2 diabetes patients. Diabetes Obesity Metabolism 2001;3:428–34.

[83] Abraira C, Colwell JA, Nuttall FQ, et al. Veterans Affairs Cooperative Study on glycemic control and complications of type II diabetes (VA CSDM): results of the feasibility trial. Veterans Affairs Cooperative Study in Type II Diabetes. Diabetes Care 1995;18: 1113–23.

[84] Johnson JL, Wolf SL, Kabadi UM. Efficacy of insulin and sulfonylurea combination therapy in type 2 diabetes. Arch Intern Med 1996;156:259–64.

[85] Landstedt-Hallin L, Adamson U, Arner P, et al. Comparison of bedtime NPH or preprandial regular insulin combined with glibenclamide in secondary sulfonylurea failure. Diabetes Care 1995;18:1183–6.

[86] Buse JB. Overview of current therapeutic options in type 2 diabetes. Diabetes Care 1999;22(Suppl 3):C65–9.

[87] Hara T, Nakamura J, Koh N, et al. An importance of carbohydrate ingestion for the expression of the effect of α-glucosidase inhibitor in NIDDM. Diabetes Care 1996;19: 642–7.

[88] Albu J, Konnarides C, Pi-Sunyer FX. Weight control. Metabolic and cardiovascular effects. Diabetes Reviews 1995;3:335–47.

[89] Clinical Guidelines on the Identification, Evaluation, and Treatment of Overweight and Obesity in Adults. The Evidence Report. 1998. NIH Publication #98–4083.

[90] Beebe CA, Pastors JG, Powers MA, et al. Nutrition management for individuals with non-insulin-dependent diabetes mellitus in the 90s: a review by the Diabetes Care and Education Dietetic Practice Group. J Am Diet Assoc 1991;91:196–207.

[91] Williams G. Obesity and type 2 diabetes: a conflict of interests? Int J Obes 1999;23(Suppl 7):S2–4.

[92] Williamson DF, Thompson TJ, Thun M, et al. Intentional weight loss and mortality among overweight individuals with diabetes. Diabetes Care 2000;23:1499–504.

[93] Leibson CL, Williamson DF, Melton LJ III, et al. Temporal trends in BMI among adults with diabetes. Diabetes Care 2001;24:1584–9.

[94] Rosenfalck AM, Hendel H, Rasmussen MH, et al. Minor long-term changes in weight have beneficial effects on insulin sensitivity and β-cell function in obese subjects. Diabetes Obes Metab 2002;4:19–28.

[95] Williams KV, Mullen ML, Kelley DE, et al. The effect of short periods of caloric restriction on weight loss and glycemic control in type 2 diabetes. Diabetes Care 1998;21:2–8.

[96] Bray GA. Drug treatment of obesity. Am J Clin Nutr 1992;55:538S–44S.

[97] Bray GA. Basic mechanisms and very low calorie diets. In: Blackburn GL, Bray GA, editors. Management of obesity by severe caloric restriction. Littleton (MA): PSG; 1985. p. 129–69.

[98] Flier JS. Obesity and lipoprotein disorders. In: Khan RC, Weir GC, editors. Joslin's diabetes mellitus. Philadelphia: Lea & Febiger; 1994. p. 351–6.

[99] Hauner H. The impact of pharmacotherapy on weight management in type 2 diabetes. Int J Obes 1999;23(Suppl 7):S12–7.

[100] Finer N, Bloom SR, Frost GS, et al. Sibutramine is effective for weight loss and diabetic control in obesity with type 2 diabetes: a randomized, double-blind, placebo-controlled study. Diabetes Obes Metab 2000;2(2):105–12.

[101] Fujioka K, Seaton TB, Rowe E, et al. Weight loss with sibutramine improves glycaemic control and other metabolic parameters in obese patients with type 2 diabetes mellitus. Diabetes Obes Metab 2000;2(3):175–87.

[102] Rissanen A. Weight loss on sibutramine treatment for 12 months improves lipid profile in obese type 2 diabetic patients [abstract]. 36th Annual Meeting of the European Association for the Study of Diabetes 2000. Available at: http://www.easd.org. Accessed September 25, 2002.

[103] Serrano-Rios M, Melchionda N. Moreno-Carreterot E. Role of sibutramine in the treatment of obese type 2 diabetic patients receiving sulfonylurea therapy. Diabet Med 2002;19:119–24.

[104] Gokcel AG, Karakose H, Ertorer EM, et al. Effects of sibutramine in obese female subjects with type 2 diabetes and poor blood glucose control. Diabetes Care 2001;24:1957–60.

[105] James WPT, Astrup A, Finer N, et al, for the STORM Study Group. Effect of sibutramine on weight maintenance after weight loss: a randomized trial. Lancet 2000;356:2119–25.

[106] Hauner H. Current pharmacological approaches to the treatment of obesity. Int J Obes 2001;25(Suppl 1):S102–6.

[107] Guerciolini R. Mode of action of orlistat. Int J Obes 1997;21(Suppl 3):S12–23.

[108] Lamotte M, Annemans L, Lefever A, et al. A health economic model to assess the long-term effects and cost-effectiveness of orlistat in obese type 2 diabetic patients. Diabetes Care 2002;25:303–8.

[109] Keating GM, Jarvis B. Orlistat in the prevention and treatment of type 2 diabetes mellitus. Drugs 2001;61(14):2107–19.

[110] Hollander PA, Elbein SC, Hirsch IB, et al. Role of orlistat in the treatment of obese patients with type 2 diabetes. A 1-year randomized double-blind study. Diabetes Care 1998;21:1288–94.

[111] Kelley DE, Bray GA, Pi-Sunyer FX, et al. Clinical efficacy of orlistat therapy in overweight and obese patients with insulin-treated type 2 diabetes. Diabetes Care 2002;25(6):1033–41.

[112] Sjöström L, Rissanen A, Andersen T, et al. Randomized placebo-controlled trial of orlistat for weight loss and prevention of weight regain in obese patients. Lancet 1998;352:167–72.

[113] Scheen AJ, Lefèbvre PJ. Antiobesity pharmacotherapy in the management of type 2 diabetes. Diabetes Metab Res Rev 2000;16:114–24.

[114] Heymsfield SB, Segal KR, Hauptman J, et al. Effects of weight loss with orlistat on glucose tolerance and progression to type 2 diabetes in obese adults. Arch Intern Med 2000;160(9):1321–6.

[115] Ritzel R, Schulte M, Pørksen N, et al. Glucagon-like peptide 1 increases secretory burst mass of pulsatile insulin secretion in patients with type 2 diabetes and impaired glucose tolerance. Diabetes 2001;50:776–84.

[116] Vilsbøll T, Krarup T, Deacon CF, et al. Reduced postprandial concentrations of intact biologically active glucagon-like peptide 1 in type 2 diabetic patients. Diabetes 2001;50:609–13.

[117] Mannucci E, Ognibene A, Cremasco F, et al. Glucagon-like peptide (GLP)-1 and leptin concentrations in obese patients with type 2 diabetes mellitus. Diabet Med 2000;17:713–9.

[118] Toft-Nielsen MB, Madsbad S, Holst JJ. Determinants of the effectiveness of glucagons-like peptide-1 in type 2 diabetes. J Clin Endocrinol Metab 2001;86:3853–60.

[119] Gutzwiller JP, Drewe J, Goke B, et al. Glucagon-like peptide-1 promotes satiety and reduces food intake in patients with diabetes mellitus type 2. Am J Physiol 1999;276: R1541–4.

[120] Naslund E, Gutniak M, Skogar S, et al. Glucagon-like peptide 1 increases the period of postprandial satiety and slows gastric emptying in obese men. Am J Clin Nutr 1998;68:525–30.

[121] Flint A, Raben A, Rehfeld JF, et al. The effect of glucagons-like peptide-1 on energy expenditure and substrate metabolism in humans. Int J Obes Relat Metab Disord 2000;24:288–98.

[122] Drucker DJ. Minireview: the glucagon-like peptides. Endocrinology 2001;142:521–7.

[123] van Dijk G, Thiele TE. Glucagon-like-peptide-1 (7–36) amide: a central regulator of satiety and interoceptive stress. Neuropeptides 1999;33:406–14.

[124] Larsen J, Hylleberg B, Ng K, et al. Glucagon-like peptide-1 infusion must be maintained for 24 h/day to obtain acceptable glycemia in type 2 diabetic patients who are poorly controlled on sulphonylurea treatment. Diabetes Care 2001;24:1416–21.

[125] Balkan B, Kwasnik L, Miserendino R, et al. Inhibition of dipeptidyl peptidase IV with NVP-DPP728 increases plasma GLP-1 (7–36 amide) concentrations and improves oral glucose tolerance in obese Zucker rats. Diabetologia 1999;42:1324–31.

[126] Doyle ME, Egan JM. Glucagon-like-peptide-1. Recent Prog Horm Res 2001;56:377–99.

[127] Johnson D, Drenick EJ. Therapeutic fasting in morbid obesity. Arch Intern Med 1977; 137:1381–2.

[128] Andersen T, Backer OG, Stokholm KH, et al. Randomized trial of diet and gastroplasty compared with diet alone in morbid obesity. N Engl J Med 1984;310:352–6.

[129] NIH Technology Assessment Conference Panel. Methods for voluntary weight loss and control. Ann Intern Med 1992;116:942–9.

[130] Sugerman HJ, Kellum JM, Engle KM, et al. Gastric bypass for treating severe obesity. Am J Clin Nutr 1992;55:560S–6S.

[131] Pories WJ, MacDonald KG, Morgan EJ, et al. Surgical treatment of obesity and its effect on diabetes: 10-y follow-up. Am J Clin Nutr 1992;55:582S–5S.

[132] Sagar PM. Surgical treatment of morbid obesity. Br J Surg 1995;82:732–9.

[133] Klem ML, Wing RR, Ho Chang CC, et al. A case-control study of successful maintenance of a substantial weight loss: individuals who lost weight through surgery versus those who lost weight through non-surgical means. Int J Obes 2000;24:573–9.

[134] Maclean LD, Rhode BM, Nohr CW. Late outcome of isolated gastric bypass. Ann Surg 2000;231:524–8.

[135] Pories WJ, Swanson MS, MacDonald KG, et al. Who would have thought it? An operation proves to be the most effective therapy for adult-onset diabetes mellitus. Ann Surg 1995;222:339–52.

[136] Balsiger BM, Kennedy FP, Abu-Lebdeh HS, et al. Prospective evaluation of Roux-en-Y gastric bypass as primary operation for medically complicated obesity. Mayo Clin Proc 2000;75:673–80.

[137] Sjostrom CD, Lissner L, Wedel H, et al. Reduction in incidence of diabetes, hypertension and lipid disturbances after intentional weight loss induced by bariatric surgery: the SOS Intervention Study. Obes Res 1999;7:477–84.

[138] Scheen AJ. Treatment of diabetes in patients with severe obesity. Biomed Pharmacother 2000;54:74–9.

[139] Khateeb NI, Roslin MS, Chin D, et al. Significant improvement in HbA1c in a morbidly obese type 2 diabetic patient after gastric bypass surgery despite relatively small weight loss. Diabetes Care 1999;22:651.

[140] Balsiger BM, Murr MM, Poggio JL, et al. Bariatric surgery. Surgery for weight control in patients with morbid obesity. Med Clin North Am 2000;84:477–89.

[141] Scopinaro N, Adami GF, Marinari GM, et al. Biliopancreatic diversion. World J Surg 1998;22:936–46.

[142] Luyckx FH, Scheen AJ, Desaive C, et al. Effects of gastroplasty on body weight and related biological abnormalities in morbid obesity. Diabetes Metab 1998;24:355–61.

[143] Pories WJ, MacDonald KG, Flickinger EG, et al. Is type II diabetes mellitus (NIDDM) a surgical disease? Ann Surg 1992;215:633–43.

[144] Consensus Development Panel. Gastrointestinal surgery for severe obesity: Consensus Development Conference statement. Ann Intern Med 1991;115:956–61.

[145] Sugerman H. The epidemic of severe obesity: the value of surgical treatment. Mayo Clin Proc 2000;75:669–72.

[146] Hsu LKG, Benotti PN, Dwyer J, et al. Nonsurgical factors that influence the outcome of bariatric surgery: a review. Psychosom Med 1998;60:338–46.

[147] Aldo VG, Mingrone G, Giancaterini A, et al. Insulin resistance in morbid obesity: reversal with intramyocellular fat depletion. Diabetes 2002;51:144–51.

[148] Pories WJ, Albrecht RJ. Etiology of type II diabetes: role of the foregut. World J Surg 2001;25:527–31.

[149] Hickey MS, Pories WJ, MacDonald KG, et al. A new paradigm for type 2 diabetes mellitus: could it be a disease of the foregut? Ann Surg 1998;227:637–44.

[150] Sjostrom CD, Peltonen M, Wedel H, et al. Differentiated long-term effects of intentional weight loss on diabetes and hypertension. Hypertension 2000;36:20–5.

[151] MacDonald KG, Long SD, Swanson MS, et al. The gastric bypass operation reduces the progression and mortality of non-insulin-dependent diabetes mellitus. J Gastrointest Surg 1997;1:213–20.

[152] MacLean LD, Rhode BM, Sampalis J, et al. Scientific papers: results of the surgical treatment of obesity. Am J Surg 1993;165:155–62.

[153] Hall JC, Watts JM, O'Brien PE, et al. Gastric surgery for morbid obesity. Ann Surg 1990;211:419–27.

[154] Sugerman HJ, Starkey JV, Birkenhauer R. A randomized prospective trial of gastric bypass versus vertical banded gastroplasty for morbid obesity and their effects on sweets versus non-sweets eaters. Ann Surg 1987;205:613–24.

[155] Sugerman HJ, Kellum JM, DeMaria EJ, et al. Conversion of failed or complicated vertical banded gastroplasty to gastric bypass in morbid obesity. Am J Surg 1996;171:263–7.

[156] Bloomgarden ZT. Obesity and diabetes. Diabetes Care 2000;23:1584–90.

[157] Buchwald H. Overview of bariatric surgery. J Am Coll Surg 2002;194(3):367–75.

[158] Campbell L, Rossner S. Management of obesity in patients with type 2 diabetes. Diabet Med 2001;18:345–54.

[159] Nehoda H, Weiss H, Labeck B, et al. Results and complications after adjustable gastric banding in a series of 250 patients. Am J Surg 2001;181:12–5.

[160] Schirmer BD. Laparoscopic bariatric surgery. Surg Clin North Am 2000;80:1253–67.

[161] Dixon JB, O'Brien PE. Health outcomes of severely obese type 2 diabetic subjects 1 year after laparoscopic adjustable gastric banding. Diabetes Care 2002;25:358–63.

[162] Higa K, Boone KB, Ho T, et al. Laparoscopic Roux-en-Y gastric bypass for morbid obesity: technique and preliminary results of our first 400 patients. Arch Surg 2000;135:1029–33.

17

Surgical Approaches to the Treatment of Obesity: A Practical Guide for the Covering Physician

Janey S.A. Pratt

George L. Blackburn

A 56-year-old woman presents to her physician's office for a routine physical. She weighs 290 lbs and is 5'5" tall; her body mass index (BMI) is 48 kg/m^2. Several times over the last decade she lost approximately 40 lbs, but she regained the weight within a few years. She was diagnosed with diabetes 2 years ago, and recently started on insulin. She suffers from gastroesophageal reflux disease (GERD), hypertension, and depression. Current medications include metformin hydrochloride (Glucophage), insulin (Humalog), omeprazole (Prilosec), hydrochlorothiazide and trimterene (Dyazide), amlodipine (Norvasc), citalopram (Celexa), and lorazepam (Ativan). She is concerned about her inability to lose weight. What should her physician recommend?

The clinical problem

Obesity is epidemic. Over 15 million Americans, 1 out of 20, have class II or III obesity (a BMI >35 kg/m^2). Medical management has failed to provide effective long-term treatment, but bariatric surgery (from the Greek root *baros*, meaning *weight*) has proven successful. It is already the most common upper gastrointestinal (GI) surgery in the United States [1]. Roux-en-Y gastric bypass (RYGB), which replaced vertical-banded gastroplasty (VBG), is the most common bariatric procedure in the United States;

laparoscopic adjustable gastric banding (LAGB) is the most common worldwide. Long-term studies from Europe show that biliopancreatic diversion also produces excellent sustained weight loss and significant improvement of comorbidities [2,3].

Surgical treatment for weight loss produces the best long-term results for patients suffering from class II and III obesity who have failed to respond to more conservative approaches [4]. Bariatric surgery should only be performed with the support of a multidisciplinary team that includes nutritionists, psychologists, physical therapists, internists, and surgeons [5]. Like other treatments for obesity, surgical weight loss requires active patient participation and significant support of friends and family during the pre- and postoperative periods [6].

Primary care physicians need to know the indications and contra-indications for surgery. This chapter will discuss how to evaluate patients with obesity and determine whether surgery is an appropriate treatment option. We will present the different surgical strategies, their risks, and expected outcomes. Patients who receive surgical treatment for obesity require long-term follow up and medical care, much like those who had transplant surgery.

Strategies and operations

Obesity surgery began in this country in 1954 with the first Jejeuno-Ileal bypass, which was performed for the management of hypercholesterolemia [1]. It quickly became apparent that this surgery could be used to induce long-term weight loss. The operation was popular for approximately 20 years until it was found to cause severe long-term side effects (eg, protein energy malnutrition [7], blind loop syndrome, biliary cholestasis, and liver failure leading to early death). These adverse outcomes were attributed to a diverted loop of small intestine that remained in place. Because of these negative early experiences—including high mortality associated with anesthesia—obesity surgery fell out of favor for several decades [8,9]. In 1997, problems with Fen-Phen brought it again to the attention of the mainstream medical community. This time, however, gastric restrictive [10] and gastric bypass [11] surgical approaches had been in development for over 20 years, and were now showing long-term success with low peri- and postoperative morbidity and mortality.

Different bariatric procedures

Several types of bariatric procedures are performed today. Many are covered by insurance, a benefit usually based on conclusions from a 1991 NIH Consensus Conference on Gastrointestinal Surgery for Severe Obesity (ie, that for patients with a BMI >40 kg/m^2 [class III obesity] or over 35 kg/m^2 [class II] with major comorbidities, surgery should be the treatment of choice [4,12]).

The NIH Consensus recommended VBG or RYGB based on data showing improvement of comorbidities and long-term maintenance of weight loss with these operations. Today, laparoscopic approaches to both operations are available, and malabsorptive and banding procedures are used as well. To date there is no way to know which procedure is best suited to which patient.

Gastric restrictive surgery: description

Gastric restrictive procedures restrict caloric intake by reducing the size of the gastric reservoir. These operations were first thought to work by physically restricting food intake. But it is now felt that they exert their major effect by altering gastrointestinal regulation of hunger and satiety. Distention of the small stomach pouch activates vagal afferent neurons that connect the stomach to the satiety centers in the brain, creating a sensation of early satiety. For patients who fail to experience the satiety-inducing effects of gastric surgery, the small pouch reinforces the need to limit food intake. Restrictive procedures, which maintain continuity of the intestines, minimize vitamin deficiencies and anemia seen in bypass procedures. Other benefits include decreased operation time, lack of an anastamosis and its associated complications, and the perceived reversibility of the procedures. Patients who plan to undergo surgery for obesity need to accept the risks of surgery and be made aware that no operation is completely reversible.

Restrictive procedures include gastric stapling, gastric banding, and use of the adjustable gastric band. Each of these approaches can be performed open or laparoscopically. In this chapter we discuss VBG and the LAGB.

Mason and Ito [10] first described gastric partitioning to create a small proximal pouch with a band-like restriction to slow the passage of food into the distal stomach in 1967—an operation made possible when the Russians developed surgical stapling devices to close wounds sustained during World War II. These devices, now quite sophisticated, can accurately place four parallel rows of staples to partition the proximal stomach from the distal stomach. Laparoscopic devices can only place staples in two to three rows on either side and divide the tissue between.

Early gastric staples were often performed horizontally, and pouch size was not well controlled. As a result, outcomes varied greatly. Mason eventually discovered that stapling vertically to create a pouch of 50 cc or less and placing a band around the outlet of the pouch to limit the stoma to 1 cm [13] produced better long-term results (Fig. 1). This operation became the most commonly performed bariatric procedure in the United States until the late 1990s, when it was supplanted by RYGB. Recently, VBG has been performed laparoscopically, but with the introduction of the LAGB to the United States market in 2001, it may soon be obsolete [14,15].

The LAGB is the culmination of a banding history that began in Europe in the 1980s. Initially, a fixed band was placed around the stomach to create

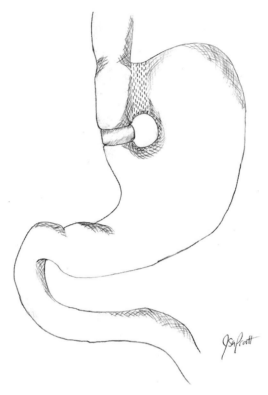

Fig. 1. Vertical banded gastroplasty (VBG). A small gastric pouch is created by staple partition or staple transection of the stomach. A band is placed around the outlet to slow food movement.

a proximal pouch and a fixed outlet into the remainder of the stomach. In Poland, the band was revised with an inflatable balloon lining the inner circumference, thereby changing the diameter of the gastric pouch outlet [16]. A port-a-cath injection port allows dynamic postoperative adjustment of the gastric outlet size (Fig. 2). Postoperative follow-up requires accessing the port-a-cath, often with fluoroscopic guidance, to inject or remove saline from the balloon to change the outlet size. This is done every 2 to 6 months for the first year, then every 4 to12 months thereafter, depending on the surgeon and the program [17].

Malabsorptive procedures: description

Jejeuno-Ileal bypass surgery, as performed in the 1960s and 1970s, gave malabsorptive operations a bad name. That procedure was different from the one developed by Scopinaro and Gianetta in 1976 [18], in which the small bowel was not defunctionalized as it continued to have flow of

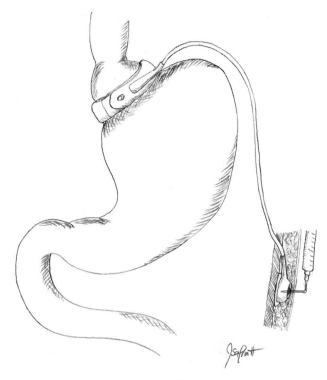

Fig. 2. Laparoscopic adjustable gastric band (LAGB). An adjustable band is placed around the top of the stomach. The diameter can be adjusted by inserting or removing saline from the reservoir, just under the skin.

hepatic and pancreatic secretions. Biliopancreatic diversion (BPD) begins by removing approximately two thirds of the stomach, leaving a 200- to 500-cc pouch. The alimentary limb is usually 100 to 250 cm in length, with the common channel 50 to 100 cm in length. The biliopancreatic limb is whatever remains (Fig. 3).

In 1998, Hess and Hess developed a hybrid malabsorptive procedure that combined BPD with a duodenal switch (DS), an operation developed by DeMeester [19] to prevent bile reflux. BPD with a DS (Fig. 4) is performed with limb lengths similar to that of BPD. Instead of a horizontal gastroplasty, however, a tube gastrectomy is performed to remove the greater curvature of the stomach [20]. Preservation of the pylorus decreased the risk of ulcers seen in 2% to 10% of patients with BPD. Both of these operations are now being done laparoscopically in selected institutions. Early studies indicate that the risks of the laparoscopic procedure in the severely obese appear to be greater than the benefits. These results, however, may be related to the difficulty of the procedure and the learning curve [21]. Randomized comparison studies are still needed.

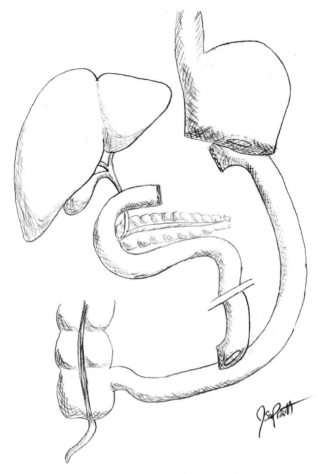

Fig. 3. Biliopancreatic diversion (BPD). Following a partial gastrectomy, the ileum is anastomosed to the stomach remnant. The intestinal limb that drains the bile and pancreatic juices is anastomosed to the terminal ileum.

Mixed operations: description

The open RYGB was descended directly from the Billroth II reconstruction following partial gastrectomy for ulcer disease. Patients who underwent this operation lost weight and could not regain it without significant intervention. Dr. Mason added the stapled gastric pouch to the RYGB to create the RYGB operation that is performed today. Although the procedure has changed over the years, data from it are now over 30 years old and show that a weight loss of greater than 50% of excess body weight is maintained by 90% of patients [22].

In 1996, two methods for performing the RYGB laparoscopically were simultaneously developed in the United States [23] and in Sweden [24]. In

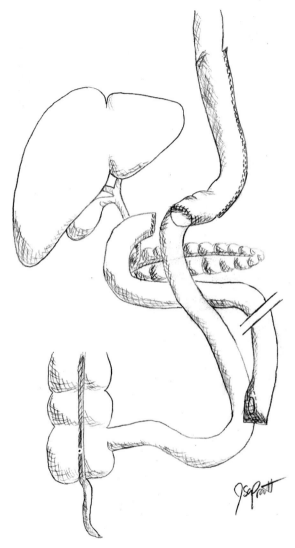

Fig. 4. Biliopancreatic diversion with a duodenal switch (BPD with DS). Similar to the biliopancreatic diversion except that a sleeve gastrectomy is done and the ileum is anastomosed to the duodendum.

the United States, these have been rapidly adopted and modified, and are now widely performed nationwide. Soon laparoscopic RYGB (LRYGB) procedures may surpass the number of open surgeries performed in the United States. Open gastric bypass traditionally involves the creation of a 30-cc gastric pouch by vertical stapling, followed by the creation of a Roux-en-Y limb which is then attached to the pouch by sewing, stapling, or a combination of the two (Fig. 5). In some cases the pouch is left attached

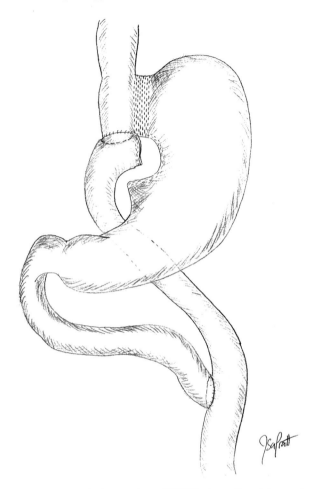

Fig. 5. Open Roux-en-Y gastric bypass (open RYGB). A small gastric pouch is created by sewing, stapling, or a combination of the two. The pouch is left "attached" to the distal stomach in this case. The pouch is anastomosed to the jejunum.

to the distal stomach; in others, it may be completely isolated. In the laparoscopic procedure, the pouch is always transected or isolated from the distal stomach; to date, there is no laparoscopic stapling device that can partition the stomach without dividing it (Fig. 6).

Another variable in these operations is the length of the small bowel limb. To bring up the Roux limb, most surgeons measure the distance from the ligament of treitz to where the small bowel is divided. The length of the biliopancreatic limb can vary from 15 to 100 cm. In most cases, a length of approximately 40 cm is used to allow a long enough mesentery on the distal limb to reach the gastroesophageal junction. The Roux (or alimentary) limb is a length of small bowel, usually jejunum, which goes to the pouch. It

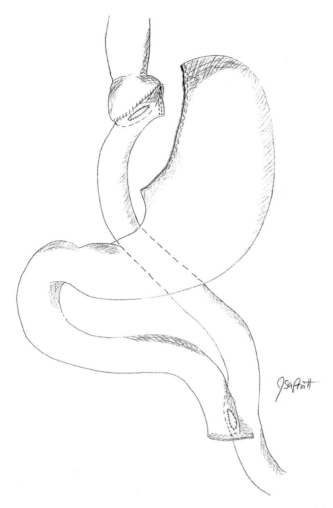

Fig. 6. Laparoscopic Roux-en-Y gastric bypass (LRYGB). A small gastric pouch is created by stapling and transecting the proximal stomach. The pouch is anastomosed to the jejunum. The length of the biliopancreatic limb can vary from 15–100 cm. The "Roux" or "Alimentary" limb can vary in length from 40–300 cm.

varies in length from 40 to 300 cm, but most surgeons use 100 to 150 cm. There is a variant of the RYGB called the long limb or distal RYGB. In this operation, the distance from the ileocecal valve is measured instead of that from the gastric pouch. In this case, the alimentary limb might be any length, while the common "channel" (ie, that part of the small bowel that sees both food and bilio-pancreatic secretions) distal to the jejunojejenostomy may be between 75 and 125 cm long [25].

Surgeons continue to debate the safety of combining a restrictive procedure with greater malabsorption. The risk of protein energy malnutrition goes up significantly with distal gastric bypass, but so does the percent of excess body weight loss maintained past 5 years. For this reason, some surgeons advocate the use of this procedure in the "super obese" (defined by a BMI >50 kg/m^2), while others prefer a purer malabsorptive procedure.

Selection criteria

Patients who can expect to gain the most benefit from surgical treatment of obesity include those with a BMI over 40 kg/m^2 or a BMI over 35 kg/m^2 who also suffer from diabetes, hypertension, GERD, arthritis, sleep apnea, or cardiovascular disease. Contraindications to bariatric surgery include end-stage organ failure, certain personality disorders, untreated major depression or psychosis, untreated eating disorders, current alcohol or drug abuse, and the inability of the patient to comply with postoperative medical, nutritional, and psychological management [26].

There is no upper age limit for surgery, but the risks may outweigh the benefits for patients over 70 years of age. Surgery on pediatric patients with comorbidities from obesity (eg, metabolic syndrome, asthma, chronic obstructive pulmonary disease, polycystic ovarian syndrome, or type 2 diabetes) is controversial. Nevertheless, protocols are being developed for teenagers with life-long obesity, who have failed behavior modification programs, and have the will and ability to follow a postoperative program [7]. Studies show that bariatric surgery in children between the ages of 12 and 18 is safe, improves self-image, and can produce excellent long-term resolution of comorbidities [27].

Obese patients have multiple medical conditions and comorbidities. Still, with today's anesthesia risk assessment, improved ventilators, shorter-acting agents, and modern surgical techniques, bariatric surgery has a very low mortality rate—less than 1% in most series [8,9]. At many bariatric surgery centers, more patients die waiting for surgery than postoperatively. For this reason, those at high medical risk (eg, status after heart or kidney transplant, status after cardiac bypass, or even severe chronic obstructive pulmonary disease) should be prioritized for surgery. Use of medically supervised preoperative weight loss to improve dysmetabolism and acute conditions is also imperative.

Only some 10% to 15% of patients fail to achieve long-term success after gastric bypass. However, there is no way to identify these individuals. Many will lose weight initially but will slowly regain it over the next 5 years. Such patients require ongoing medical monitoring and treatment. Some also need intense diet, exercise, and lifestyle behavior change as well as adjunctive weight control medications.

There are no data yet on which procedures work best for which patients. Most surgeons choose procedures based on expertise, specific exclusion criteria, and acceptable levels of invasiveness. Insurance coverage may also be a factor. Most patients succeed regardless of approach. The exceptions are those with Prader-Willi syndrome, a genetic disorder of hyperphagia following failure to thrive in early infancy; in most cases, this syndrome fails to respond to any type of bariatric surgery.

Gastric restrictive surgery: patient selection

VGB is usually covered by insurance and can be performed open or laparoscopically depending on the surgeon's training. For menstruating women, it eliminates vitamin deficiencies and reduces incidence of anemia. Because it makes no use of the small bowel, it is also an alternative for patients who have had prior small bowel procedures or have adhesions from earlier surgery. Disadvantages are long-term complications and problems with weight regain [28]. It was once thought that "sweet eaters," or patients who migrated to carbohydrates, would have less success with a purely restrictive operation due to lack of "dumping." Recent data, however, show otherwise [29–31].

Few data are available on whether the adjustability of the LAGB produces better long-term results than the VBG. One 3-year follow up study showed continued weight loss after the first 2 years, a phenomenon not often seen with other "fixed" bariatric procedures [32]. Other studies described removal and revision rates from 10% to 38%, with long-term success rates of 50% [17].

Specific selection criteria apply to the Lap-Band (INAMED Health, Santa Barbara, California) adjustable gastric band. It is not recommended in patients with Crohn's disease, hiatal hernia, cirrhosis, portal hypertension, connective tissue disease, prior gastric ulcers, or chronic steroid use. It is also not covered by many insurance companies.

Malabsorptive procedures: patient selection

Many surgeons using BPD and BPD with a DS in the super obese population are finding a greater percent of weight loss and long-term success [33–35]. Some recommend the procedures for all patients with a BMI over 50 k/mg^2 to 60 k/mg^2. However, there are significant risks associated with the malabsorption they induce. Anemia, protein energy malnutrition, diarrhea, and long-term osteoporosis are generally more severe in BPD than in RYGB [36]. Because patients who undergo BPD (with or without DS) are at higher risk of severe vitamin and protein deficiencies, it is critical that they understand the operation and the necessity for postoperative compliance. Major contraindications include: Crohn's disease, severe liver disease, or portal hypertension. Many insurance carriers do not cover this operation because it was not recommended in the 1991 consensus or its 1996 addendum [4,12].

Mixed operations: patient selection

The RYGB operation is the most effective way to achieve sustained weight loss in patients with moderate to severe obesity with the least risk of complications. In most cases, it is also covered by insurance. For these reasons, RYGB is the most commonly performed surgery for obesity in the United States today. There are very few contraindications to this operation, though many surgeons are selective in their choice of laparoscopic candidates. Prior surgery, BMI over 55 k/mg^2, weight over 400 lbs, increased age, and male sex have been associated with a higher complication rate in both open and LRYGB [37]. In one surgeon's experience, the most common reasons for conversion to an open procedure were male sex, prior surgery, and fatty liver disease with a dominant left lobe.

Comparative outcomes

Treatment outcome is measured by percent of excess body weight lost. Still, outcome measurements for bariatric surgery are controversial. If success is defined as greater than 50% of excess body weight lost over a certain period of time, bariatric surgery is clearly effective—it is the only treatment that succeeds in 70% to 90% of patients. If success is expressed as an average percent of excess body weight lost, malabsorptive procedures produce better results than restrictive ones (Table 1). Rather than weight loss, however, many bariatric surgeons argue that the most important outcome is improvement in comorbidities.

Bariatric surgery resolves type 2 diabetes in 75% to 85% of patients, with significant improvement in 95% [38]. It normalizes lipid profiles and improves ventricular function (100%), significantly decreasing cardiac risk factors and medication requirements (80% to 92%). In almost all cases,

Table 1
Treatment outcome excess body weight loss

Outcomes of bariatric operations	Reference	2 years excess body weight lost	4–10 years excess body weight lost
Laparoscopic adjustable gastric band	Dixon and O'Brien [57]	52% EBW	57% EBW (5 years)
Vertical-banded gastroplasty	Suter [27]	66% EBW	55% EBW (9 years)
Roux-en-Y gastric bypass	Multiple sources	62% EBW (estimate)	60% EBW (estimate over 15 years)
Laparoscopic Roux-en-Y gastric bypass	Wittgrove and Clark [58]	80% EBW	75% EBW (5 years)
Biliopancreatic diversion	Scopinaro and Gianetta [18]	78% EBW	78% EBW (10 years)
Biliopancreatic diversion with duodenal switch	Hess and Hess [19]	80% EBW	70% EBW (8 years)

Abbreviation: EBW, excess body weight.

obstructive sleep apnea is improved to the point of eliminating the need for continuous positive airway pressure (CPAP), with no apnea in 40% of patients and minimal episodes in 60% [39].

Symptoms of increased intra-abdominal pressure—including congestive heart failure, hypoventilation, venous stasis disease, gastroesophageal reflux, urinary stress incontinence, and pseudotumor cerebri—resolve relatively quickly following surgery [40–45]. Urinary stress incontinence is improved in 81% to 97% of patients. After gastric bypass surgery, gastroesophageal reflux is improved in 77% to 98% of patients; purely restrictive procedures, however, may worsen reflux despite resolution of intra-abdominal pressure. Significant weight loss improves osteoarthritis in most patients. It also resolves pain from rheumatoid arthritis, though it often recurs after a brief respite. Obesity is an independent risk factor for many types of cancer, including breast, endometrial, prostate, and gallbladder; weight loss reduces the risk of these and other cancers.

The two most important outcomes of bariatric surgery are improved quality of life and reduced risk of premature death. Quality of life measures consistently show improvement following weight loss from any type of bariatric surgery [39]. Risk of premature death rises significantly with increasing BMI. Several recent studies show that patients live longer with surgery than without it [39]. MacDonald et al [46] followed patients approved for surgery who did not undergo it; they found 28% mortality over 6 years without surgery versus 9% with it. As mentioned earlier in this chapter, more patients die waiting for bariatric surgery than following it. There are two reasons for this: a very low (<0.5%) risk of perioperative death and a longer life expectancy after resolution of comorbidities. Patients, even when they suffer complications from surgery, report 90% to 98% satisfaction.

Clinical recommendations

Our 56-year-old patient with a BMI of 48 k/mg^2 and a history of type 2 diabetes, hypertension and GERD would be an excellent candidate for surgery. In the United States, the most likely operation would be RYGB. The patient could expect to live longer with surgery than without it. She would decrease her risk of premature death from 4% per year to 1% per year. It would be important for her to undergo an extensive preoperative evaluation and learning program. Preoperative weight loss, behavior modification, and education are important for long-term success following bariatric surgery. Postoperatively, the patient would be monitored at 2, 6, 9, and 12 months, then annually for complications from surgery. She would be required to take a multivitamin—iron, B_{12}, and calcium—for the rest of her life.

At 18 months after surgery you would expect the patient in this case to have an average BMI of 30. She should see sustained resolution of her diabetes and GERD and improvement in her hypertension. One could expect her to no longer need metformin hydrochloride (Glucophage), insulin (Humalog), omeprazole (Prilosec), hydrochlorothiazide and trimterene (Dyazide), or lorazepam (Ativan), though she may need to continue taking amlodipine (Norvasc) and citalopram (Celexa) in addition to her vitamin supplements. She would eat small meals 3 times per day, eat one snack per day, and no longer feel that her weight and life were out of control.

This case illustrates the importance of surgery in the treatment of obesity. If the patient were of childbearing age, she would be discouraged from becoming pregnant for 18 months following surgery or until her weight had stabilized [47]. Evidence suggests an increased risk of neural tube defects if pregnancy occurs earlier. Preoperative evaluation, informed consent, and education about postoperative eating and behavior modification are critical.

Preoperative evaluation

Most bariatric surgeons support a multidisciplinary team approach and consider it imperative to long-term success following surgery [6]. The team is involved in evaluating the patient before surgery and in the education and treatment of the patient after surgery. The team also supports preoperative weight loss in those with super obesity (BMI > 50 kg/m^2), and development of a lifestyle compatible with gastric restrictive surgery. The ideal evaluation has four components: nutritional, psychological, medical, and surgical. The nutritionist preoperatively assesses eating disorders, evaluates eating patterns or triggers, and documents prior weight loss attempts. The psychologist or psychiatrist assesses for untreated binge eating disorder, depression, readiness to make behavioral changes, and ability to comply with long-term follow-up. The internist evaluates the patient for obesity-related comorbidities and clears the patient for anesthesia from cardiovascular and pulmonary standpoints [48].

The most common"newly diagnosed" comorbidities discovered in preoperative evaluation are: abnormal liver enzymes (ALT and AST), steatohepatitis, abnormal sleep lab and obstructive sleep apnea, and hypothyroidism. Preoperative weight loss, CPAP, and medications, in that order, should be used to treat these disorders before surgery. The surgeon evaluates the patient's motivations and expectations, explains different surgical options and their associated risks, and chooses an appropriate surgical approach for each patient.

Although it is possible to handle all required assessments, evaluations, treatments, and informed consent in a bariatric surgeon's office, comprehensive weight control centers are ideal for initial evaluations. In these centers, evaluations are performed by bariatric specialists—nutritionists, psychologists, internists or surgeons—who then meet as a team to discuss medical, behavioral, and surgical options. Programs offering multiple weight loss therapies are able to provide most patients with appropriate treatments; for example, a patient with a binge eating disorder may need a behavior modification and medication program before surgery. It is also important that each patient have strong support from family, friends, or significant others. Support group meetings encourage patients to bring their supporter to preoperative education programs and provide educational materials for them.

Postoperative follow-up

Postoperative diet recommendations depend on the type of surgery and the program; however, all have certain points in common. Patients are usually started on a liquid diet. Clear liquids may continue for 2 to 7 days; after that, protein shakes, yogurt, high protein smooth soups, and milk are started and continue for 2 to 21 days. Patients who are doing well are transitioned to soft solids. All patients are counseled to eat protein first and drink plenty of liquids.

Most programs start patients on chewable vitamins and calcium immediately following surgery; some prescribe B_{12}, iron or vitamin D as well. Patients are often told to avoid carbonated beverages, though little is known about the effects of drinking such beverages after bariatric surgery.

Most surgeons and bariatric nutritionists teach patients to avoid getting too hungry by eating every 5 hours. Patients should be taught to eat only until they feel full, perhaps one or two bites at first. With restrictive and mixed procedures, they need to chew their food well, eat slowly, and avoid drinking until 1 to 2 hours after meals. This allows food to stay in the pouch without washing through and produces a feeling of sustained satiety. Patients should cut food into very small portions, and put their fork down between bites. Those who successfully maintained long-term weight loss after gastric bypass surgery displayed six primary characteristics (Box 1) [49].

Box 1. Habits of successful patients following Roux-en-Y gastric bypass

1. Eat three balanced meals and two snacks per day.
2. Drink 40 to 64 oz per day; 58% avoid carbonation.
3. 92% take vitamins, 68% take calcium, 39% take iron.
4. Sleep 7 hours per night on average.
5. Exercise four times per week for at least 40 minutes.
6. 69% weigh themselves weekly and take personal responsibility for their weight loss.

Success was defined by 72% excess body weight lost. Out of 100 patients surveyed, 97% viewed their gastric bypass as successful.
Adapted from Cook CM, Edwards C. Success habits of long-term gastric bypass patients. Obes Surg 1999;9:80–2; with permission.

The most common causes of nausea early on are pain medications, vitamins, and dehydration. Rehydration sometimes resolves the problem. If patients vomit early on, it is usually because they do not understand how to eat. Eating too fast, or not chewing or cutting food sufficiently, can result in vomiting. Once vomiting has started, the patient may develop some swelling in the pouch and narrowing at the anastamosis, which leads to more vomiting. This can usually be amended by returning to a full liquid diet for a period of 2 to 3 days, then restarting solids with more mindful eating techniques.

To assess for adjustment problems, early follow-up with the psychologist or psychiatrist is imperative. For patients with prior abuse histories, eating disorders, depression, or significant emotional eating, the postoperative adjustment period can be very difficult. Psychological support and medical intervention, if needed, can be essential for well being. Patients should join a monthly or biweekly support group where they can share knowledge about eating patterns, coping mechanisms, and exercise plans. These groups are available around the country and on-line, and may be important to long-term outcomes.

Exercise will often have to be limited to walking for the first 6 to 12 weeks. Often consultation with a physical therapist or personal trainer is beneficial, and some bariatric centers may have them on staff. To obtain the best possible compliance, it is important to define a convenient, comfortable, and fun form of exercise. The most successful RYGB patients exercise for 40 minutes 4 or more times per week.

Evaluation and treatment of complications

Depending on the operation and the level of compliance, postoperative complications occur in 10% to 50% of patients. These are usually defined as early (<4 weeks), midterm (1–6 months), and late (>6 months). A table of complications by operation should give an overview of possible adverse events (Table 2). It's important for patients to know the signs and symptoms of postoperative complications because early recognition and treatment can lessen their physical and emotional impact.

Early complications

Depending on the type of operation and any postoperative complications, patients may be discharged from hospitalization after only 1 to 7 days. They should be seen and have their weight monitored at least 2 to 4 times in the first 6 weeks postopertively to assure adequate hydration, and to assess for early postoperative complications such as wound infections, DVT, nausea, vomiting, and diarrhea or constipation. A leak from the gastro-

Table 2
Complications of different bariatric operations[a]

Operation[b]	Mortality	Leak	Pulmonary embolism	Bleeding	Wound infection	Band complication	Revisional surgery	Stenosis	Marginal ulcer	Incisional hernia	Staple line dehissance	Bowel obstruction	Protein calorie malnutrition
1	0					18%-25%	18%-25%						
2	0.5%					2%	30%	20%		13%	11%		
3	0.5%	0%-1.5%	0.5%	1%	2%		5%-15%	5%-16%	5%-13%	20%	2%-11%		
4	0%-0.5%	0%-4%	0.7%	0.5%-3%	0%-8%			2%-5%	0.5%-10%	0.5%		0.5%-6%	
5	0.5%	0.5%	0.5%		1%		3%-12%		3%	8%-10%		1%	3%-12%
6	0.5%	0.5%	0.5%	3%			4%	0.5%	0			2%	4%

[a] Results are compiled from multiple published and unpublished studies of over 500 patients for each operation.
[b] Name of operation corresponds to number in this column. 1, laparoscopic adjustable gastric band; 2, vertical banded gastroplasty; 3, Roux-en-Y gastric bypass; 4, laparoscopic Roux-en-Y gastric bypass; 5, biliopancreatic diversion; 6, biliopancreatic diversion with duodenal switch.

jejeunal, gastro-duodenal, or jejeuno-jejeunal anastamoses is the most serious and life-threatening complication. The leak rate is higher in the early learning curves of most surgeons who perform these operations laparoscopically. Leaks usually occur during hospitalization, with sustained tachycardia the most sensitive indicator.

Other signs and symptoms include increased pain, fever, rigors, desaturation, or hypotension. Treatment in the stable patient may involve diagnosis by barium swallow followed by nothing by mouth (NPO), total parenteral nutrition (TPN), and antibiotic therapy with or without percutaneous drainage of any associated collection. In the unstable patient, immediate reoperation for repair, drainage, and G- or J-tube is indicated. Bleeding, which usually occurs from a staple line, may have similar symptoms and can be followed expectantly if the patient is stable [50]. Serial hematocrits and transfusion are appropriate in the stable patient because symptoms most often resolve spontaneously.

The most common cause of death following bariatric surgery is pulmonary embolism. Preoperative screening for risk factors (including family history of clotting disorders, personal history of deep vein thrombosis (DVT) or pulmonary embolism (PE), venous stasis disease, or a history of cancer) can allow for aggressive treatment in perioperative prophylaxis. Pneumatic compression boots, sq heparin (Hep-Lock), sq low molecular weight heparin (Fragmin), dextran (Gentran), and inferior vena cava filters (Kimray-Greenfield filter) have all been used. Postoperative immobility and dehydration increase risk of DVT. In some cases, DVT and pulmonary embolism can occur 1 to 2 weeks postoperatively. It may be difficult to assess the obese patient for either DVT or PE; however, even if patient size or hospital resources limit diagnostic studies, postoperative heparinization lowers the threshold for early intervention and treatment and is not contraindicated in most cases. Wound problems are more common in open bariatric procedures than in laparoscopic ones, occurring 5% to 20% of the time versus 0% to 5%, respectively [51]. Cellulite near the wound is often from underlying abscesses and should always be evaluated by the primary surgeon. Diarrhea in the early postoperative period is most commonly from a new onset of lactose intolerance. This occurs much more frequently than was previously thought [52].

Diarrhea, bloating, and gas usually resolve almost immediately after stopping milk products or switching to enzymatically treated milk products. If diarrhea does not resolve, other diagnoses should be considered, such as dumping syndrome (treated with octreotide [Sandostatin] if severe), *c difficile* colitis (treated with metronidazole [Flagyl], or postcholecystectomy bile acid malabsorption (treated with cholestyramine resin [Questran]). In BPD and BPD with DS, diarrhea may be normal in the early postoperative period but should improve as the intestine adjusts to the new configuration. Because of prolonged postoperative diarrhea in 25% of patients, the risk of hemorrhoids is 2% to 10%. Constipation is more common than diarrhea in

LAGB, VBG, and RYGB due to narcotic pain medication, decreased mobility, and dehydration.

It is extremely important to monitor patient comorbidities in the early postoperative period. Many preoperative medications will need to be adjusted or even stopped. For example, a diabetic, hypertensive patient who is sent home on the same medications he or she was admitted with would be hypoglycemic and hypotensive within 24 hours. Oral hypoglycemics should be held postoperatively, and insulin should be given only on a sliding scale basis. These may be restarted based on glucometer readings over the first 2 weeks. Accordingly, antihypertensives, especially diuretics, should also be held. Blood pressure and hydration status should be checked at each visit, and medications should be adjusted accordingly.

Midterm complications

The most common midterm complications seen in RYGB and BPD are gallstones, stomal stenosis, marginal ulcers, dumping, and nausea [53]. Gallstones can be prevented with a 6-month course of ursodiol (Actigall, Urso) given orally in doses of 600 mg daily [54]. Some surgeons perform prophylactic cholecystectomies in all patients, while others select only patients with preoperative documentation of cholelithiasis. Narrowing of the gastro-jejeunostomy can be dilated endoscopically, and marginal ulcers can be treated medically with antisecretory drugs, proton pump inhibitors (eg, omeprazole [Prilosec] or lansoprazole [Prevacid]), H_2-receptor antagonists (eg, cimetidine [Tagamet], ranitidine [Zantac], famotidine [Pepcid], nizatidine [Axid]), or cytoprotective agents (eg, sucralfate [Carafate]).

In LAGB, mid-term complications include band slipping, food intolerance, and port problems. Newer techniques for pouch creation (with a 15-cc proximal pouch) have reduced the incidence of slipping and of food intolerance to less than 5% in most series. Port problems are also decreasing with minor modifications of the band design. VBG complications usually involve recurrent vomiting. Sometimes this is a result of noncompliance, but stenosis of the band should always be ruled out. Some of the earlier Marlex bands tended to scar down over time, leading to food intolerance.

One major reason for weight regain after gastric restrictive procedures is recurrent vomiting. Patients tend to adjust their diets to foods that are best tolerated. Unfortunately, this can lead to a diet of shakes, cookies in milk, or other high-calorie liquid foods. The healthier proteins, vegetables, whole grains, and fruits get caught at the outlet and tend to induce vomiting. In some cases, the outlet can be endoscopically dilated to allow for better passage of food. If this is not successful, however, a bariatric specialist or registered dietitian can be particularly effective in the development of pureed foods (eg, "smoothies"), steamed vegetables, and new chewing and digestive habits to achieve healthy eating and weight management. If the patient is still unable to adjust and has persistent vomiting, then surgical revision to a gastric bypass will allow the patient to eat and keep food down.

Dumping is the response of the jejunum to a large amount of undigested carbohydrate. The release of enteroglucagon and other GI hormones cause the influx of fluid into the lumen of the small intestine; runny nose, salivation, nausea and syncope, vomiting, and diarrhea usually follow [55]. Dumping is often mild and is controlled by avoiding certain foods. When severe, it can be controlled by injection of somatostatin or octreotide (Sandostatin) before meals. Nausea is often related to ketosis and dehydration, and resolves, as the patient is able to take in more liquids. If persistent vomiting occurs, one must be acutely aware of the risk of B-1 thiamine deficiency leading to the development of Wernicke Korsakoff syndrome.

Lifetime complications

The most common complications following any bariatric procedure are vitamin and mineral deficiencies. Long-term follow up should involve careful evaluation of vitamin levels, including B_{12}, iron, folate and vitamin D. If these nutrients are not followed and replaced, severe neurological disorders, anemia, and bone mineral loss can result. Some patients may require high-dose oral B_{12} or iron, while others will require intramuscular or intravenous supplementation. Complete blood count should be tracked to assess for anemia. A follow-up sleep study in patients with sleep apnea should be considered; likewise with liver function tests (LFT)s and liver biopsy in patients with steatohepatitis. Periodic assessment of bone density may also be advisable.

Formation of hernias and staple-line dehiscence leading to gastro-gastric fistula are two long-term complications. Risk of these is reduced in LRYGB. Hernia is quite common in open RYGB (7%–25%) but is uncommon in the laparoscopic approach (2%–5%). The breakdown of the gastric partitioning staple line can happen with or without transection; however, this is more common in the untransected stomach (2%–15%) and is therefore rarely seen in the laparoscopic approach (<1%).

In malabsorptive procedures, protein energy malnutrition can be as high as 26% and should be carefully followed by checking quarterly serum albumin levels. If protein energy malnutrition cannot be treated by significant oral protein supplementation, then short-term TPN and possible surgical revision need to be considered. Bowel obstruction from adhesions or internal hernia can present with vomiting or severe abdominal pain without vomiting. In both RYGB and BPD, bypassed segments can become obstructed, leading to pain and perforation without the usual symptoms associated with small bowel obstruction (SBO).

The American Academy of Neurology described a post–weight loss surgery syndrome known as APGARS (acute post gastric reduction surgery neuropathy) neuropathy. It is most common in patients with persistent vomiting, and symptoms include weakness and paresthesias. This entity appears to be distinct from B_1 thiamine deficiency seen in those with intractable vomiting who develop Wernicke Korsakoff syndrome.

Pregnancy should be avoided in the first 18 months following surgery; the rapid weight loss, dehydration, and vitamin deficiency may cause a higher than normal risk of neural tube defects, which have been associated with low folate levels. After 18 months, many patients will have lost most of their excess weight. At this stage, patients may have severely sagging skin and request surgical intervention. The excess skin can cause interdiginous dermatitis, especially on the abdominal wall. It may also hinder patient mobility when on the legs and lower abdomen. A plastic surgeon should be consulted for evaluation and management of these problems.

Summary

The absence of effective, long-term behavioral or pharmacological options for most patients with obesity has led to renewed appreciation of surgical treatments. The most common operation to induce weight loss—RYGB—is now the most frequently performed upper GI surgical procedure in the United States and is the fastest growing of all general surgical procedures. Surgical therapy should be considered for patients with class II or III obesity who have major medical complications from their obesity, have not succeeded with more conservative approaches, and have a critical need to lose weight and maintain the weight loss long-term.

Sustained weight loss after bariatric surgery is strongly facilitated by postoperative behavior modification therapy. With surgery alone, 5-year success is approximately 50%; addition of an intensive postoperative lifestyle change program increases the success rate to 80%. More than 95% of patients who maintain weight loss for 5 years subsequently maintain it for an additional 10 years [26]. The long-term effectiveness of bariatric surgery has provided strong evidence that most comorbidities of obesity are reversible with significant weight loss. In fact, following bariatric surgery even before significant weight loss there is a 75% to 100% resolution of diabetes, urinary incontinence, GERD, arthritis, asthma, hypertension, and obstructive sleep apnea.

Complications occur in 3% to 35% of patients following bariatric surgery and need to be evaluated and treated similar to other medical procedures and medications. Vitamin and mineral levels need to be monitored at least annually, the abdominal wall should be evaluated for hernias, LAGBs need to be adjusted at appropriate intervals, and occasionally (2%–5%) surgical revision is required. Despite these drawbacks [56], surgery offers patients improved quality of life [51], decreased risk of premature death [46], and improvements in self-image [27]. Although surgery is invasive and associated with some risks, for most patients the risks of continued obesity far outweigh those of bariatric surgery.

Acknowledgments

We acknowledge with gratitude the administrative and medical editing assistance of Barbara Ainsley, Rita Buckley and Jessica Prescott.

References

[1] Buchwald H, Buchwald JN. Evolution of operative procedures for the management of morbid obesity 1950–2000. Obes Surg 2002;12:705–17.

[2] Nanni G, Balduzzi GF, Capoluongo R, et al. Biliopancreatic diversion: clinical experience. Obes Surg 1997;7:26–9.

[3] Marceau P, Hould FS, Potvin M, Lebel S, Biron S. Biliopancreatic diversion (duodenal switch procedure). Eur J Gastroenterol Hepatol 1999;11:99–103.

[4] Brolin RE. Update: NIH consensus conference. Gastrointestinal surgery for severe obesity. Nutrition 1996;12:403–4.

[5] Blackburn GL, Greenberg I. Multidisciplinary approach to adult obesity therapy. Int J Obes 1978;2:133–42.

[6] Balsiger BM, Murr MM, Poggio JL, Sarr MG. Bariatric surgery. Surgery for weight control in patients with morbid obesity. Med Clin North Am 2000;84:477–89.

[7] Blackburn GL, Bistrian BR. Surgical techniques in the treatment of adolescent obesity. In: Collipp PJ, editor. Childhood obesity. Acton MA: Pub Science Group, Inc; 1975. p. 117–30.

[8] Schroder T, Nolte M, Kox WJ, Spies C. Anesthesia in extreme obesity. Herz 2001;26: 222–8.

[9] Sabers C, Plevak DJ, Schroeder DR, Warner DO. The diagnosis of obstructive sleep apnea as a risk factor for unanticipated admissions in outpatient surgery. Anesth Analg 2003;96:1328–35.

[10] Mason EE, Ito C. Gastric bypass in obesity. Surg Clin North Am 1967;47:1345–51.

[11] Maini BS, Blackburn GL, McDermott WVJ. Technical considerations in a gastric bypass operation for morbid obesity. Surg Gynecol Obstet 1977;145:907–8.

[12] NIH Conference. Gastrointestinal surgery for severe obesity. Consensus Development Conference Panel. Ann Intern Med 1991;115:956–61.

[13] Mason EE. Vertical banded gastroplasty for obesity. Arch Surg 1982;117:701–6.

[14] Magnusson M, Freedman J, Jonas E, Stockeld D, Granstrom L, Naslund E. Five-year results of laparoscopic vertical banded gastroplasty in the treatment of massive obesity. Obes Surg 2002;12:826–30.

[15] Ren CJ, Horgan S, Ponce J. US experience with the LAP-BAND system. Am J Surg 2002;184:46S–50S.

[16] Kuzmak LI, Yap IS, McGuire L, Dixon JS, Young MP. Surgery for morbid obesity. Using an inflatable gastric band. AORN J 1990;51:1307–24.

[17] Busetto L, Segato G, De Marchi F, et al. Postoperative management of laparoscopic gastric banding. Obes Surg 2003;13:121–7.

[18] Scopinaro N, Gianetta E. Biliopancratic diversion for obesity at eighteen years. Surgery 1996;119:261–8.

[19] DeMeester TR, Fuchs KH, Ball CS, Albertucci M, Smyrk TC, Marcus JN. Experimental and clinical results with proximal end-to-end duodenojejunostomy for pathologic duodenogastric reflux. Ann Surg 1987 Oct;206(4):414–26.

[20] Hess DS, Hess DW. Biliopancreatic diversion with a duodenal switch. Obes Surg 1998;8:267–82.

[21] Ren CJ, Patterson E, Gagner M. Early results of laparoscopic biliopancreatic diversion with duodenal switch: a case series of 40 consecutive patients. Obes Surg 2000;10:514–23 [discussion: 524].

[22] Mun EC, Blackburn GL, Matthews JB. Current status of medical and surgical therapy for obesity. Gastroenterology 2001;120:669–81.

[23] Wittgrove AC, Clark GW. Laparoscopic gastric bypass, Roux-en-Y: experience of 27 cases, with 3–18 months follow-up. Obes Surg 1996;6:54–7.

[24] Lonroth H, Dalenback J, Haglind E, Lundell L. Laparoscopic gastric bypass. Another option in bariatric surgery. Surg Endosc 1996;10:636–8.

[25] Brolin RE, LaMarca LB, Kenler HA, Cody RP. Malabsorptive gastric bypass in patients with superobesity. J Gastrointest Surg 2002;6:195–203.

[26] Cummings SM, Pratt JSA, Kaplan LM. Obesity and its complications. In: Carlson K, Eisenstat S, editors. Primary care of women, 2nd edition. New York: Mosby. 2002. p. 141–9.

[27] Sugerman HJ, Sugerman EL, DeMaria EJ, et al. Bariatric surgery for severely obese adolescents. J Gastrointest Surg 2003;7:102–8.

[28] Suter M, Jayet C, Jayet A. Vertical banded gastroplasty: long-term results comparing three different techniques. Obes Surg 2000;10:41–6 [discussion: 47].

[29] Hudson SM, Dixon JB, O'Brien PE. Sweet eating is not a predictor of outcome after Lap-Band placement. Can we finally bury the myth? Obes Surg 2002;12:789–94.

[30] Lindroos AK, Lissner L, Sjostrom L. Weight change in relation to intake of sugar and sweet foods before and after weight reducing gastric surgery. Int J Obes Relat Metab Disord 1996;20:634–43.

[31] Sugerman HJ, Londrey GL, Kellum JM, et al. Weight loss with vertical banded gastroplasty and Roux-Y gastric bypass for morbid obesity with selective versus random assignment. Am J Surg 1989;157:93–102.

[32] Rubin M, Spivak H. Prospective study of 250 patients undergoing laparoscopic gastric banding using the two-step technique. Surg Endosc 2003;17:857–60.

[33] Skroubis G, Sakellaropoulos G, Pouggouras K, Mead N, Nikiforidis G, Kalfarentzos F. Comparison of nutritional deficiencies after Roux-en-Y gastric bypass and after biliopancreatic diversion with Roux-en-Y gastric bypass. Obes Surg 2002;12:551–8.

[34] Baltasar A, Bou R, Bengochea M, et al. Duodenal switch: an effective therapy for morbid obesity—intermediate results. Obes Surg 2001;11:54–8.

[35] Gawdat K. Bariatric re-operations: are they preventable? Obes Surg 2000;10:525–9.

[36] Sugerman HJ. Bariatric surgery for severe obesity. J Assoc Acad Minor Phys 2001;12: 129–36.

[37] Livingston EH, Ko CY. Assessing the relative contribution of individual risk factors on surgical outcome for gastric bypass surgery: a baseline probability analysis. J Surg Res 2002;105:48–52.

[38] Pories WJ, MacDonald KGJ, Morgan EJ, et al. Surgical treatment of obesity and its effect on diabetes: 10-y follow-up. Am J Clin Nutr 1992;55:582S–5S.

[39] Choban PS, Jackson B, Poplawski S, Bistolarides P. Bariatric surgery for morbid obesity: why, who, when, how, where, and then what? Cleve Clin J Med 2002;69: 897–903.

[40] Sugerman HJ. Effects of increased intra-abdominal pressure in severe obesity. Surg Clin North Am 2001;81:1063–75.

[41] Sugerman HJ, Sugerman EL, Wolfe L, Kellum JM Jr, Schweitzer MA, DeMaria EJ. Risks and benefits of gastric bypass in morbidly obese patients with severe venous stasis disease. Ann Surg 2001;234:41–6.

[42] Sugerman HJ, Felton WL 3rd, Sismanis A, Kellum JM, DeMaria EJ, Sugerman EL. Gastric surgery for pseudotumor cerebri associated with severe obesity. Ann Surg 1999;229:634–40 [discussion: 640–2].

[43] Sugerman H, Windsor A, Bessos M, Wolfe L. Intra-abdominal pressure, sagittal abdominal diameter and obesity comorbidity. J Intern Med 1997;241:71–9.

[44] Sugerman HJ, Felton WL 3rd, Salvant JB Jr, Sismanis A, Kellum JM. Effects of surgically induced weight loss on idiopathic intracranial hypertension in morbid obesity. Neurology 1995;45:1655–9.

[45] Bump RC, Sugerman HJ, Fantl JA, McClish DK. Obesity and lower urinary tract function in women: effect of surgically induced weight loss. Am J Obstet Gynecol 1992;167:392–7 [discussion: 397–9].

[46] MacDonald KGJ, Long SD, Swanson MS, et al. The gastric bypass operation reduces the progression and mortality of non-insulin-dependent diabetes mellitus. J Gastrointest Surg 1997;3:213–20.

[47] Wittgrove AC. Pregnancy following gastric bypass for morbid obesity. Obes Surg 1998;8:461–4 [discussion: 465–6].

[48] Pasulka PS, Bistrian BR, Benotti PN, Blackburn GL. The risks of surgery in obese patients. Ann Int Med 1986;104:540–6.

[49] Cook CM, Edwards C. Success habits of long-term gastric bypass patients. Obes Surg 1999;9:80–2.

[50] Nguyen NT, Rivers R, Wolfe BM. Early gastrointestinal hemorrhage after laparoscopic gastric bypass. Obes Surg 2003;13:62–5.

[51] Nguyen NT, Goldman C, Rosenquist CJ, et al. Laparoscopic versus open gastric bypass: a randomized study of outcomes, quality of life, and costs. Ann Surg 2001;234:279–89 [discussion: 289–91].

[52] Gudmand-Hoyer E, Asp NG, Skovbjerg H, Andersen B. Lactose malabsorption after bypass operation for obesity. Scand J Gastroenterol 1978;13:641–7.

[53] Schneider BE, Villegas L, Blackburn GL, Mun E, Critchlow JF, Jones DB. Laparoscopic gastric bypass surgery: outcomes. The Journal of Laparoendoscopic & Advanced Surgical Techniques, in press.

[54] Sugerman HJ, Brewer WH, Shiffman ML, et al. A multicenter, placebo-controlled, randomized, double-blind, prospective trial of prophylactic ursodiol for the prevention of gallstone formation following gastric-bypass-induced rapid weight loss. Am J Surg 1995;169:91–7.

[55] Kellum JM, Kuemmerle JF, O'Dorisio TM, et al. Gastrointestinal hormone responses to meals before and after gastric bypass and vertical banded gastroplasty. Ann Surg 1990;211:763–70.

[56] Mitka M. Surgery for obesity: demand soars amid scientific, ethical questions. JAMA 2003;289:1761–2.

[57] Dixon JB, O'Brien PE. Selecting the optimal patient for LAP-BAND placement. Am J Surg 2002;184:17S–20S.

[58] Wittgrove AC, Clark GW. Laparoscopic gastric bypass, Roux-en-Y-500 patients: technique and results, with 3–60 month follow-up. Obes Surg 2000;10:233–9.

Index